Drug Formulation Design

Edited by Rahul Shukla,
Aleksey Kuznetsov and Akbar Ali

Published in London, United Kingdom

Drug Formulation Design
http://dx.doi.org/10.5772/intechopen.105307
Edited by Rahul Shukla, Aleksey Kuznetsov and Akbar Ali

Contributors
Zakio Makuvara, Asmita Gajbhiye, Debashree Das, Shailendra Patil, Raju R Thenge, Vaibhav Adhao, Gautam Mehetre, Pavan Chinchole, Nikesh Tekade, Nilesh Mahajan, Rakesh Patel, Ritesh Popat, Rahul Darakhe, Nishant Chopade, Bhaskar Mohite, Nandu Kayande, Prashant Deshmukh, Aleksey Kuznetsov, Akbar Ali, Muhammad Ibrahim, Azhar Abbas, Nadia Akram, Tahir Maqbool, Ushna, Rahul Shukla, Kailash Ahirwar, Sreeram Sudhir, Amritha Pozhaiparambil Sasikumar, Nagib Qarah, Ezzouhra El-Maaiden, Siamak Javani, Atiyeh Nomani, Anvarsadat Kianmehr, Shahriyar Abdoli, Samit Kumar, Amit Kumar, Dinesh K. Mishra, Rahul Soman, Sabna Kotta, Devika Sivakumar, Rakhi Raju, Y.T. Kamal, Shahana Salam, Ushasi Das, Dilip Kumar Panda, Sanchita Mandal, Madhavi Kasturi, Jagruti Desai, Ashwini Patel, Tapan Desai, Smita Kumbhar, Manish Bhatia

First published in London, United Kingdom, 2023 by IntechOpen
IntechOpen is the global imprint of INTECHOPEN LIMITED, registered in England and Wales, registration number: 11086078, 5 Princes Gate Court, London, SW7 2QJ, United Kingdom

British Library Cataloguing-in-Publication Data
A catalogue record for this book is available from the British Library

Additional hard and PDF copies can be obtained from orders@intechopen.com

Drug Formulation Design
Edited by Rahul Shukla, Aleksey Kuznetsov and Akbar Ali
p. cm.
Print ISBN 978-1-83768-471-7
Online ISBN 978-1-83768-472-4
eBook (PDF) ISBN 978-1-83768-473-1

For EU product safety concerns:
IN TECH d.o.o., Prolaz Marije Krucifikse Kozulić 3, 51000 Rijeka, Croatia,
info@intechopen.com or visit our website at intechopen.com.

Meet the editors

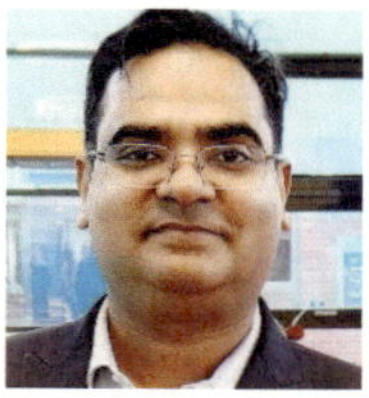

Dr. Rahul Shukla is an assistant professor in the Department of Pharmaceutics, National Institute of Pharmaceutical Education and Research, Raebareli, India, and a visiting researcher at the University of Central Lancashire, UK. He obtained his Ph.D. from the Council of Scientific & Industrial Research, Central Drug Research Institute (CSIR-CDRI) and Jawaharlal Nehru University (JNU), New Delhi, India. He also holds an MPharm and BPharm from the Indian Institute of Technology (BHU) Varanasi, India, and Jamia Hamdard, New Delhi, India, respectively. His experience includes being a research scientist at Dr. Reddy's Laboratories, Hyderabad, India, and a D.S. Kothari postdoctoral fellow at Panjab University, Chandigarh, India. Dr. Shukla has more than 10 years of research and academic experience. He has more than 100 publications in peer-reviewed journals and books to his credit and he has edited several books. He holds seven patents and one copyright. His research interests include targeted drug delivery systems for neurodegenerative diseases, particle engineering, and solubilization and bioavailability enhancements.

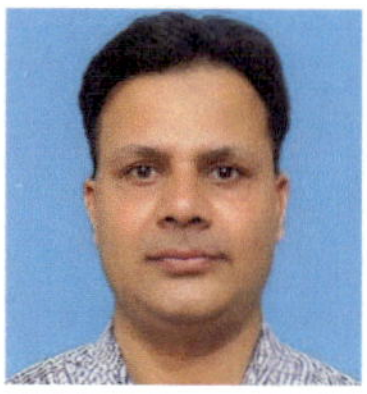

Dr. Akbar Ali is an assistant professor in the Department of Chemistry, Government College University Faisalabad, Pakistan. Previously, he was an assistant professor at the Institute of Chemistry, University of Sargodha, Pakistan. Dr. Akbar Ali obtained his Ph.D. in Synthetic Organic Chemistry from Federal University of Sao Carlos, Brazil, and Leibniz Institute of Plant Biochemistry (IPB), Germany. He has more than eighty publications to his credit. His interests include organic synthesis, click chemistry, green and photo chemistry, asymmetric organocatalysis, multicomponent reactions, and co-crystals synthesis.

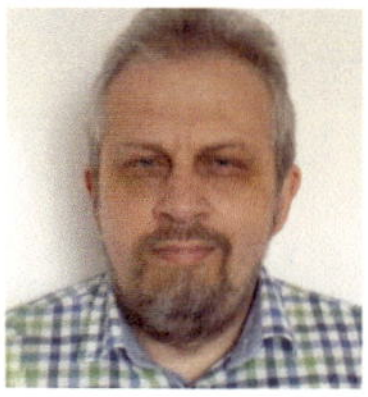

Dr. Aleksey Kuznetsov obtained his Ph.D. in Physical Chemistry from the Department of Chemistry and Biochemistry, Utah State University, USA. He graduated in 2003, after 3 years of doctorate studies, with a specialization in computational/theoretical chemistry. In 2019, after several postdoctoral and visiting professor positions in Germany (including an Alexander von Humboldt fellowship stay), the United States, and Brazil, he acquired a permanent faculty position at the Department of Chemistry, Technical University Federico Santa Maria, Chile, where he has been working on the computational design of various complexes of porphyrins, including core-modified porphyrins, with nanoparticles, fullerenes, and graphenes, along with computational studies of transition metal complexes, organic compounds with pharmacological applications, metal–fullerene complexes, compounds with anticorrosive properties, and more.

Contents

Preface

Drug formulation design has evolved from simple and traditional systems to more modern and complex novel dosage forms. Formulation development is a tedious process and requires an enormous amount of effort from many different people. Effective drug delivery systems are used to optimize the therapeutic properties of drugs and render them safe, effective, and reliable. Such delivery systems offer numerous advantages compared to conventional dosage forms, including improved efficacy, reduced toxicity, and improved patient compliance and convenience. This improvement can increase the therapeutic activity compared to the side effects, reducing the number of drug administrations required during treatment. Moreover, the attached drugs can be targeted to specific organs, tissues, or cells. In recent years, emerging trends in the design and development of drug products have indicated the increasing need for integrated characterization and an in-depth understanding of their roles in drug delivery applications.

Written by worldwide experts in the field, this book discusses innovative aspects of drug design and formulation. It studies, analyzes, and upholds the pillars of drug design, crystal engineering, and formulation. Moreover, it describes a systematic methodology for formulating drug products so that they perform according to one's goals, providing formulation scientists with a fast track to the implementation of the methodology. This book is a vital tool for researchers and students in pharmaceutical science, as it gives incredible insights into emerging trends and concepts.

Dr. Rahul Shukla
Department of Pharmaceutics,
National Institute of Pharmaceutical Education
and Research-Raebareli,
Lucknow, India

Dr. Akbar Ali
Department of Chemistry,
Government College University Faisalabad,
Faisalabad, Pakistan

Dr. Aleksey Kuznetsov
Department of Chemistry,
Technical University Federico Santa Maria,
Santiago, Chile

Section 1

Preformulation

Chapter 1

Preformulation Studies: A Versatile Tool in Formulation Design

Kailash Ahirwar and Rahul Shukla

Abstract

The physicochemical properties of pharmacological molecules have a tremendous effect on safety and efficacy. Poor physicochemical properties can often make it hard to set up a reliable structure-activity relationship (SAR) with no prominent efficacy in preclinical and clinical models. This can lead to more variability in capability and higher drug development costs in the entire development process, and in the worst case, even to stop the clinical trials in the later period. Understanding the basic physicochemical properties makes it possible to separate and untangle investigational observations hence poor molecular properties can be changed or fixed during the design phase. This makes it more likely that the molecule will make it through the long and difficult development process. The decline in innovator pharmacotherapeutics number registrations decline each year and the industry is under even more pressure than in the past to speed up the drug development process. This reduces the length of time required for development and introduces innovative pharmaceutical products. To do this, it is imperative to proceed with an organised approach and act appropriately the first time. The current chapter aims to focus on the important physicochemical properties of the selected molecule, along with how those properties are evaluated and implicated in both discovery enablement and final dosage form development.

Keywords: conventional drug delivery, novel drug delivery, new chemical entities, generics, biopharmaceutical

1. Introduction

Preformulation studies are synonymously known as "Learning before doing". The Preformulation concept emerged between 1950 and 1960 and since then the pharmaceutical product development emphasis has transformed. Therefore, preformulation studies are required for the early step of data collecting relating to the physicochemical properties of the therapeutic molecule, assessing possible salts and excipient appropriateness. Hence, preformulation is the interface between new chemical entities (NCE) and the formulation development phase therefore it is the sole study to provide a complete pathway of drug formulation development [1]. These studies are most and much important before formulation development and they give us an idea about the stages of drug formulation development related to the physicochemical properties of new chemical entities (NCEs) or any drug substances [2–4]. During drug development stages, the physical and chemical properties are categorised and standardised to establish the optimum mark for formulation development and ensure that these properties are helpful for formulation development [5, 6]. Key preformulation factors are thermal particle size, shape, dissociation and partition coefficient, drug/API stability, absorption behaviour, and solid-state characters like polymorphism. Furthermore, the structural, degradable, biophysical, and physicochemical characteristics of the macromolecules are also evaluated at the preformulation stage [3, 7].

Characterisation of the drug at the initial stage is the most important step for an early stage of drug product development to have the understanding and behaviour of drug molecules at the entry level in the cycle of drug development (**Figure 1**). Hence, the preformulation studies are the optimum available tool for API and drug product development. It comprises a set of physicochemical parameters and biopharmaceutical principles to design and develop appropriate drug delivery systems [8, 9]. Therefore, the experimental confirmation of the interaction of drug molecule and excipients are well studied at the preformulation level hence it gives an idea about their interaction and adduct formulation results in intelligent selection of drug molecules and excipients. The primary drug degradation profile is also studied to guide the formulation stability and storage conditions for final dosage forms leads the quick development of desired dosage forms [10].

Post-drug discovery with strong basic knowledge of the physicochemical behaviour of candidate molecules, solid state, and relevant powder characteristics of drug molecules are required to develop the most appropriate intended form of formulation to be administered to humans. Each drug molecule proceeds through various physical and chemical checkpoints before being developed into a final dosage form. Furthermore, these properties are helpful to get information about the combination of drug molecules and ingredients. Preformulation studies were performed for NCEs or any extracted compounds to get information about toxicity, pharmacokinetics, drug distribution, degradation process, adverse conditions, and finally bioavailability [11].

Deep understanding and thorough information of physicochemical and related biopharmaceutical properties of the drug direct scientists to design optimum and appropriate formulation delivery methods to get strong proof of concept (POC) and

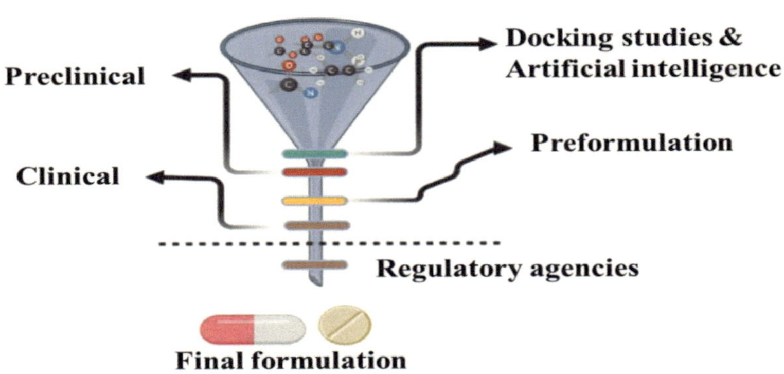

Figure 1.
Stages of preformulation studies.

pre-clinical studies to have a clear understanding of active pharmaceutical ingredients (API) characters and relevant additives that might affect the final formulation and drug performance [5].

Preformulation studies performed post-scientific literature survey of some type of drug molecules to recognise the following parameters [2, 12–14]:

- Chemistry of API, the synthetic pathway of API, drug product manufacturing processes.
- Degradation process and metabolites.
- Development of analytical methods.
- Distribution kinetics and bioavailability of same kind molecules.
- Toxicity profile of candidate drug.
- Preformulation influences, drug candidate selection, formulation adjuvants.
- Optimum storage containers and conditions selection.

Preformulation studies provide a path for formulation development and drug product development in respect of drug form, adjuvants, composition, physical structure, and chemistry of drug molecules, facilitating pharmacokinetic and biopharmaceutical properties evaluation, adjustments, and their implementation to get an appropriate end product, product process development support for Process Analytical Technology to get qualified products, harvest essential and suitable scientific facts for analytical method development and validation [15]. Preformulation research is performed to generate data related to biopharmaceutical, physicochemical, and physic-mechanical properties of molecules, and adjuvants (**Figure 2**) [16, 17]. These analytical investigations inspire formulation strategies and manufacturing methods for drug substances and drug products [18].

Various regulatory guidelines like the ICH and US-FDA support and recommend basic concepts for preformulation development. Preformulation studies are advised by NDA, IND, and ANDA and released by the ICH and the US FDA regulatory agencies. ICH guidelines state that all technical requirements for drug approval applications should be submitted in a standardised e-CTD format. This format, known as QOS-QbR, is even more comprehensive technically and is used by the US-FDA. Additionally, the Quality by Design method, which improves the effectiveness of the FDA review process, is the foundation of the QbR format.

There are various scientific and regulatory descriptions available for acquiring preformulation data that are helpful for the predetermination of the final dosage form. These are 1. Setting up drug product specifications for clinical supply preparations and toxicological testing. 2. Creating initial specifications for clinical supplies and their formulation. 3. Provide scientific evidence to support the creation of dosage forms and assessments of the effectiveness, quality, stability, and bioavailability of products. 4. Review of the stability of early dosage formulations produced. 5. Meeting the CMC section's requirements for the IND and any subsequent NDAs or ANDAs submissions [19, 20].

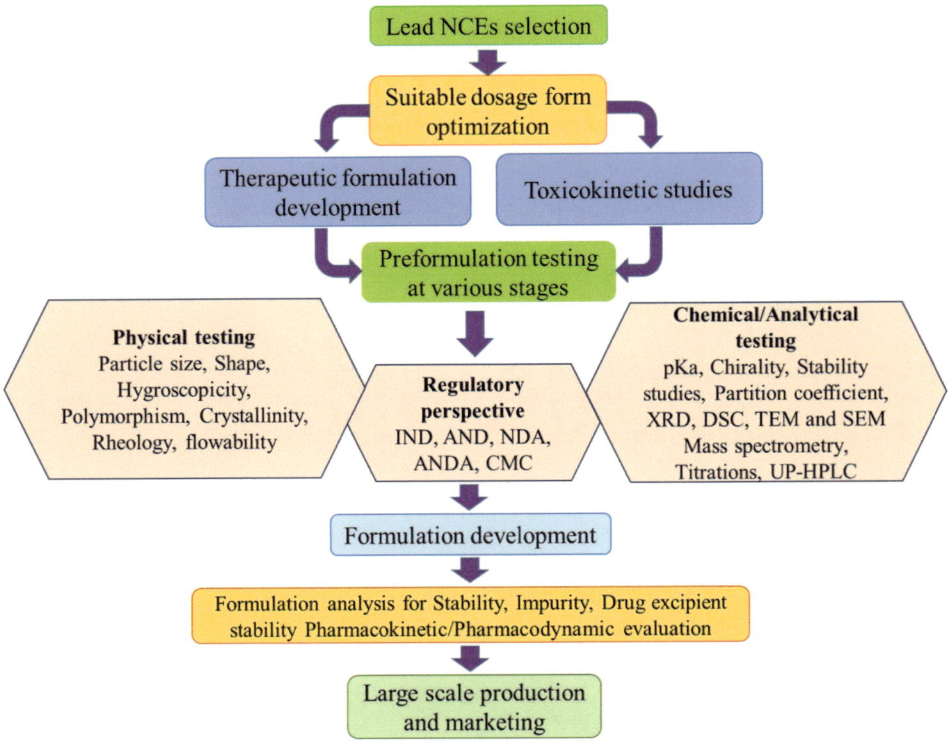

Figure 2.
Preformulation study schematic representation.

2. Overview of preformulation studies

2.1 Preformulation studies: an essential concept in formulation development

Preformulation is the vital concept for final formulation dosage form development intended to target disease as a result preformulation studies are carried out to generate usable data and uncover crucial information that innovators and industry professionals may utilise to produce dosage forms that are stable effective and safe for end users patients it is the main step toward the creation of final dosage form it encompasses comprehensive knowledge of physicochemical aspects of the drug and mixing with appropriate adjuvants to the final design of effective, safe and stable drug delivery system [21]. But it is noteworthy to have data evidence about the basic properties of the drug molecule, its stability information, pharmacokinetic data of lead drug molecules or the same kind of molecule available in the market and bioavailability profile, and feasible route of drug administration before preformulation studies [22]. Additionally, it includes the molecular optimization of the API to change its dissolution and solubility behaviour, for example, salt production techniques have been commonly used to boost solubility, its rate of dissolution (diclofenac sodium salt) and prodrug approach (Levodopa and Enalapril). Also, it determines the connection between physicochemical variables and the kinetic profiles of a novel drug moiety and investigation several aspects of an API's bulk, solubility, stability and compatibility of drug and excipients [23, 24].

Biotherapeutics (Vaccine, proteins and peptides preformulation studies) development into a drug candidate has many difficulties associated with a drug's clinical effectiveness in patients depending on the unique physicochemical and biological features of a given biotherapeutic molecule, including stability, viscosity, manufacture ability, bioavailability, and immunogenicity. To overcome these challenges before being developed a final dosage form is covered under preformulation studies for monoclonal antibodies, peptides, and proteins. The methods used to analyse the candidate macromolecules' primary, secondary, and tertiary structures, along with tests to determine the types and concentrations of contaminants, are the first steps in the process. Then, for the best possible potential to develop the intended biological products, the functions of the various compounds are evaluated using various screening procedures, along with research on their solubility and stability [25]. As a result, it will eventually open the door for the creation of dosage forms that are acceptable to patients and have high levels of stability, safety, efficacy, and are low-cost affordable dosage forms for the patients.

2.2 Pharmaceutical drug product life cycle

Nowadays the century of the internet and artificial intelligence have changed things very fast. For pharmaceutical industry considerations, drug discovery and data mining tools have made the industrial process quick to reach. This is a kind of opportunity used by the scientists working in various research and development teams of the pharmaceutical industry are working at foremost for generating the new drug concept and brand development for the industry [18]. Using modernised data science tools, the entire product life cycle is being transformed by this technology like discovery biology and medicine research and development, production, and validation. Industrial operations must show that the process is compliant with the specified, validated acceptable limits for both isolated process parameter control strategies and comprehensive production control strategies once the process has been validated. ICH recommendations specify in ICH-Q12 that technological and legal aspects of pharmaceutical product lifecycle management should be taken into account [26].

The key funding from product life cycle management:

- Provide comprehensive and detailed knowledge of the product to the company's product pipeline.
- Determine the product specifications continuously within the purview of the regulatory framework and know about product specifications.
- Determine batch variability by trend analysis resulting from differences in the raw materials and ageing of the equipment, and establish the proper preventive maintenance and corrective action and preventive action.
- Manage post-commercialization data related to regulatory approvals, change management, data publication from other sources and sales.

2.3 Preformulation: objectives

The preformulation tool can be viewed as a decisive tool for making decisions during the drug discovery and development phases. Thorough knowledge of physicochemical characteristics and how they affect biological performance enables the choice of possible lead molecules and related drug delivery challenges detection [3, 27].

- To produce the helpful data required for the development of desired, convenient, stable, efficacious, and products produced at a large level.
- Establish a fine understanding of the physicochemical properties of new drug substances before being developed into a final dosage form.
- Physical characteristics establish the selection of the appropriate form of a drug substance.
- Selection of accurate excipients and additives which are compatible with drug substances.

2.4 Preformulation: goals

- The establishment of the physicochemical properties leads to a drug candidate.
- Establish pharmacokinetics and biodistribution profile of selected drug molecule.
- Establishment of drug molecule common excipients compatibility.
- Significant roadblocks to the development of successful pharmaceutical products

2.5 Preformulation study challenges and mitigation

There are various hurdles associated with successful drug product development. That's why a question that comes around scientists working in pharmaceutical product development is Why do 90% of drug development fail at the clinical stage, and what can be done to change that? [11]. The baseline difficulties related to drug candidate evaluation at the research and development level like market potency of a drug candidate, poor project plan, pre-submission challenges, drug development timelines, and cost of drug product development and thereafter the regulatory filing need to be investigated carefully [28]. Drug development starting from discovery is a long and costly process with high chances of failure. Generally, molecules failed to make a place in the market because they do not perform well in clinical phases II and III (40–50%), show unmanageable toxicity (30%), poor drug-like properties and strategic planning (10–15%), and fewer business opportunities (10%). Some of the drug discovery and developmental challenges are listed in **Table 1** [35].

3. Physical characteristics

3.1 Organoleptic properties

Organoleptic properties of new chemical entity preformulation start with a detailed description of drug substances' organoleptic properties including colour, odour, flavour, texture, and taste and these properties should be recorded at the

Discovery team	Developmental challenges	Strategies to overcome drug discovery challenges	Reference
Drug discovery	Poor drug-like properties	Use of "Lipinski rule of 5" for chemical structure design of candidate drug. Robust selection criteria with certain cut-off values for solubility, stability, permeability, protein binding, and in vitro permeability of more than 2–3 × 10^6 cm/s are favoured for oral drug absorption, and in vivo pharmacokinetic parameters.	[22]
Discovery unit	Poor drug potency and specificity	Apply SAR to get drugs with low IC50 (nmol/L) values for lower toxicity and improved effectiveness. STR-mediated structural modifications are useful for clinical efficacy, and safety dose selection in clinical studies.	[29]
Clinical	Lack of clinical efficacy	The top leading candidate for clinical trials is identified by the ratio of their IC50 value and kinase profile selectivity which is 10-fold higher for disease vs. other kinases.	[11]
Safety (clinical toxicity)	Off-target toxicity	Toxicogenomics as a tool for early toxicity determination	[30, 31]
Safety (clinical toxicity)	On-target toxicity	Inhibition of disease-related targets and required titration of dose, toxicogenomics used for early assessment of potential toxicity.	[32, 33]
Business development	Poor strategic planning	Industries have a multidisciplinary business development team which make a detailed roadmap and milestone for new compound development from laboratory to market authorization. Nowadays, Artificial Intelligence with the help of large data analytics enables pharma industries to quickly choose emerging disease areas, and new disease diagnoses cost-effectively.	[34]

Table 1.
List of drug product development challenges and strategies to overcome the challenges.

preformulation stage and also described using expressive terminology. These properties vary as vendor changes and hence they are evaluated with reference standards to confirm the API purity. Further, once these organoleptic properties are established, they may analyse for batch-to-batch consistency mentioned in **Table 2** [14, 20].

3.2 Bulk properties and characterisation: physical, analytical, and physicochemical

3.2.1 Solid-state properties

They include crystallisation, salt formation, polymorphisms, and solvates that profoundly impact solubility, stability, permeability, and finally bioavailability. These are the most crucial parameters of drugs that are necessary for the effective development of drug candidates for patients [36]. For example, powders are masses of solid particles encased in the air (or another fluid), these two systems are significantly bearing on the bulk properties of the powders. The fluid content and other variable parameters are associated with the powder formulations that may affect flow

Organoleptic properties	Characters	Challenges	Mitigations/acceptance
Colour	Off-white, cream yellow, tan, shiny, yellowish white	In the case of low-dose coloured API, maintaining colour homogeneity in the finished uncoated tablets is particularly challenging	Uncoated tablets need to be coated for colour uniformity
Odour	Pungent, sulphurous, fruity, aromatic, odourless	API with bad odour	Use a flavouring agent or capsules/coated tablets to mask the odour
Taste	Acidic, bitter, bland, intense, sweet, tasteless	API with unpalatable taste should not consider for mouth-dissolving or chewable tablets	Sweeteners or flavours are added to get taste-masking properties by covering the entire surface (capsule or coated tablet)

Table 2.
List of various organoleptic properties.

performance which is impacted by the physical features of particles like shape, size, size inconsistency, angularity, and rigidity. Some outside factors including humidity, aeration, vibration, and conveying environment intensify the problem [37].

3.2.2 Flow properties

The flow characteristics of powders are essential to successful tabletting operations. For effective mixing and tolerable weight consistency for the compressed tablets, an optimum flow of granules/powders is required. Suppose, at the preformulation stage a drug is categorised as "poor flowable" therefore the proper selection of excipients can resolve this problem. Precompression and granulation methods are utilised for powder drugs to improve their flow behaviour. A preformulation test of the granule mass for the measurement of flow properties is performed with the help of the angle of repose, flow through an orifice, Hausner ratio, bulk and tapped density, inter-particle porosity, Carr's index and ideal flowability. Generally, a uniform shape or large crystal displays a narrower angle of repose and a low Carr's index resulting from changes in particle size and shape [38].

The angle of repose can be understood as the maximum angle formed between the free-standing surface of the powder heap and the horizontal plane of the powder at the base. It may use to evaluate the interparticle force of powder particles and bulk characterisation of solids.

The range of angle of repose can vary from 0° to 90°, the angle of repose value below 25° represents excellent flow properties however, on the other if the angle of repose value ranges between 25° and 45°, the flow is considered poor, the values of angle of repose indicated in **Table 3**. The formula for the calculation of the angle of repose is as follows [39].

$$\mathrm{AOR} : \tan \theta^{-1} \left(2\,\mathrm{h} / \mathrm{d}\right) \tag{1}$$

h is heap height, and d is the horizontal base diameter.

Preformulation test name	Formula	Observations	Properties	Reference
The angle of repose (flow behaviour of granule)	AOR = $\text{Tan}\theta^{-1}(2\,h/d)$	<20	Excellent flow	[39]
		20–30	Free-flowing	
		30–34	Passable flow	
		>40	Poor flow	
Bulk density (individual particle arrangement)	Pb = M/Vo	> 0.5 g/ml (high value)	Limitation to flow	[39]
Tapped density (degree of powder packing, cohesiveness)	Pt = M/Vt	High density	Better flow	[40]
Inter-particle porosity (Ie)	Ie = {(Pb – Pt)/(Pb × Pt)}			[41]
Carr Index (CI%, strength, stability, and compressibility)	CI = ((Pb – Pt)/Pt)	<0.10	Excellent flow	[42]
		0.26–0.31	Poor flow	
Hausner ratio (HR, inter-particulate friction, and compressibility)	HR = Pt/Pb	1.00–1.11	Free-flowing	[43]
		1.35–1.45	Poor flow	

Vo: volume, M: known weight of the granule's mixture, Vt: tapped volume in measuring cylinder, Pb: bulk density, Pt: tapped density, AOR: angle of repose

Table 3.
Preformulation tests for measurement of granule flow properties.

3.2.3 Particle size distribution

The particle size of dosage form affects the physicochemical properties and biopharmaceutical behaviour of drug substances. Drug solubility is frequently inversely proportional to the particle size; for example, a smaller particle size dosage form has a large surface area, similarly surface area to volume ratio as well. A stronger contact between the surface area and the solvent increases the solubility. Particle size reduction methods like milling and grinding frequently subject the drug product to high levels of physical stress, which could lead to degradation [43]. Moreover, micronization is the conventional technique used to make particles smaller and increase the surface area of drugs thereby enhancing solubility and dissolution.

However, micronization milling techniques (rotor-stator colloid mill, and jet mill) are not appropriate for drugs because they do not change the saturation solubility.

Griseofulvin, progesterone, phenacetin, and fenofibrate are examples where smaller particle with large surface area enhances drug bioavailable concentration [44]. Spray drying, active compound milling, and grinding are common methods of particle size reduction. These techniques frequently subject the therapeutic product to severe physical stress, which could lead to degradation.

3.2.4 Compressibility

Compressibility is the ability of drug powders to decrease in volume under pressure and compress into tablet dosage forms with specific tensile strength. It is calculated by the Hausner ratio and Carr's index (formula mentioned in **Table 3**) to determine the flow behaviour of powder-based drugs to calculate the density at the preformulation stages [45].

3.2.5 Crystallinity and polymorphism

Polymorphism and crystalline behaviour of solid-state drugs are important for formulators because most of the drugs exist in the solid states and are suitable for the intended use. In a solid state, drugs may exist in salt form, cocrystals, hydrates, polymorphs, amorphous form, solid solutions, and eutectics. Liquid states drugs like valproic acid and general anaesthetics as gaseous phases. In a crystal, lattice atoms are arranged in a unique pattern and they are highly ordered arrangement based on this arrangement they are categorised as crystalline or amorphous. Both forms show different physical and chemical properties, therefore, they have different solubility and stability performances which influence the delivery system and activity of the drug [38].

When the crystalline and amorphous drug substances are analysed and confirmed that they show different X-ray patterns, vapour pressure, melting point, crystal shape, density, hardness, dissolution, solubility, and bioavailable concentration at the site of action. Furthermore, other properties also fluctuate from their standard values for example limited free energy, high melting point and decrease in solubility behaviour can be considered for stable polymorph. A metastable polymorph has a lower melting point, increased solubility, and is more bioavailable than a stable polymorph. Crystals and polymorphs are analysed by advanced techniques such as the X-ray diffraction method, FTIR, NMR, Optical crystallography, hot stage microscopy, SEM/TEM, and differential scanning calorimetry [46, 47]. The polymorphism and crystal habit behaviour affect solubility, for example, anhydrous Carbamazepine has three different polymorphic forms and these forms are different in their physicochemical properties hence, they show different solubility behaviour at different conditions of temperature and melting points. However, the hydrous form of Carbamazepine as such will not have any polymorphic forms. The melting point may also significantly impact the selection of polymorphic forms like most stable form is polymorph III [44].

3.2.6 Hygroscopicity and deliquescence

Hygroscopicity can be demonstrated as the potency of a drug or salt to gain moisture or water vapour. Compounds can be interacted with moisture by retaining it in bulk or absorbing it on the surface, capillary condensation, and chemical reactions. Atmospheric conditions and the surface area of drug substances are responsible for the amount of moisture absorption. Moisture level variation highly affects the stability, compressibility, and flow properties that's why these attributes should be studied cautiously.

The moisture uptake measurement is done by Karl Fischer titration, Thermogravimetric analysis (TGA), and gas chromatography techniques. As per European Pharmacopoeia, four separate grades of hygroscopicity are defined when a drug substance is stored at 80% relative humidity and a temperature of 25°C for 24 h. The four classes of hygroscopicity are described here as per the above-mentioned storage conditions [48, 49].

Class I: Non-hygroscopic drug substances, when no moisture is detected below 90% relative humidity condition.

Class II: Slightly hygroscopic drug substances are those when their weight increases between 0.2% but less than 2% w/w in presence of moisture.

Class III: Hygroscopic drug substances produces weight increases between 0.2% and less than 15% w/w.

Class IV: Very hygroscopic when the weight increases more than 15% w/w.

Moisture is a significant element that may have an impact on the stability of potential medications and their formulations. Hydrolysis is frequently seen by the adsorption of water molecules onto a potential medication (or excipient). Water molecules have hydrogen bonds and high polarity, this property of water made it absorb the surface of drug substances and affects crystal habit properties, compaction, flow properties, dissolution rate, lubricity, and drug permeability across biological membranes. Therefore, to get rid of the hygroscopicity problems it is necessary to select an appropriate adjuvant, stabile drug compounds, and optimum storage conditions during the preformulation phase. The substances absorb moisture to the highest quantity and liquefy themselves. Deliquescent substance absorbs moisture to a greater extent and liquefies themselves hence, they dissolve solids and leave a thin water film on their surface. This process is linked with relative humidity conditions, this condition measured by vapour diffusion and heat transport rates [18].

3.2.7 Pseudo-polymorphism

Pseudopolymorphism refers to the phenomenon in which the drug molecules get incorporated into the crystal lattice of solids. The solids can exist in different crystal forms known as pseudo polymorphs and the process is pseudopolymorphisms. These forms contain a secondary heterostructure within the crystal lattice, with the same chemical makeup (examples are water, solvent, co-former, etc.). These forms are also known by other names like hydrates, solvates, and cocrystals, and FDA considered them polymorphs [50].

3.3 Preformulation solubility parameters

A significant barrier to product development is solubility. Poor drug solubility (shown in **Table 4**) is a common cause of medication discovery and development failure.

Insufficient solubility can hinder the molecule's capacity to be developed since it can make it difficult to design assays and negatively affect how the compound behaves in vivo. Therefore, inadequate solubility may prove to be a barrier to therapeutic development. In general, drug solubility is influenced by several factors such as lattice energy, molecular arrangement, bond strength, weak bonding forces, lipophilicity, ionisation potential, pH, cosolvency, additives, dielectric constant, solubilisation by surfactant, hydrotrophy, complexation, temperature, pressure, and molecular volume. If these factors have been studied well during preformulation studies, they can be useful for final formulation development with fewer chances of drug failure [51].

In summary, the variables that might alter a drug's solubility profile include the temperature, pH conditions, diluents, additives, solvent system, and the physical condition of drug molecules. The common ion releases in the medium in presence of

BCS Class	Solubility	Permeability	Formulation strategies	Examples
I	High	High	Solid oral conventional dosage forms	Metoprolol, Paracetamol
II	Low	High	Increase solubility by nano-crystallisation, surfactant and co-solvents	Glibenclamide, Bicalutamide
III	High	Low	Permeability enhancers	Cimetidine, Acyclovir
IV	Low	Low	Both class II&III applies here	Chlorothiazide, Furosemide

Table 4.
BCS classification system for solubility and permeability.

solubilising agents responsible for drug molecules crystallisation [52, 53]. Solubility, particularly water solubility, is a crucial physical-chemical property of a medicinal ingredient. For a medication to be therapeutically effective in the physiological pH range of 1–8, considerable water solubility is required.

If a drug substance's solubility is less than ideal, consideration must be paid to increasing it. 10 mg/ml is considered as poor solubility which may result in irregular or partial drug absorption from 1 to 7 pH range at 37°C. But for novel molecules, an understanding of two fundamental qualities is necessary [14].

3.3.1 pH measurement during the preformulation stage

The negative logarithm of hydrogen ion concentration of drug substances is known as pH. The formula for calculation of pH is pH = – Log [H+] and based on the pH scale it is categorised as an acidic drug with 1–7 pH, ±7 is a neutral drug, and 7–14 pH is alkaline/basic drugs.

Most of the drugs are available in salt form or they are either weak bases or acids. Therefore, it is very important to have a complete understanding of molecule ionisation behaviour at specific pH values. Hence, at the preformulation stage, the effect of drug ionisation, ionic strength, pH, and temperature are simultaneously studied to understand dosage form stability, solubility, bioavailability, and efficacy of drug molecules [54].

Importance of pH in preformulation

1. Injectable formulation should be in the range of pH 3–9 to prevent tissue damage and pain at the injection site.

2. Oral syrups cannot be formulated too acidic for palatability reasons.

3. More alkali formulations may attack the glass container.

4. If the drug is susceptible to degradation in acidic pH, then its delayed-release formulation is to be prepared.

5. The pH of the formulation must not sensitise the site of application. For example pH for buccal application should be in the range of 6.6 to 6.8. 6. GIT shows a variety of pH ranges like pH 1.2 for the stomach, pH 6.6 buccal, and pH 7–8 for

the small intestine throughout its length from the oral cavity to the colon. As a key point note, the drug formulation should be stable at the pH intended for the target site of absorption [55, 56].

3.3.2 Dissociation constant (pKa) assessment

pKa is the dissociation constant of a drug and they are available as weak bases or acids in the solution, hence drugs can exist in the ionised or un-ionised form at particular pH. The aqueous solubility of drugs depends on the ionisation and fraction of ionised to the unionised form of the drug. The un-ionised form of drugs is lipophilic, thus permeating through the bilayer membrane however, the ionised substances are lipid insoluble hence permeation is slow. Three parameters that are crucial for absorption are the ionisation constant, which is the un-ionised form of drug at the gastrointestinal tract site available for absorption to show its efficacy [57].

The degree of ionisation depends on the Henderson-Hasselbalch equation and can be determined by UV spectroscopy, potentiometric titration, and titrimetric methods from intrinsic solubility data. A parameter that also considers a compound's ionisation state is the ionisation constant (pKa). Understanding pKa is crucial for predicting the absorption route of weakly acidic or basic medications [3, 58].

The equations for basic and acidic compounds are mentioned below:

$$\text{For acidic drugs}: \text{pH}=\log \text{pKa}+\text{ratio of un}-\text{ionised to ionised drug} \quad (2)$$

$$\text{For basic drugs}: \text{pH}=\log \text{pKa}+\text{ratio of ionised to un}-\text{ionised drug} \quad (3)$$

$$\%\text{Ionisation} = 10(\text{pH-pKa})/1+10(\text{pH-pKa}), \text{where } Ka \text{ is the dissociation constant} \quad (4)$$

Weakly acidic drugs with around 4 pKa value are absorbed fast from the stomach because drug molecules available here in an un-ionised state at this pKa value in the stomach. Similarly, basic drugs with an 8 pKa value are available in an unionised form and easily absorbed from the intestine [58]. Various methods used for the determination of the partition coefficient are a shake-flask method, chromatographic determination, microelectrometric titration, counter current and filter probe. pKa determination at the preformulation stage is important because of the following reasons [59].

- Based on the pKa value, particular pH can be selected to obtain optimum solubility and suitable salt form to get improved bioavailability, and stability.
- pKa is helpful for a selection of buffer, temperature, ionic strength, and co-solvent.
- The extent of drug dissociation can be determined.

3.3.3 Partition coefficient (Log P) assessment

The ratio of unionised drugs dispersed in the aqueous and organic phases is known as the partition coefficient. This is helpful to predict drugs' ability to cross the bilayer. Lipinski's Rule of 5 has been used to predict solubility and permeability.

The log P can be determined with the formula log P=(oil/water) at equilibrium. (5)

A compound's lipophilicity is represented by its Log P value, 0 log P value indicates that the drug substance is similarly soluble in both n-octanol and water. While 2 Log P values indicate the hydrophilic nature of the drug and 5 indicates the lipophilic nature. A suitable absorption profile ranges between log P values of 1 and 3, while a Log P value of less than 1 and more than 6 indicates poor permeability. The software tools are nowadays very helpful for Log P value determination for example Molecular Modelling Pro™ 6.27 software [60].

3.3.4 Distribution coefficient (Log D)

Log D provides an approximation of the lipophilicity of drug molecules in blood plasma at pH 7.4. It can be determined by correlating the drug retention time compared with a similar compound with a known log P value. Log D values consider the possibility of drug molecules in an ionic state [3, 14].

3.3.5 Thermal effect (enthalpy of solution)

The effect of heating on drug solubility can be measured in the form of heat of solution. The heat released or absorbed during the dissolution of a mole of solute in a large volume of solvent is referred to as the heat of the solution. The ideal temperature range should typically include 5, 25, 37, and 50°C. For the endothermic process, the heat of the solution is considered positive and negative for exothermic. Positive heat of solution with an increase in temperature leads to an increase in the drug solubility hence at the preformulation stage, with the use of the heat of solution formula, the optimum drug solubility can be determined. The heat of solution between 4 and 8 kcal/mol indicates un-ionised forms of weak bases and acidic drugs dissolved in water [36].

3.3.6 Common ion effect (Ksp)

Pre-formulation evaluation performed for solubility determination must not avoid the common ion effect since the common ions are responsible for salt solubility reduction.

Le Châtelier's principle states that when an equilibrium is out of balance, the reaction will change to put it back in balance. An equilibrium between a weak acid or base and a common ion will shift in favour of the reactants. The common ions suppress the ionisation of a weak acid in the presence of a weak base or acid by producing more comparable product ions [61]. Hence, adding common ions to the solution may shift the reaction toward the reactant to dismiss excess product stress in the form of precipitation leading to a decrease in the solubility. For example, the solubility of weakly basic drugs in acidic (HCl) solution is diminished when they are administered as HCl salts due to Cl common ions. Hydrochloride salt's intrinsic dissolution rate evaluation between water, and water containing 1.2% w/v NaCl, and 0.9% w/v NaCl in 0.05 M HCl medium suggest a common ion interaction pathway. Following this, if the drug's solubility has not decreased, the drug can suitable to administer as a chloride salt; otherwise, it should be discarded. Hence, to get optimum solubility common ions effect must be avoided [14].

3.3.7 Dissolution

The dissolution rate is defined as the quantity of drug substances dissolve per unit of time with specific circumstances of temperature and solvent conditions for liquid or solid interface. The process is termed dissolution. The dissolution rate can be determined with the help of the Noyes-Whitney Equation. The dissolution rate is the rate-limiting step at the site of absorption for drugs in solution. At the preformulation stage, scientists understand, how excipients, surface area, and particle size affect the dissolution behaviour of drug substances and ascertain whether the rate-limiting behaviour is dissolution mediated. The drug dissolution is followed by reaching into the systemic circulation and is dependent on the type of dosage forms like solid oral (tablets, capsules, and suspensions) and intramuscular (pellets or suspensions); the rate-limiting factor governs which type of drug administration route is optimum for a selected dosage form [3, 14].

3.4 Permeability assessment at the preformulation stage

After dissolution, when a drug is present in the physiological fluids, such as in gastric juices, the small intestine or in plasma, it must have to penetrate cells and tissues to reach the intended site for action. Drug penetration is mediated by various transport mechanisms both passive and active. The drug must diffuse through aqueous pores in tissues or partition with the lipid components of cells to cause passive diffusion, however, active diffusion requires energy. The early drug development process; involves the in vitro models to forecast drug permeation because they offered a simple, repeatable way of monitoring drug absorption rate and mechanism with a favourable cost-benefit ratio. Some of the drug permeability assessment models are listed here.

In-vitro permeability assessment models:

- Caco-2 cells assay for oral permeability assessment
- Parallel Artificial Membrane Permeability Assay
- Madin-Darby canine kidney cells assay
- Franz diffusion cells model

Artificial intelligence-based models (In silico):

- Corneal PAMPA-based in-silico models
- Hierarchical support vector regression (HSVR) scheme

The human epithelial colorectal carcinoma cells-based model is known as the Caco-2 monolayer assay for permeability assessment. This is a diversified in-vitro permeability assay that covers P-glycoprotein efflux transporters, a variety of enzymes like esterases and peptidases, and tight cellular junctions that resemble the small intestine. These in-silico methods are applied to assess drug permeability with the ability to filter massive amounts of sample data while producing precise and accurate results quickly and accurately. Caco-2 cell permeability approach can be used for in-vitro pharmacokinetic research for oral dosage forms. This cell-based assay is suitable for P-glycoprotein efflux and intestinal enzyme metabolism studies [62].

3.5 Stability analysis as per ICH guidelines

According to ICH (International Conference on Harmonisation) Q1A (R2) regulatory guidelines, the purpose of these guidelines is to test drug substances under different stress conditions such as long-term stability testing, accelerated stability testing for a minimum three different time points, and sometimes the intermediate testing also done for some special cases. These stability testing depend upon the climatic zones where the testing is to be done and follow the criteria of that particular zone. The testing includes the effect of pH temperature, humidity, and photolysis under stress conditions. Stability studies during the preformulation stage are most important to check chemical stability and product degradation for the solid-state and liquid-state formulations [2]. Furthermore, some drugs which are prone to degradation produce toxic substances hence it is important to determine the conditions under which this drug degradation happens. This degradation pattern of the drug substance can suggest a way to mitigate or stabilise or to determine the optimum storage, climatic and shelf-life improvement conditions. The physical observation at product development to check, caking, liquefaction, discolouration, odour, and gel formation. After physical observation, degradation can be identified by mass spectroscopy, HPLC or DSC, NMR, FTIR or other relevant sophisticated analytical techniques.

3.5.1 Photostability

The photostability standard conditions are well mentioned in ICH-Q1B guidelines. The photostability of drug substances and drug products must be understood to specify handling, packaging, labelling, adverse effects analysis, and to consider innovative formulation strategies. The optimum exposure for simulation during drug manufacture is casually 1.2 million lux as per the European Federation of Pharmaceutical Industries Expert Working Group. Further, during drug/API manufacture, the cumulative exposure of the compounds can be accepted as 100 Klux of visible light without UV exposure, however, the ICH guideline is not applicable here and this data may be helpful for internal audits.

3.5.2 Solid-state stability

When it comes to solid-state stability, environmental elements including temperature, light, and moisture, as well as the packing materials that come into contact with the dosage form, are the first to have an impact on drug stability. Excipients may affect different chemical interactions with the drug/formulation if selected improperly. The excipients' bound or free moisture, pH, and microclimate can start the deterioration of the dosage forms. Therefore, excipients with low moisture content and low hygroscopicity are preferred for medications that are resistant to hydrolysis-induced deterioration. Various physical properties of the drug molecules like particle shape, size, and surface area, morphology, presence of impurities can play a significant responsibility in drug degradation, either alone or in the presence of excipients [63]. For heat-sensitive drug substances, the processing conditions should maintain at low-temperature conditions to escape from drug degradation. It is possible to use a variety of unique formulation techniques, such as multi-layer particles in capsules or tablets, tablets with moisture-proof coatings, compression coating, tablets inside tablets, or tablets inside capsules. Stressed settings, such as high-temperature studies, high humidity, exposure to high wetness, and high-intensity light environments, can be used to assess the solid-state stability of an active substance. It provides an early warning of stability issues that could affect product development [61].

As a case study, published by Carney et al. the degradation pattern of Ciclosidomine in solution due to temperature, buffer constituents, and ionic strength are described. The first-order hydrolysis rate appears in absence of light, again at pH 3.0, 5.0, and 6.0 with the absence of light and in presence of air or nitrogen, reported drug degradation. Hence, optimum light and air conditions should be maintained during small-scale and manufacture stages [14].

3.5.3 Solution state stability studies

Compared to solid-state reactions, liquid-state reactions are simpler to spot. The methodologies for detecting unidentified liquid incompatibilities are the same as for solid dosage forms. For suspensions and solutions formulations of bulk drugs, the investigations include listed conditions and they must be evaluated as per FDA stability guidelines, these conditions are higher nitrogen and oxygen environment, alkaline/acidic pH conditions, and the existence of chelating agents and stabilisers [64]. The results of stability studies can help guide stabilisation strategies, giving feedback to the chemistry team on how to modify labile groups to improve stability, assisting researchers in determining the compound's developability, and providing instructions on how to handle and store compounds [2].

3.5.4 Drug-excipients compatibility

The medicine is in close contact with one or more excipients in the tablet dosage form; they could have an impact on the drug's stability. Therefore, understanding how drugs and excipients interact helps the formulator choose the best excipients. It's possible that this knowledge already exists for well-known drugs. The preformulation scientist must produce the necessary data for new medications or excipients. Binders, disintegrants, lubricants, and fillers are typically found in tablets [65]. A new drug's compatibility screening must take into account two or more excipients from each class. The preformulation scientist has a great deal of control over the medication-to-excipient ratio employed in these studies. The following conclusions are made from the drug-excipient compatibility studies [9].

- DECS data submission is essential for new formulation as per FDA regulatory agencies.
- Provide ideas for long-term drug stability.
- Mitigation of difficulties before formulating the final dosage form.
- Determine any chemical and physical interactions with the drug and excipient and how they can affect the stability and bioavailability of the formulation.

Various sophisticated analytical techniques are used to detect drug-excipient compatibility are differential FT-IR spectroscopy, scanning calorimetry, fluorescence spectroscopy, differential thermal analysis, osmometry, diffuse reflectance spectroscopy, high-pressure liquid chromatography, radiolabelling [66].

4. Chemical properties optimization

4.1 Hydrolysis

Hydrolysis reactions are very commonly observed chemical reactions responsible for drug degradation due to the high dipolar water molecules availability which binds to the drug molecules and leads to hydrolysis. It involves nucleophilic reaction the of the labile group [67]. The PH can be adjusted to stop hydrolysis. Since the majority of drugs are weak acids or bases in compositions. Formulate the drug solution so that it has a pH that will ensure its stability, add a water-soluble solvent to the formulation, use the optimal buffer concentration to prevent ionisation, or add a surfactant to stabilise against enzyme catalysis. Drug solubility decreased by creating less soluble salts or esters of the drug which are susceptible to ester hydrolysis. The carbonyl functional groups of esters, lactones, amides, lactams, carbamates and imides are susceptible to hydrolysis. By adjusting the pH conditions of liquid dosage form its shelf life can be lengthened however, stability and solubility should not be compromised.

The hydrolysis problem can be prevented by different approaches, such as drug hydrolysis should be checked to stop drug degradation and this can be achieved with the addition of bulky alkyl groups near the functional group by chemical modifications to hinder the action of a nucleophile or enzyme and decreases drug hydrolysis. Similarly, the labile ester functional group is replaced with urethane or amide can increase chemical and metabolic stability [68].

4.2 Oxidation

A high-oxygen environment can be used to examine a drug's oxidation sensitivity. Rapid evaluation is typically feasible in an atmosphere with 40% oxygen. Samples are kept in desiccators with three-way stop cocks, which are then alternately evacuated and submerged in the desired environment. To ensure the desired environment is created, the method is repeated three or four times. The outcomes could be used to decide if the formulation needs an antioxidant or whether the final drug product has to be packaged in an inert environment [67].

4.3 Reduction

Reduction is a more prevalent mechanism for drug metabolism. Nicotinamide adenine dinucleotide phosphate is necessary for hepatic microsomes to perform a variety of reductive chemical reactions. Cytochrome P450 catalyses the reduction of azo and nitro compounds. Alcohol dehydrogenase converts chloral hydrate to its active metabolite, trichloroethanol. The active metabolite hydrocortisone is produced when prednisolone and cortisone are reduced. Azo dyes are used as colouring additives in drug products or food items and this can be degraded by liver and intestinal flora to create amines [48].

4.4 Chirality

The chirality determination at the preformulation stage is considered during the drug development strategy. The undesirable enantiomer should be removed from the therapeutic formulation since, in most cases, one of the enantiomers lacks the necessary pharmacological characteristics. When a separation method is available, the inactive form should be eliminated from considerations of cost. Optical activity evaluation for drug molecules is an essential analysis performed during the early discovery process for NCEs. This would suggest the active enantiotropic form of drug molecules. The drug must be in the enantiopure form as it is a legal requirement for IND filing. Therefore, choosing the appropriate enantiomeric form for the market product must be made before IND filling or a patent. As a case study, the Sirolimus [20] branded as Rapamune in liquid solution was marketed by Pfizer and approved in 1999 by the FDA for immunosuppression. Sirolimus contains Phosal 50-PG active ingredient and polysorbate 80 as an inactive ingredient which is nonaqueous. Further, in solid-state Sirolimus is a chiral compound, however, in aqueous solutions, this drug is found in A, B, and C isomers hence the nonaqueous vehicle is selected for drug product development [69].

5. Preformulation studies for biopharmaceuticals development: proteins, peptides, and vaccines

The concept of recombinant DNA technology and clustered regularly interspaced short palindromic repeats (CRISPR) associated protein 9 is flourishing for biopharmaceutical product development. These technologies when coupled with artificial intelligence gel large genome data for the proper designing of peptide, protein, and vaccine products [70]. Proteins are classified into secondary, tertiary, and quaternary structures based on their kinds, which in turn affects each structure's molecular size. With the help of the prodrug approach, the vulnerable peptide backbones undergone proteolytic cleavage can be mitigated. Therefore, peptides can be chemically altered to create more stable and high plasma-concentration prodrugs. The prodrug can be produced by chemical modification and substitution reactions like dehydroamino acid substitution, D-amino acid substitution, thio-methylene modification, carboxyl reduction, and PEG-amino acid joining [71].

Preformulation studies are facilitated the right path of selecting the appropriate adjuvants and other formulation conditions required during manufacture. For example, the stability profile of a live attenuated Ty21a bacterial typhoid vaccine performed by spectroscopic techniques provides time-dependent real-time high throughput information at a broad range of temperatures (10–85°C) and pH (4–8). The above information is useful during preformulation studies of other similar type of peptide drugs. An empirical phase diagram, which was created using data from circular dichroism and fluorescence techniques suggests Ty21a cells exist in various physical states and the most stable state occurs at pH 6–7 below 30°C. Among other potential stabilisers, 10% sucrose and 0.15 M glutamic acid show the strongest protective properties, increasing Ty21a cells' transition temperature by roughly 10°C each. Foam-dried formulations have also been the subject of preliminary research as a potential alternative strategy for further stabilising Ty21a cells. Additionally, in-process stability can be improved by 10% sucrose and trehalose solutions [20, 72].

6. Role of artificial intelligence in preformulation studies

A large, multidisciplinary discipline known as artificial intelligence gives machines the ability to think, learn, and reason. Artificial intelligence has two subsets: machine learning and deep learning. Scientists frequently integrate computer-added drug design tools with artificial intelligence, powered decision-making at crucial stages of drug discovery programs [1, 73]. Deep learning-based artificial neural networks and machine learning-based expert systems are currently very well-liked for predicting interactions between drugs and their targets as well as physicochemical properties, quality, stability, toxicity, safety, and biological activity of formulations. Medical diagnostics, epidemic breakouts, and individualised treatments are all examples of how AI is used in the healthcare industry [34]. The healthcare industry pursues exceptional advancements with the help of AI tools for example Adaptive neuro-fuzzy inference system (ANFIS) performance is satisfactory for excipients selection hence the AI-based algorithms made drug research simple and shorten the drug discovery and development timelines. In-silico models found their way as successful tools for determining drugs' aqueous solubilities. These factors include molecular size, molecular shape, and hydrogen bonding capacities [74].

7. Preformulation studies: a regulatory perspective

A preformulation report for a novel molecule includes information on stability, excipient compatibility tests, solid-state characteristics, physicochemical characters, biopharmaceutical features, thermal behaviour, mechanical properties, and analytical profiling. In the area of the IND devoted to CMC/pharmaceutical development, these drug substance features have to be highlighted. For example, the medicine must be in the enantiopure form as it is a legal requirement for IND filing. Therefore, choosing the appropriate drug enantiomeric form should be indicated with its activity before filing an IND or a patent [75].

The characteristics of a specific drug material must now be thoroughly explored early in the initial development process, and the findings from these investigations must be provided in the CMC part of an IND. As part of robust regulatory guidelines, the drug excipient additives, manufacturing procedures, and storage conditions, utilised to make the drug substance and drug product are all included in the CMC section. This data is analysed to make sure that the business can effectively manufacture and supply the drug consistently. Nowadays, regulatory agencies have made a common format of documents for submission as indicated by ICH guidelines to harmonise CMC requirements for global marketing. A common technical document that will harmonise CMC regulatory requirements for global development and marketing. The creation of CMC sections by European Union and American standards yields two formally distinct NDAs. The CMC sections of the EU Marketing Authorization Applications and the US-FDA largely share the same components [33].

8. Preformulation studies for nano-based therapeutics

Nano-based therapeutics are suitable formulation strategies for the delivery of active drug ingredients because of their harmonious morphological design and features. The novel drug delivery systems are [76]. The objectives of the preformulation study for nano-based formulations are to design and demonstrate kinetic profile, acceptability with the other substances, physicochemical parameters, and polymorphism of the new drug entity to design an elegant dosage form [77]. At the preformulation stage, the shape, size, amorphous or crystal structure, and size variability are some of the important features which are evaluated for nano-based delivery systems hence the synthesis of nano-based therapeutics systems is truly based on the physiochemical characteristics [78]. The diluents and solvents also play a significant role in inhomogeneity, size and shape in the nanoprecipitation methods. The profiling of active moieties is crucial in terms of their solubility studies, melting point, thermal properties, and pKa behaviour. In the preformulation phase, physiochemical properties and the compatibility of the drug with excipients of the formulation are regulating the nano-system behavioural selected for the final formulation design. Preformulation studies are conducted to create an appropriate dosage form by establishing the pharmacokinetics and pharmacodynamic profile parameters [79, 80]. Moreover, the dissolution profile, polymorphic forms, the pharmacokinetics of the drug, and its bioavailability, details on the drug's deterioration process, undesirable drug-related conditions, and pharmacodynamic effects are also an important part of preformulation studies which are provided by physicochemical properties of the drug. The nano-based formulations can be used for topical, transdermal, injectable and oral deliveries for compound development, screening, therapeutic, imaging and diagnostic purposes therefore they are novel systems for targeting cancer, inflammatory diseases and autoimmune disorders [81, 82]. For example, these considerations are helpful for justification for the preparation of nanoparticles, lipid-based nanoparticles, polymeric nanoparticles, concerning polymer, adjuvant selection, crucial formulation profiling, preparatory techniques, process-related variables optimization for favourable formulation parameters, nanoparticle characterisation, stability profiling and entrapment efficiency enhancement [28].

9. Conclusion

Preformulation studies are all about selecting a good drug candidate with the help of various supporting parameters. The utmost requirements are starting from the optimum drug candidate selection, API form of drug, compatible excipients, drug manufacturing process, stability studies as per regulatory guidelines, container and closure selection, solubility parameters, pharmacokinetics and biopharmaceuticals behaviour, and safety strategies all come up in physical and chemical properties optimization as per current industrial regulatory perspectives. Preformulation studies provide a strong and optimum scientific background of a drug molecule concerning "proof of concept" implementation in drug development, public safety concerns, new technologies of dosage forms, improvement of quality standards, and regulatory perspectives. All the preformulation parameters are should be studied for biological drug candidates and NCEs as well in every dimensional approach to have fewer chances of molecule failure. This review chapter summarises the path of drug candidate development facilitated by preformulation studies.

Acknowledgements

The authors acknowledge the Department of Pharmaceuticals, Ministry of Chemical and Fertilizers, Govt. of India for support. The NIPER-R communication number for the review article is NIPER-R/Communication/404.

Conflict of interest

The authors declare no conflict of interest among themselves.

Abbreviations

ANDA	abbreviated new drug application
API	active pharmaceutical ingredient
CADD	computer aided drug design
CMC	chemistry, manufacturing, and controls
eCTD	electronic common technical documents
FT-IR	Fourier transform infrared spectroscopy
HCl	hydrochloric acid
HSVR	hierarchical support vector regression
IC50	inhibitory concentration
ICH	international conference on harmonisation
IND	investigational new drug
Ksp	solubility product constant
Log D	distribution constant
Log P	partition coefficient
NaCl	sodium chloride
NDA	new drug application
PAT	Process Analytical Technology
pH	potential of hydrogen
pKa	dissociation constant
QbR	question-based review
QoS-QbR	quality overall summary-question-based review
RP-UHPLC	reverse-phase ultra-high performance liquid chromatography
SAR	structure-activity relationship
TGA	thermogravimetric analysis
US-FDA	United states food and drug administration

Author details

Kailash Ahirwar and Rahul Shukla*
Department of Pharmaceutics, National Institute of Pharmaceutical Education and Research-Raebareli, Lucknow, India

*Address all correspondence to: rahulshuklapharm@gmail.com

References

[1] Higgins J, Cartwright ME, Templeton AC. Progressing preclinical drug candidates: Strategies on preclinical safety studies and the quest for adequate exposure. Drug discovery today. 2012 Aug 1;**17**(15-16):828-836

[2] Jones TM. Preformulation studies. In: Tovey GD, editor. Pharmaceutical Formulation: The Science and Technology of Dosage Forms. Croydon, UK: The Royal Society of Chemistry; 2018. p. 1-19

[3] Kumar P, Desu PK, Vaishnavi G, Divya K, Lakshmi U, Kumar DP. An overview on preformulation studies. Indo American Journal of Pharmacetical Sciences. 2015;**2**(10):1399-1407

[4] Gopinath R, Naidu RS. Pharmaceutical preformulation studies. Current Review. International Journal of Pharmaceutical & Biological Archives. 2011;**2**(5):1391-1400

[5] Patel P. Preformulation studies: An integral part of formulation design. In: Pharmaceutical Formulation Design—Recent Practices. London, UK: IntechOpen; 2020:1-19

[6] Ebube NK, Owusu-Ababio G, Adeyeye CM. Preformulation studies and characterization of the physicochemical properties of amorphous polymers using artificial neural networks. International Journal of Pharmaceutics. 2000;**196**(1):27-35

[7] Younis US, Vallorz E, Addison KJ, Ledford JG, Myrdal PB. Preformulation and evaluation of tofacitinib as a therapeutic treatment for asthma. AAPS PharmSciTech. 2019;**20**:1-11

[8] Borhade V, Pathak S, Sharma S, Patravale V. Clotrimazole nanoemulsion for malaria chemotherapy. Part I: Preformulation studies, formulation design and physicochemical evaluation. International Journal of Pharmaceutics. 2012;**431**(1-2):138-148

[9] Liu M, Sharma M, Lu GL, Yin N, Gailani M, Sreebhavan S, et al. Preformulation studies of l-glutathione: Physicochemical properties, degradation kinetics, and in vitro cytotoxicity investigations. Drug Development and Industrial Pharmacy. 2020;**46**(5):717-731

[10] Sripetch S, Ryzhakov A, Loftsson T. Preformulation studies of dovitinib free base: Solubility, lipophilicity and stability. International Journal of Pharmaceutics. 10 May 2022;**619**:121721

[11] Sun D, Gao W, Hu H, Zhou S. Why 90% of clinical drug development fails and how to improve it? Acta Pharmaceutica Sinica B. 2022;**12**(7):3049-3062

[12] Segall AI. Preformulation: The use of FTIR in compatility studies. Journal of Innovations in Applied Pharmaceutical Sciences. 2019;**4**:1-6

[13] Srinivasarao J, Gopinath C. Preformulation studies of nifedipine. International Journal of Pharmaceutical Research. 2020;**12**(3):71-85

[14] Desu PK, Vaishnavi G, Divya K, Lakshmi U. An overview on preformulation studies. Indo American Journal of Pharmaceutical Sciences. 2015;**2**(10):1399-1407

[15] Rathod D, Fu Y, Patel K. BRD4 PROTAC as a novel therapeutic approach for the treatment of vemurafenib resistant melanoma: Preformulation studies, formulation development and in vitro evaluation. European

Journal of Pharmaceutical Sciences. 2019;**138**:105039

[16] Shahwal VK, Dubey BK, Bhoumick M. Preformulation study of levofloxacin. International Journal. Advances in Pharmaceutics. 2013;**1**(1):1-8

[17] Aodah A, Pavlik A, Karlage K, Myrdal PB. Preformulation studies on piperlongumine. PLoS One. 2016;**11**:3

[18] Acharya PC, Shetty S, Fernandes C, Suares D, Maheshwari R, Tekade RK. Preformulation in drug research and pharmaceutical product development. Dosage Form Design Considerations. 2018;**I**:1-55

[19] Lance PT, Greenaway RV, Edwards B. An Assessment of Concerns Regarding New Regulatory Guidance for Combination Products: A review of the submissions made to the FDA regarding their proposed draft new guidance on human factors studies for a combination product in an abbreviated new drug application. Therapeutic Innovation & Regulatory Science. 2019;**53**(2):254-263

[20] Bandopadhyay S, Bandyopadhyay N, Deb PK, Singh C, Tekade RK. Preformulation studies of drug substances, protein, and peptides: Role in drug discovery and pharmaceutical product development. Dosage Form Design Considerations. 2018;**I**:401-433

[21] Ahmad N, Alam MA, Ahmad R, Umar S, Jalees AF. Improvement of oral efficacy of irinotecan through biodegradable polymeric nanoparticles through in vitro and in vivo investigations. Journal of Microencapsulation. 2018;**35**(4):327-343

[22] Hageman M. Preformulation designed to enable discovery and assess developability. Combinatorial Chemistry & High Throughput Screening. 2010;**13**(2):90-100

[23] Stephenson A, Wu Z, Yuan X. The preformulation stability studies of a proline prodrug of methotrexate. Medicinal Chemistry. 2012;**8**(4):622-628

[24] Gualdesi MS, Ravetti S, Raviolo MA, Briñón MC. Preformulation studies of novel 5′-O-carbonates of lamivudine with biological activity: Solubility and stability assays. Drug Development and Industrial Pharmacy. 2014;**40**(9):1246-1252

[25] Alsharabasy AM. Concise review: Considerations for the formulation, delivery and administration routes of biopharmaceuticals. Archives of Biotechnology and Biomedicine. 2017;**1**(1):033-053

[26] ICH Official web site: ICH

[27] Amarji B, Abed SN, Bairagi U, Deb PK, Al-Attraqchi O, Choudhury AA, et al. Four stages of pharmaceutical product development: Preformulation, prototype development and scale-up, biological aspects, and commercialization. Dosage Form Design Considerations. 2018;**I**:637-668

[28] Dhapte V, Pokharkar V. Nanosystems for drug delivery: Design, engineering, and applications. Green Synthesis, Characterization and Applications of Nanoparticles. Amsterdam, Netherlands: Elsevier Inc., 2019:321-345. DOI: 10.1016/B978-0-08-102579-6.00013-7

[29] Ashizawa K. Physicochemical profiling and preformulation studies at the drug discovery stage. Nihon Yakurigaku Zasshi. 2006;**127**(3):213-216

[30] Gomis-Tena J, Brown BM, Cano J, Trenor B, Yang PC, Saiz J, et al. When

does the IC50 accurately assess the blocking potency of a drug? Journal of Chemical Information and Modeling. 2020;**60**(3):1779-1790

[31] Gomase V, Tagore S. Toxicogenomics. Current Drug Metabolism. 2008;**9**(3):250-254

[32] Pippa N, Stangel C, Kastanas I, Triantafyllopoulou E, Naziris N, Stellas D, et al. Carbon nanohorn/liposome systems: Preformulation, design and in vitro toxicity studies. Materials Science & Engineering. C, Materials for Biological Applications. 2019:105

[33] Bharate SS, Vishwakarma RA. Impact of preformulation on drug development. Expert Opinion on Drug Delivery. 2013;**10**(9):1239-1257

[34] Patel V, Shah M. Artificial intelligence and machine learning in drug discovery and development. Intelligent Medicine. 2022;**2**(3):134-140

[35] Sigfridsson K, Nilsson L, Ahlqvist M, Andersson T, Granath AK. Preformulation investigation and challenges; salt formation, salt disproportionation and hepatic recirculation. European Journal of Pharmaceutical Sciences. 2017;**104**:262-272

[36] Ledeţi A, Vlase G, Vlase T, Bercean V, Murariu MS, Ledeţi I, et al. Solid-state preformulation studies of amiodarone hydrochloride. Journal of Thermal Analysis and Calorimetry. 2016;**126**(1):181-187

[37] Huang LF, Tong WQ. Impact of solid-state properties on developability assessment of drug candidates. Advanced Drug Delivery Reviews. 2004;**56**(3):321-334

[38] Baldelli A, Power RM, Miles REH, Reid JP, Vehring R. Effect of crystallization kinetics on the properties of spray dried microparticles. Aerosol Science and Technology. 2016;**50**(7):693-704

[39] Harahap U, Marianne M, Yuandani Y, Laila L. Preformulation study of Pugun Tano (Curanga fel-terrae [lour.] Merr) Ethanolic extract granule mass in capsule as Hepatoprotective drug. Open access Maced. Journal of Medical Sciences. 2019;**7**(22):3729-3732

[40] Akseli I, Hilden J, Katz JM, Kelly RC, Kramer TT, Mao C, et al. Reproducibility of the measurement of bulk/tapped density of pharmaceutical powders between pharmaceutical laboratories. Journal of Pharmaceutical Sciences. 2019;**108**(3):1081-1084

[41] Antonio A, Júnior S, Carbinatto FM, Castro O. Preformulation studies of Gymnema sylvestre extract powder formulation for hard gelatin capsules. Revista de Ciências Farmacêuticas Básica e Aplicada. 2011;**32**(2):175-180

[42] Moravkar KK, Korde SD, Bhairav BA, Shinde SB, Kakulade Sv, Chalikwar SS. Traditional and advanced flow characterization techniques: A platform review for development of solid dosage form. Indian Journal of Pharmaceutical Sciences. 2020;**82**(6):945-957

[43] Szunyogh T, Ambrus R, Szabóné RP. Importance of particle size decrease in the preformulation. Acta Pharmaceutica Hungarica. 2011;**81**(1):29-36

[44] Quodbach J, Kleinebudde P. A new apparatus for real-time assessment of the particle size distribution of disintegrating tablets. Journal of Pharmaceutical Sciences. 2014;**103**(11):3657-3665

[45] Nachajski MJ, Bazela A, Zarzycka M, Broszczyk A, Kołba A,

Kołodziejczyk MK. Effect of API on powder flowability, direct compression and properties of orally disintegrating tablets: A preformulation study. Indian Journal of Pharmaceutical Sciences. 2019;**81**(3):489-495

[46] Gao Z, Rohani S, Gong J, Wang J. Recent developments in the crystallization process: Toward the pharmaceutical industry. Engineering. 2017;**3**(3):343-353

[47] Burger A, Lettenbichler A. Polymorphism and preformulation studies of lifibrol. European Journal of Pharmaceutics and Biopharmaceutics. 2000;**49**(1):65-72

[48] Patel C, Suthar D, Patel H, Movaliya V, Parejiya P. Preformulation study of glimepiride: An insight for formulation and development of parenteral formulation. Journal of Pharmaceutical Research International. 2022;**34**(15b):38-49

[49] Kesharwani R, Ansari MS, Patel DK. Novel technology used in the preformulation study: A review. Journal of Drug Delivery and Therapeutics. 2017;7(4):20-33

[50] Bashir Alsirawan MHD, Paradkar A. Impact of the polymorphic form of drugs/NCEs on Preformulation and formulation development. In: Bachhav Y, editor. Innovative Dosage Forms: Design and Development at Early Stage. Wiley. 2019:1-47

[51] Makoni PA, Ranchhod J, WaKasongo K, Khamanga SM, Walker RB. The use of quantitative analysis and Hansen solubility parameter predictions for the selection of excipients for lipid nanocarriers to be loaded with water soluble and insoluble compounds. Saudi Pharmaceutical Journal. 2020;**28**(3):308-315

[52] Wang X, Wei L, Kotra LP. Cyanocobalamin (vitamin B12) conjugates with enhanced solubility. Bioorganic & Medicinal Chemistry. 2007;**15**(4):1780-1787

[53] Tahvanainen M, Rotko T, Mäkilä EA, Santos H, Neves D, Laaksonen T, et al. Tablet preformulations of indomethacin-loaded mesoporous silicon microparticles. International Journal of Pharmaceutics. 2012;**422**(1-2):125-131

[54] Di L, Kerns EH. Drug-Like Properties. Amsterdam: Elsevier; 2016. DOI: 10.1016/B978-0-12-801076-1.00023-X

[55] Pramar Y, Gupta V, das, Bethea C, Zerai T. Stability of cefuroxime axetil in suspensions. Journal of Clinical Pharmacy and Therapeutics. 1991;**16**(5):341-344

[56] Parasrampuria J, das Gupta V. Preformulation studies of acetazolamide: Effect of pH, two buffer species, ionic strength, and temperature on its stability. Journal of Pharmaceutical Sciences. 1989;**78**(10):855-857

[57] Dudzinski J, Lachman L, Shami E, Tingstad J. Preformulation studies I: Molindone hydrochloride. Journal of Pharmaceutical Sciences. 1973;**62**(4):622-624

[58] Davis DG, Perlman ME, London RE. Direct measurements of the dissociation-rate constant for inhibitor-enzyme complexes via the T1 rho and T2 (CPMG) methods. Journal of Magnetic Resonance. Series B. 1994;**104**(3):266-275

[59] Bharate S, Kumar VA, Vishwakarma R. Determining partition coefficient (log P), distribution coefficient (log D) and ionization constant (pKa) in early drug discovery. Combinatorial Chemistry

& High Throughput Screening. 2016;**19**(6):461-469

[60] Thumma S, Majumdar S, ElSohly MA, Gul W, Repka MA. Preformulation studies of a prodrug of Delta9-tetrahydrocannabinol. AAPS PharmSciTech. 2008;**9**(3):982-990

[61] Chikezie Ayogu P, Ezugwu MI, Ifeanyi EF. Principle of common-ion effect and its application in chemistry: A review. Journal of Chemistry Letters. 2020;**1**(2):77-83

[62] Chang J, Leong RW, Wasinger VC, Ip M, Yang M, Phan TG. Impaired intestinal permeability contributes to ongoing bowel symptoms in patients with inflammatory bowel disease and mucosal healing. Gastroenterology. 2017;**153**(3):723-731.e1

[63] Majee SB, Biswas GR. Computational methods in preformulation study for pharmaceutical solid dosage forms of therapeutic proteins. Physical Sciences Reviews. 2019;**2**(6):19-19

[64] Chaudhary P. Preformulation studies for ayurveda drugs: A review. International Research Journal of Pharmacy. 2019;**10**(3):19

[65] Egart M, Janković B, Srčič S. Application of instrumented nanoindentation in preformulation studies of pharmaceutical active ingredients and excipients. Acta Pharmaceutica. 2016;**66**(3):303-330

[66] Verma G, Mishra MK. Pharmaceutical Preformulation studies in formulation and development of new dosage form: A review. International Journal of Pharma Research & Review. 2016;**5**(10):12-20

[67] Waterman KC, Adami RC, Alsante KM, Hong J, Landis MS, Lombardo F, et al. Stabilization of pharmaceuticals to oxidative degradation. Pharmaceutical Development and Technology. 2002;7(1):1-32

[68] Lieberman H, Vemuri NM. Chemical and Physicochemical Approaches to solve formulation problems. In The Practice of Medicinal Chemistry. Academic Press. 2015:767-791

[69] Kahan BD, Napoli KL, Kelly PA, Podbielski J, Hussein I, Urbauer DL, et al. Therapeutic drug monitoring of sirolimus: Correlations with efficacy and toxicity. Clinical Transplantation. 2000;**14**(2):97-109

[70] Tenchov R, Bird R, Curtze AE, Zhou Q. Lipid nanoparticles from liposomes to mRNA vaccine delivery, a landscape of research diversity and advancement. ACS Nano. 2021;**15**(11):16982-17015

[71] Thapa RK, Winther-Larsen HC, Diep DB, Tønnesen HH. Preformulation studies on novel garvicin KS peptides for topical applications. European Journal of Pharmaceutical Sciences. 2020;**151**:105333

[72] Vilegave K, Vidyasagar G, Chandankar P. Preformulation studies of pharmaceutical new drug molecule & products: An overview. American Journal of Pharmacy and Health Research. 2013;**1**(3):1-20

[73] Chawla R, Rani V, Mishra M, Kumar K. Computer simulation and Modeling in pharmacokinetics and pharmacodynamics. Computer Aided Pharmaceutics and Drug Delivery. Singapore: Springer Nature; 2022:217-254

[74] Nainwal N, Bahuguna R, Banerjee S, Saharan VA. Historical developments on computer applications in pharmaceutics. Computer Aided Pharmaceutics and Drug Delivery. 2022:39-72. ISBN: 978-981-16-5179-3

[75] A Al-Achi · Integrated Pharmaceutics - Applied Preformulation, Product Design, and Regulatory Science, 2nd Edition (Hardcover Book) (2022.

[76] Tyagi RK, Garg N, Shukla R, Bisen PS, editors. Role of Novel Drug Delivery Vehicles in Nanobiomedicine. BoD–Books on Demand. 26 Feb 2020

[77] Shukla R, Handa M, Lokesh SB, Ruwali M, Kohli K, Kesharwani P. Conclusion and future prospective of polymeric nanoparticles for cancer therapy. In: Polymeric Nanoparticles as a Promising Tool for Anti-cancer Therapeutics. Academic Press; 1 Jan 2019:389-408

[78] Shahwal VK. Preformulation studies and preperation of dithranol loaded solid lipidnanoparticles. International Journal of BioMed Research. 2012;**3**(7):343-350

[79] Senthila S, Manojkumar P, Venkatesan P. Characterisation of preformulation parameters to design, develop and formulate silymarin loaded plga nanop articles for liver targeted drug delivery. Research Journal of Pharmacy and Technology. 2021;**14**(10):5508-5514

[80] Castro SR, Ribeiro LNM, Breitkreitz MC, Guilherme VA, Rodrigues da Silva GH, Mitsutake H, et al. A pre-formulation study of tetracaine loaded in optimized nanostructured lipid carriers. Scientific Reports. 2021;**11**(1):21463

[81] Chaurasia G. A review on pharmaceutical preformulation studies in formulation and development of new drug molecules. International Journal of Pharmaceutical Sciences and Research. 2016;**7**(6):2313-2320

[82] Majid H, Puzik A, Maier T, Eberhard D, Bartel A, Mueller HC, et al. Exploring the transmucosal permeability of cyclobenzaprine: A comparative preformulation by standardized and controlled ex vivo and in vitro permeation studies. International Journal of Pharmaceutics. 2021;**601**:120574

Section 2

Formulation Design and Approaches

Chapter 2

Formulation by Design: An Overview

Ushasi Das, Dilip Kumar Panda and Sanchita Mandal

Abstract

Quality is the most important and necessary attribute for pharmaceutical product development, and it has become the focus of regulatory bodies in order to approve safe, efficacious, stable, patient-compliance, and cost-effective drug delivery systems. QbD-based formulation development is discovered to be an immerging technique in this context. FbD is a formulation development concept that aims to create more effective, safe, robust, cost-effective, and patient-compliant drug delivery systems. This chapter will provide an overview of Formulation by Design (FbD), different terminologies, design of experiment (DoE) and quality by design (QbD), types of experimental design, QbD applications, and FbD methodology along with benefits.

Keywords: formulation by design (FbD), quality by design (Qbd), Design of Experiment (DoE), drug delivery systems, pharmaceutical product development

1. Introduction

Quality is the most crucial and essential attribute for pharmaceutical product development, and it has become the thrust area for the regulatory bodies to approve safe, efficacious, stable, patient-compliance and economical drug delivery systems. It is important to recognize that "The Quality cannot be tested into products; i.e., quality should be build in by design". In this context, QbD-based formulation development is found to be an immerging technique. Pharmaceutical cGMPs for the 21st Century - A Risk-Based Approach, published in 2004, describes the Quality by Design approach, which was approved by the FDA. Detailed specifications for pharmaceutical product quality are provided in International Conference on Harmonization (ICH) Q8 pharmaceutical development, Q9 quality risk assessment, and Q10 pharmaceutical quality system. QbD and DoE strategies aid in the implementation of ICH/Q8 and ICH/Q9 [1]. Pharmaceutical Quality by Design (QbD) begins the systematic development of product(s) and process(es) with desired quality based on the Juran's Quality philosophy. The QbD philosophy, which is a patient-centric approach, prioritizes patient safety by designing drug products with enhanced quality and decreased manufacturing costs by planning quality early to prevent quality crises [2]. ICH guidance Q8 (R2) describes QbD as, "a systematic approach to pharmaceutical development that begins with predefined objectives and emphasizes product and process understanding and process control, based on sound science and quality risk management" [3]. Quality by design is an approach that aims to ensure the quality of medicines by employing statistical, analytical and risk-management methodology in the design, development and manufacturing of medicines. The identification, justification, and management of all sources of variability impacting a process are some of the objectives of quality by design. This enables the finished medicine to consistently meet its predefined characteristics from the start - so that it is 'right first time' [4]. The OFAT-method (one-factor-at-a-time) was the conventional strategy for ensuring and sustaining product quality. It was an empirical technique based on trial and error and built on the *ceteris paribus* principle. This method included the risk of accounting for the potential occurrence of unanticipated, out-of-specification results due to inadequate product and process understanding, both during process optimization and at the validation stage [5]. In these OVAT experiments, the first variable is fixed at a specified value, and each subsequent variable is investigated until no more improvement in the response variable is shown (s). In a summary, the OVAT technique has shown to be insignificant in terms of effort, time, and money as well as unable to offer the true answer by correcting the errors; the results continue to be unpredictable and sometimes even unsuccessful [6]. Recently, whether in industrial practice or in the research milieu, a comprehensive and rigorous approach of pharmaceutical quality by design (QbD) has become popular throughout drug product development [3, 6–9]. **Table 1** provides a brief representation of the advantages of FbD over OVAT methodology. DoE along with QbD having much wider applicability in recent trends in the Pharma industrial as well as in the research milieu, an appropriate term has evolved specifically in development of pharmaceutical dosage form, that is, "Formulation by Design (FbD)". The FbD methodology, therefore, tends to encompass in its purview a rational usage of DoE approach to design more efficacious, safe, robust, economical and patient-compliant Drug Delivery System to accomplish the QbD objectives. The FbD technique is remarkable for its ability to forecast formulation performance as well as

Attributes	OVAT	FbD
Choice of optimum formulation	May result only in sub-optimal solutions	Produces the optimum formulation possible.
Interaction among the ingredients	Inept to reveal possible interactions	Estimates any synergistic or antagonistic interaction among constituents
Scale-up and postapproval changes	Extremely challenging to design formulations that just slightly deviate from the ideal formulation, especially after Level II	All response variables are quantitatively controlled by a set of input variables, making it simple to incorporate changes in the optimal formulation
Resource economics	Highly resource-intensive, as it leads to unnecessary runs and batches	Economical, as it furnishes information on product/process performance using minimal trials
Time economics	Incredibly time-consuming because each product must have its performance analyzed independently	Can use model equations to simulate the behavior of the product or process

Table 1.
Comparison of OVAT (one-factor-at-a-time) and FbD (formulation by design) methodology.

identify and calculate potential interactions and synergy between variables. FbD helps to fully comprehend the formulation system, and can trace and rectify a "problem" in a remarkably easier manner. As a result, the FbD technique frequently includes a reasonable application of the DoE approach to create high-quality drug products in an efficient and economical manner, endeavoring ultimately to achieve the QbD objectives [10].

2. FbD Teminology

During FbD practice, specific terminology, both technical and non-technical, is usually used. Important terms have been compiled in **Table 2** to facilitate better understanding of FbD of oral DDS precepts. Prior to applying FbD, it is critical to be familiar with FbD terminology and have prior multidisciplinary knowledge on various possible products and process variables. Therefore, it is necessary to separate a "knowledge space," or a whole worth exploring area, from the potential large ocean of scientific material based on prior knowledge. As a result, a "knowledge space" includes all the product and process variables that could even slightly affect the final product's quality. A "design space" must be defined as a subset construct of a "knowledge space" to ensure the best possible performance of a process or product using a "chosen few" key variables. This "design space" is used to further derive the "control space," which is the experimental area reserved for in-depth research when studies are conducted within narrower ranges of input variables. It is also known as "control tactic" on occasion. The knowledge space is transformed into the control space using a methodical strategy on archived data in the "design space" [11]. For relatively complex DDSs, extensive experimentation may be required to eliminate uncertainty and justify a design space greater than that needed for traditional formulation systems like tablets. Working within the design space would not begin any post-approval change process in accordance with federal regulations because it is not regarded as a "change" [3]. **Figure 1** depicts the order of importance in the knowledge, design, and control spaces.

3. FbD methodology

The theme of FbD optimization methodology provides thorough and thought-through information on diverse aspects, organized in a five-step sequence, as schematically depicted in **Figure 2**.

- **Step I: Ascertaining Drug Product Objective(s):** A quality target product profile (QTPP) is embarked upon encompassing the fundamental information of the product to be prepared or aspired as "goal-setting" exercise through brain storming among the team members cutting across industrial disciplines. Various critical quality attributes (CQAs), or response variables, which pragmatically epitomize the objective(s), are earmarked for the purpose. All the independent product/process variables are also listed likewise.

- **Step II: Prioritizing Input Variables for Optimization:** The critical material attributes (CMAs) and critical process parameters (CPPs), which directly influence the CQAs, represent the product quality are prioritized. Prioritization

Term	Definition
Antagonism	Undesired negative change due to interaction among factors.
Blocks	A set of relatively homogenous experimental conditions, wherein every level of the primary factor occurs the same number of times with each level of nuisance factor.
Categorical variables	Qualitative variables which cannot be quantified.
Coding (or normalization)	Process of transforming a natural variable into a non-dimensional coded variable.
Confounding	Lack of orthogonality.
Constraints	Restrictions imposed on the factor levels.
Contour plot	Geometric illustration of a response obtained by plotting one independent variable against another, while holding the magnitude of response and other variables as constant.
Control space	Domain of design space selected for detailed controlled strategy.
Control strategy	A planned set of controls that ensures process performance and product quality and is derived from current product and process information. Controls may include facility and equipment operating conditions, in-process controls, finished product specifications, and the associated methods and frequency of monitoring and control. They may also include parameters and attributes related to drug substance and drug product materials and components.
Critical Formulation Attributes	Formulation parameters affecting critical quality attribute.
Critical Process Parameters	A process parameter whose variability has an impact on a critical quality attribute and therefore should be monitored or controlled to ensure the process produces the desired quality.
Critical Quality Attributes	A physical, chemical, biological or microbiological property or characteristic that should be within an appropriate limit, range, or distribution to ensure the desired product quality.
Design Matrix	Layout of experimental runs in matrix form as per experimental design.
Design Space	The demonstrated multidimensional combination and interaction of process factors (such as material qualities) and input variables that can guarantee quality. Change is not regarded as occurring when working within the design space. Exiting the design space is seen as a change and ordinarily starts a regulatory post-approval change process. The applicant submits a design space proposal, which is subject to regulatory review and approval.
Effect	The magnitude of the change in response caused by varying the factor level(s).
Empirical Model	Mathematical model describing factor–response relation using polynomial equations.
Experimental Domain	Part of the factor space, investigated experimentally for optimization.
Factors	Independent variables, which tend to influence the product/process characteristics or output of the process.
Factor Space	Dimensional space defined by the coded variables.
Formal Experimental Design	A structured, organized method for determining the relationship between factors affecting a process and the output of that process. Also known as "Design of Experiments".
Independent Variables	Input variables, which are directly under the control of the product development scientist.

Term	Definition
Interaction	Lack of additivity of factor effects
Knowledge Space	Scientific elements to be considered and explored on the basis of previous knowledge as product attributes and process parameters.
Levels	Values assigned to a factor.
Lifecycle	All phases in the life of a product from the initial development through marketing until the product's discontinuation.
Main Effect	The effect of a factor averaged over all the levels of other factors.
Nuisance Factors	Uncontrollable factors which complicate the estimation of main effect or interactions.
Optimize	Make as perfect, effective or functional as possible.
Optimization	Implementation of systematic approaches to achieve 'the best' combination of product and/or process characteristics under a given set of conditions using Formulation by Design and computers.
Orthogonality	A condition where the estimated effects are due to the main factor of interest, but independent of interactions.
Process Analytical Technology (PAT)	A system for planning, evaluating, and managing production through timely measurements of key performance and quality characteristics of raw and in-process materials and processes, with the aim of ensuring the quality of the finished product.
Process Robustness	Ability of a process to withstand material variability, changes in the process, and equipment modifications without negatively affecting quality.
Proven Acceptable Range	A defined range of a process parameter that, when used while maintaining other parameters constant, would produce materials that fulfill the necessary quality standards.
Quality	The suitability of either a drug substance or a drug product for its intended use. This term includes such attributes as the identity, strength, and purity.
Quality by Design (QbD)	A systematic approach to development that begins with predefined objectives and emphasizes product and process understanding and process control, based on sound science and quality risk management.
Quality Target Product Profile (QTPP)	A future summary of the qualities of a drug product that should be attained to assure the intended quality, taking into account the product's safety and efficacy.
Quantitative Variables	Variables that can take numeric values.
Resolution	The measure of the degree of confounding.
Response Surface	Graphical depiction of the mathematical relationship.
Response Surface Plot	3D graphical representation of a response plotted between two independent variables and one response variable.
Response Variables	Characteristics of the finished drug product or the in-process material.
Runs or Trials	Experiments conducted according to the selected experimental design.
Synergism	Desired positive change due to interaction between factors.

Table 2.
Important terms used in the formulation by design of pharmaceutical drug delivery:

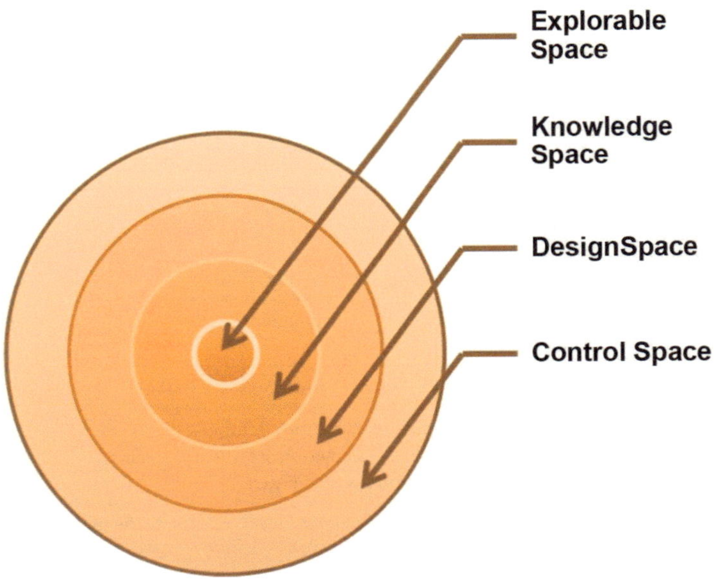

Figure 1.
Inter-relationship among knowledge, design and control spaces.

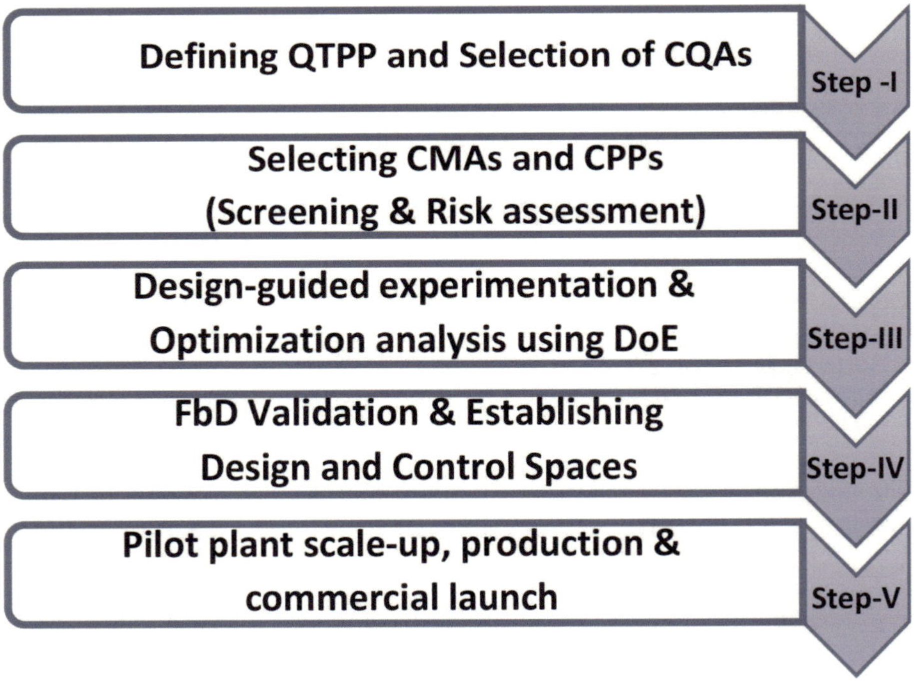

Figure 2.
Schematic representation of FbD optimization methodology.

may be accomplished by carrying out the risk assessment and quality risk management (QRM) approach by earmarking the severity of risk, its frequency of occurrence and detectability associated with each input variable. For that, the moderate to high risk factors are chosen from patient perspectives through brainstorming among the team members using techniques like risk estimation matrix (REM), failure mode effects analysis (FMEA). These techniques help in identifying and sorting the potential risk associated with each CMA as applicable to the identified CQAs. Selection of "vital few" influential factors among the "possible many" input variables is invariably conducted using experimental designs through a process, popularly termed as factor screening. In a nutshell, screening exercise tends to help the scientist in opting the "leader" variables, while weeding out the "idler" ones. By and large, low-resolution first-order designs (like full-factorial and fractional factorial, Plackett-Burman, Taguchi designs) suffice the purpose of screening of a large number of experimental parameters. Experimental studies are also undertaken to define the broad range of factor levels. Apt use of screening designs, in this regard, helps to identifying the potential CMAs actually affecting the CQAs and reducing their number.

- **Step III: Design-guided Experimentation & FbD Analysis:** An experimental design constitutes the pivot of the entire FbD exercise esp. for RSM analysis. A suitable experimental design is worked out to map the responses on the basis of the study objective(s), CQAs being explored, number and the type of factors, and factor levels viz. high, medium or low. Out of several experimental designs, the factorial, Box-Behnken, composite, optimal and mixture designs are most extensively and frequently to optimize various drug products esp. those capable of handling second order nonlinear responses. For the purpose of directing the drug delivery scientists, a design matrix—a matrix-based architecture of experimental runs—is afterwards created. The design matrix is followed in the experimental preparation of the medication formulations, and the selected response variables are carefully assessed.

- **Step IV: FbD Modelization & Validation:** The quantitative dependence of a response variable on the independent variables is defined by a model, which can be expressed mathematically or graphically. Primarily, first, second, and very infrequently third order polynomials are used as models. Response surface methodology (RSM) uses the interaction of RSM polynomials, the required constraints/criteria for optimum search, and the design constraint to connect a response variable to the levels of input variables. Additionally, 2D-contour and 3D-response surface plots, which are incredibly helpful in revealing the pertinent scientific nitpicking and interactions between the input variables, are used in the Response surface modeling and analysis. As a component of knowledge and an explorable space, a design space is entered into in order to find the best formulation composition.

- **Step V: FbD Validation, Scale-up and Production:** The FbD methodology's validation is an important milestone in determining how well the polynomial models under investigation can predict the future. Different drug formulations are chosen from the many experimental domain regions, created, and tested following with the standard operating procedures established for the formulations created earlier, usually described as checkpoints or confirmatory runs. The residual analysis is then carried out after comparing the findings from these checkpoints with those that were projected.

The optimum formulation is scaled up through a pilot plant, an exhibit, and production scale to confirm FbD performance. This phase is carried out in an industrial setting to guarantee that the performed drug product optimization study is reliable and reproducible. The entire process results in a thorough grasp of the product and process at the production and/or commercial scale, in addition to the final product being made available in an "optimized" form compatible with product excellence and federal compliance. A comprehensive and adaptable "control plan" is painstakingly developed and put into practice, ultimately leading to the objective of "continuous improvement" of drug delivery.

3.1 Experimental designs used during FbD of oral DDS

An experimental design serves as the basis of the FbD exercise. In systematic FbD optimization of DDS, a thorough "screening" of crucial variables is followed by a study of the experimental design-based response surface. Out of all experimental designs, oral DDS has been widely optimized using factororial and central composite designs [12–17]. The main experimental approaches used for oral DDS optimization are compared in **Table 3**, along with their advantages and disadvantages. Full factorial designs (FDs), including two-level and three-level FDs, fractional factorial designs (CCD), Box-Behnken designs (BBD), Plackett-Burman designs (PBD), Taguchi methods, and mixture designs, are among the several types of experimental designs (**Figure 3**) [19].

Advantages of Experimental Designs (ED) (Figure 4)

- Increased innovation as a result of process improvement.
- Fewer batch errors.

Design	Description	Diagrammatic representation
1. Full Factorial Designs (FDs): a. two-level full FDs; b. three-level full FDs	A factorial experiment is one in which all of the levels (x) of a particular factor (k) are coupled with all of the levels of every other factor in the experiment, with xk total experiments. **Merits:** • Maximizing the use of data while being effective in estimating major effects and interactions **Demerits:** • In a 2-level architecture, curvature reflection is not conceivable • Additional trials are needed.	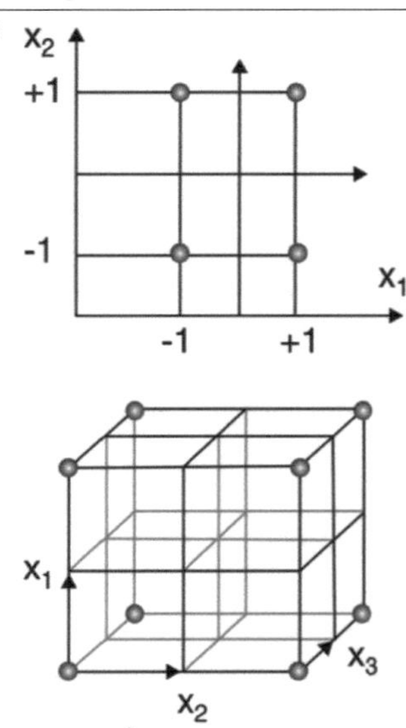 a. 2^2 FD; b. 2^3 FD

Design	Description	Diagrammatic representation
2. Central Composite Design (CCD) or Box-Wilson Design	CCDs are most typically employed for nonlinear responses needing second order models. A (2 k) FD or (2 k-r) FFD is embedded in the "composite design," which is further enhanced by a group of star points (2 k) and a "centre" point. 2 k + 2 k + 1 equal the total number of factor combinations in a CCD. **Merits:** • Combines the benefits of star and FD designs. • Enables the work to be done in stages; for example, if a linear 2-level FD is unable to effectively fit the data, a centre point may be added to the design. • Requires fewer tests. **Demerits:** • Fractional value (α) practice is challenging.	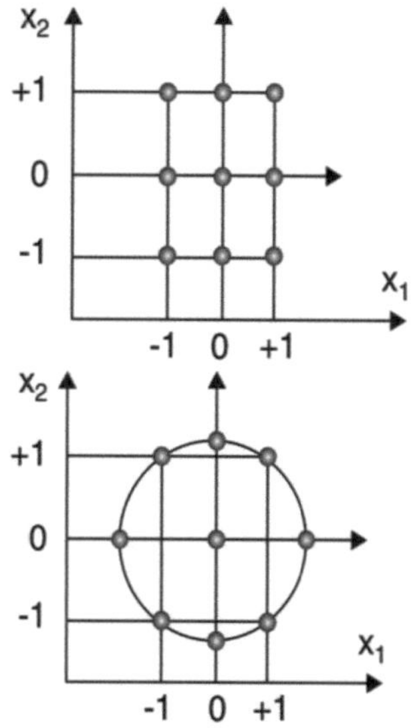 a. CCD (rectangular) with $\alpha = 1$; b. CCD (spherical) with $\alpha = 1.414$
3. Box-Behnken Design (BBD)	A specially made design, the BBD, requires only three levels for each factor, i.e., –l, 0 and + 1. A BBD is an economical alternative to CCD	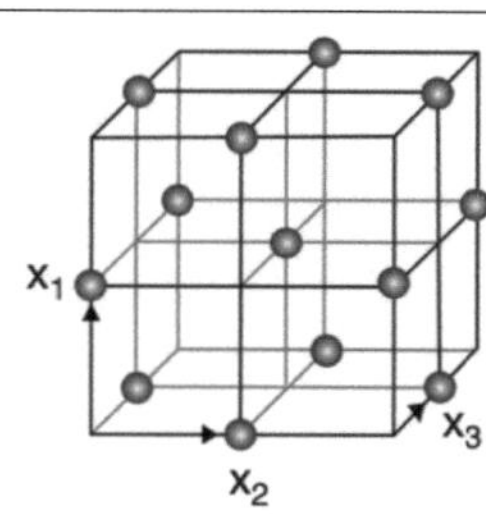 BBD for three factors
4. Plackett- burman Designs (Hadamard Design)	PBDs are unique two-level FFDs that are typically employed for K factor screening, or N-1 factor screening, where N is a multiple of 4. The designs, which are also known as Hadamard designs or symmetrically reduced 2 k-r FDs, are simply created with a few numbers of attempts. **Merits:** Suitable for a very broad range of factors, including those requiring a large number of experiments for FFDs **Demerits:** Design structure is complicated as a result of aliasing.	
5. Taguchi Designs	Used to create processes or products that are resilient to natural variability. Because it is a technique for assuring successful performance throughout the creation of products or processes, the design is also known as experimental design as "off-line quality control."	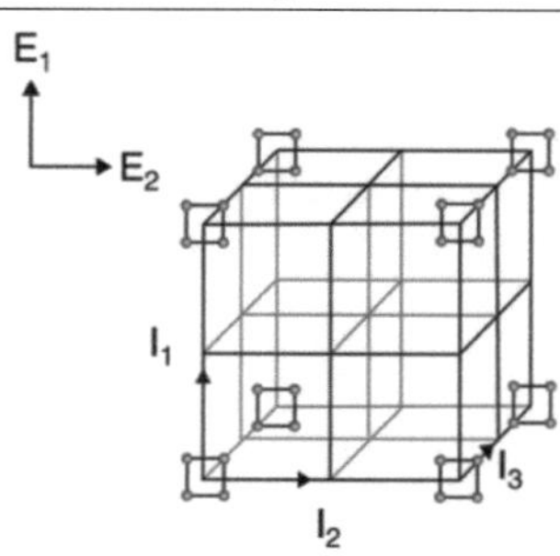 Inner 2^3 and outer 2^2 arrays of Taguchi design

Design	Description	Diagrammatic representation
6. Mixture Designs	The properties of the final product in DDS containing numerous excipients typically depend more on the quantities of the ingredients than their individual amounts. In these circumstances, mixture designs are highly advised. Only one factor level can be individually varied in a two-component combination, but only two factor levels can be freely varied in a three-component mixture. **Merits:** Ideal for formulations where a constraint is placed on a certain combination of factor levels. **Demerits:** Understanding the polynomials produced by mixture design is challenging. Quadratic effects and interactions are not estimated.	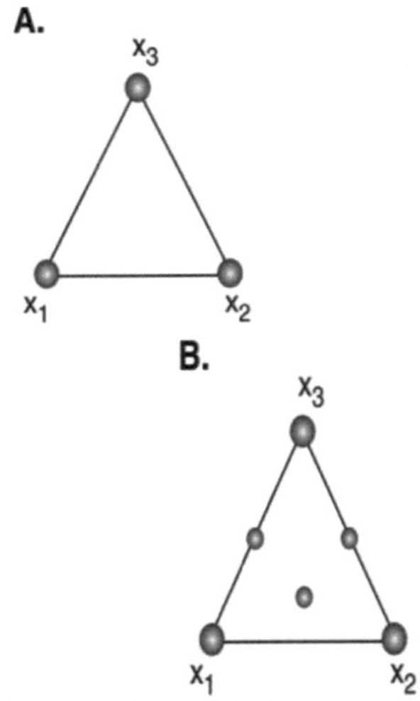 Mixture Design (a) linear model; (b) quadratic model.
7. Optimal Designs	The adoption of optimal designs is possible when the domain has an irregular form. These are the non-traditional custom designs produced by a computer exchange programme. These unique designs are typically created using an optimality criterion, such as the D-, A-, G-, I-, or V- optimality criteria. **Merits:** Can be applied even if the experimental domain is asymmetrical. **Demerits:** Uses a comparatively complicated model.	
8. Equiradial Design (Erd)	ErDs are first-degree response surface designs, consisting of N points on a circle around the center of interest in the form of a regular polygon.	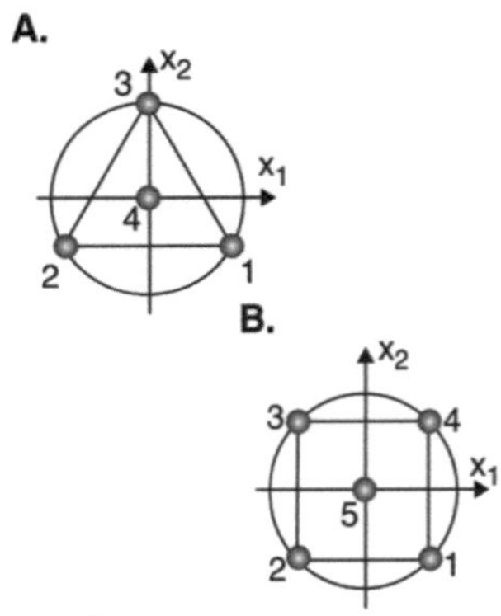 Two-factor ErD (a) triangular four-run design; (b) square fiverun design
9. Screening designs: Fractional Factorial design (FFD)	It is possible that the highest order interactions have no discernible impact when there are several elements at play. As a result, the quantity of experiments can be decreased in a methodical manner. The resulting designs are known as FFDs or occasionally partial factorial designs. An FFD is a discrete portion (1/xr) of a full or complete FD, where xk-r is the total number of necessary experiments and r is the degree of fractionation. **Merits:** Compatible with a wide range of factors or factor levels.	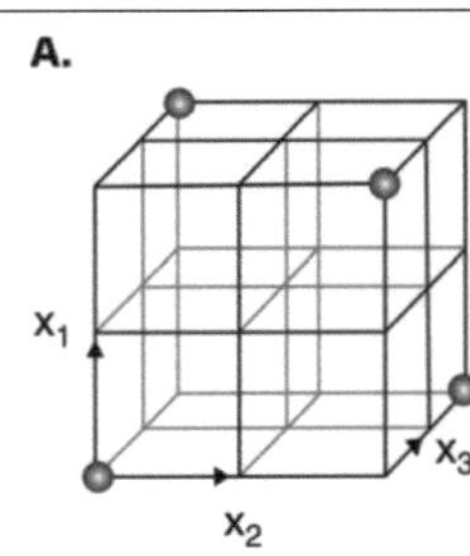

Design	Description	Diagrammatic representation
	Demerits: Effects are difficult to build, cannot be assessed in a singular manner, and are muddled by interaction terms.	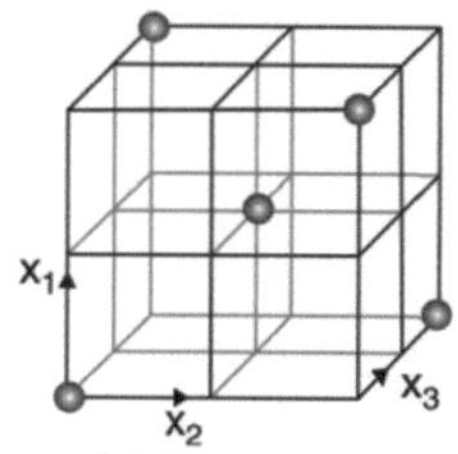 (a) 2^{3-1} FFD with design points as spheres (b) 2^{3-1} FFD with added center point.

Table 3.
Experimental designs used during formulation by design (FbD) [18].

- A higher level of regulator confidence in durable products.
- More effective manufacturing technology transfer.
- Results are acquired with replications.

Uses of Experimental Designs (ED).
It is used to discover the causes behind the variance in the response, to identify the circumstances in which the desired (maximum or minimum) response is obtained, to contrast responses at various levels of controlled variables, and to create a model for predicting response.

4. Selection of experimental design

The quantity of resources available and the degree of control desired by the experimenter over making poor decisions (i.e., Type I and Type II errors for testing hypotheses) determine which design is chosen among the numerous sorts of alternatives. For the objective of a more straightforward screening of many experimental factors, low-resolution designs like FFDs, Plackett Burman designs (PBDs), or Taguchi designs are sufficient. Only linear replies are supported by screening designs. Therefore, a more complicated design type is required if a nonlinear response is observed or if a more precise depiction of the response surface is needed. Therefore, response surface designs that can detect curvatures are used when the investigator is interested in estimating interaction and even quadratic effects or intends to have an idea of the local shape of the response surface [20]. In a nutshell, the important factors to take into account when choosing an experimental design are as follows:

- All designs can be applied for optimization of product characteristics, but SMD and EVD should not be used for process optimization.
- For screening studies, any design from 2 k FD, xk FD, FFD, PBD, or TgD may be used. The exception to this rule is all 2-level designs.

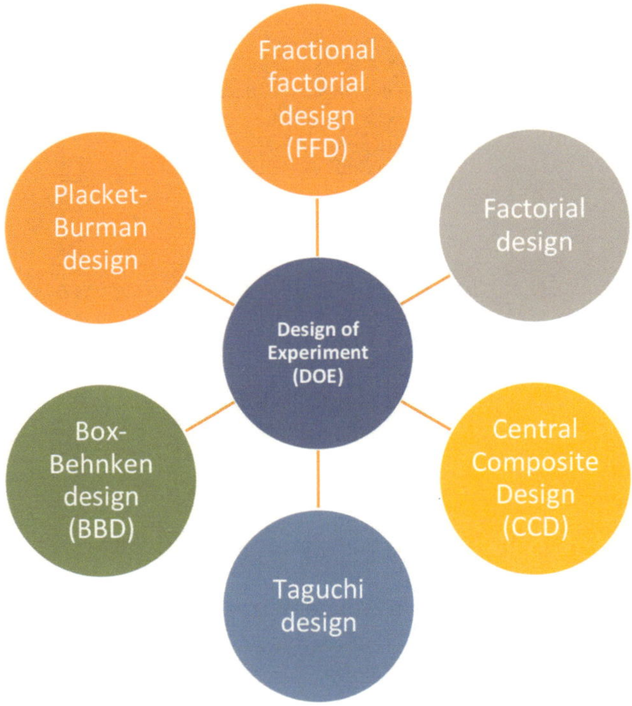

Figure 3.
Classification of Design of Experiments techniques.

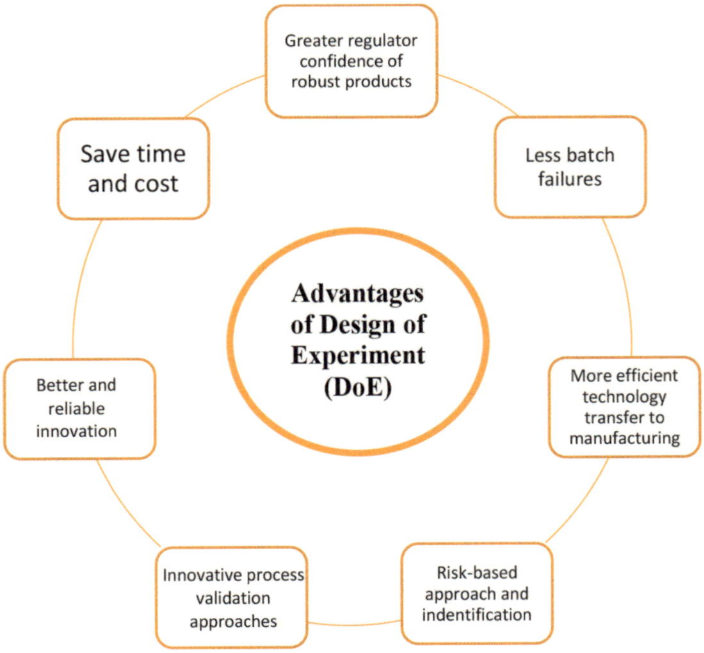

Figure 4.
Advantages of Design of Experimentation techniques.

- PBD is an option. However, screening using FFD, PBD, or Taguchi design should be used first for higher number of factors (> 6).

- Any 2 k FD, FFD, PBD, or mixture design can be used if there are only two factor levels. However, CCD, Box-Behnken (BBD), equiradial, simplex centroid, and optimal designs are preferred when there are more than three factor levels.

- xk FD, CCD, BBD, or equiradial design are preferred for quadratic models.

5. Model development

A model is an expression that shows how quantitatively dependent the independent variables are on a response variable. Both theoretical and empirical numerical models are possible. A way to explain the relationship between factors and responses is through an empirical model. It is typically a collection of polynomials of a certain order or degree. First, second, and sporadically third order polynomials are the models most frequently used to describe the response(s). The initial hypothesis is a first order model. Higher order models are used if a simple model is found to be insufficient for explaining the phenomenon.

Using regression analysis, the coefficients for quantitative factors can be estimated. Regression analysis is not used in the case of qualitative factors, however, because interpolation between discrete (i.e., categorical) factor values is meaningless. Multiple linear regression analysis (MLRA) is typically preferred for situations where there are more factors, interactions, and higher order terms. When the factor-response relationship is nonlinear, multiple nonlinear regression analysis is advised. The techniques of partial least squares (PLS) or principal component analysis can also be used for regression in multivariate studies where there are numerous variables [21]. When there are fewer observations than there are predictor variables, PLS, an extension of MLRA, is used. ANOVA, Student's t test [22], predicted residual sum of squares, and Pearsonian coefficient of determination When there are fewer observations than there are predictor variables, PLS, an extension of MLRA, is used. ANOVA, Student's t test [22], predicted residual sum of squares, and Pearsonian coefficient of determination are all taken into account when conducting model analysis (r2) are all taken into account when conducting model analysis. The essential stages required in developing and examining a mathematical model is outlined in the narrative that follows [23]:

- The data are meticulously checked for any anomalies and evident issues. The results are presented in a variety of graphs, including response distributions, responses vs. time order scatter plots, responses versus factor levels, main effects plots, and normal or half-normal plots of the effects.

- Remainder graphs are used to test the model's presumptions. ANOVA is used if none of the model presumptions are broken. If possible, the model is further condensed.

- Model transformation is suggested and a new model is developed if model assumptions are broken.

- The model's findings are used to determine critical elements, identify ideal conditions, and other things.

6. FbD models testing and revision

The main variables for evaluating and improving a FbD model are:

- Response versus predictions: These charts show how the independent variables interact or are involved.
- Residual lag plots: These graphs can be used to determine how random the data are. In a perfect world, the plots would have no specific structures. In the absence of any random patterns, interactions or other errors are likely. Latency plots can be produced for any arbitrary lag, with "lag 1" being the most typical. A plot comparing the values of Yi versus Yi-1 is known as a "lag 1" plot.
- Residuals histogram: A univariate data set's distribution is graphically summarized by a residuals histogram. The histogram visually represents the data's distribution, skewness, outliers, and many nodes.
- Normal probability plot of residuals: The normal probability plot evaluates the data's distribution pattern, whether normal or not, in a visual way. These graphs plot data against a hypothetical normal distribution so that the dots should roughly form a straight line. This straight line is a good indicator of deviations from normality.

7. Search optimization

The optimization of a single answer or the simultaneous optimization of several responses from the thus chosen models must be carried out graphically, numerically, with artificial neural networks (ANNs), and/or by extrapolation outside the domain.

7.1 Graphical optimization

The goal of graphical optimization is to choose the optimum formulation from a feasible factor space region. To do this, the factor values are screened in accordance with the desired limits of the response variables. A combination of the following approaches can be used to optimize graphics: ANNs, canonical analysis, overlay plots, brute-force searches, and mathematical optimization are further methods for optimizing numerous replies.

7.1.1 Brute-force search

The simplest and most precise optimization search technique is brute-force search, commonly referred to as exhaustive search because it involves looking at every single point in the function space. Here, the response variables of the formulations that can be created by practically every feasible arrangement of independent factors are filtered [24]. Then, by further reducing the possible region, the acceptable boundaries are established for these responses, and a thorough search is once more carried out. The final viable space (also known as the grid search), which satisfies the most requirements established during experimentation, is searched for the optimum formulation. The benefit of using this thorough approach is that there is very little risk of missing the actual best formulation.

7.1.2 Overlay plots

To visually find the optimal compromise, the bi-dimensional response contour plots are stacked over one another. An overlay plot or integrated contour plot is what this is known as. The permissible range of objective values is defined with minimum and maximum values. The area that contains all acceptable responses is highlighted. By balancing several reactions, an optimum is found within this region.

7.1.3 Canonical analysis

According to canonical analysis, each of the extracted components from the criterion set of variables may be predicted from the corresponding components from the predictor set of variables [25–29]. The method is restricted to single response optimization. A saddle point is a stationary point that is not a local extremum in the domain of a function of two variables. The surface at such a location typically resembles a saddle that curves up in one direction or down in another (like a mountain pass). A saddle point on a contour line is typically identified by what appears to be an intersection of the contour with the line. The method is restricted to single response optimization. Additionally, there are additional crucial techniques for graphically locating the best formulation, including Pareto-optimality charts.

7.2 Mathematical optimization

Typically, when there is only one response, a graphic analysis is deemed sufficient. But when there are several responses, it is typically wise to perform mathematical or numerical optimization first to identify a workable area.

7.2.1 Desirability function

Desirability function is a method of getting around the challenge of having various, occasionally conflicting, responses [20]. Each response in this strategy has a unique partial desirability function [30, 31]. The ideal point is the one with the highest value for desirability [32]. The experimenter should combine contour plots of the most significant replies with an analysis of the contour plot of the desirability surface surrounding the optimal. Strong formulation or a combination of processing circumstances will be indicated by a big area or volume of high desirability. Although the method necessitates the use of certain computer software, it is a very helpful and practical approach to optimization. DDS has also been numerically optimized using the "objective function" and "sequential unconstrained minimization technique" techniques.

7.3 Artificial neural networks (ANN)

Machine-based computational methods called Artificial Neural Networks (ANNs) aim to imitate some of the neurological processing capabilities of the human brain. Because of their nonlinear processing power and capacity to simulate complex systems, ANNs have special advantages [33–37]. The results are equivalent with superior prognostic capabilities when compared to other optimization techniques. However, they are rather challenging to apply to more levels or elements, and no statistical criterion is made clear to indicate the level of applicability of the model.

7.4 Extrapolation outside the domain

For first order designs, steepest ascent (or descent) methods are direct optimization techniques [38], particularly when the optimum is external to the domain and needs to be reached quickly. The optimum path method, which is employed for extrapolating the optimum outside of the experimental region, is just like the steepest ascent approach. Several industrial processes use the evolutionary operations technique, which allows the production procedure (formulation and process) to evolve to the best possible state through careful planning and repeated repetition.

8. Benefits of FbD implementation during product development

- High-quality drug product development.
- Improved product and process understanding.
- Astute planning with a team approach.
- Decreased resource use.
- Shortened time to reach the market.
- Few product recalls and rejects.
- A quicker regulatory product review process.
- Excellent returns on investment.
- Decreased consumer-generic skepticism.
- Efficient regulatory oversight.
- Fewer post approval changes.
- Dynamic control technique that increases operational flexibility.

- Complementation with federal question-based reviews (QbR).
- Wide operating ranges.
- End-product testing done solely for validation.

9. Overall FbD approach for drug delivery development

A comprehensive plan can be used to outline the overall strategy for carrying out a FbD study in oral DDS [24, 39]. The key steps in this FbD method include the following:

- **Definition of the problem:** The FbD problem is fully understood and defined.
- **Factor selection and factor levels:** Among the quantifiable and easily controllable variables, the independent factors are found.
- **Design of experimental protocol:** A suitable experimental design is chosen, and the number of experimental runs is determined, based on the independent factors and response variables chosen.
- **Formulating and evaluating the dosage form:** Different drug delivery formulations are created in accordance with the selected design and tested for the desired outcome(s).
- **Prediction of the best formulation:** A mathematical model is created using experimental data, and then the best formulation is found using graphical and/or numerical methods.
- **Validation of optimization:** Responses are assessed when the expected optimal formulation is generated. If results are confirmed, they are then transferred via scale-up methods and activities at pilot plants to the production cycle.

Figure 5 is a flow chart that shows the several key processes that make up a FbD approach as a whole.

10. Software usage in FbD optimization

FbD optimization approaches have several benefits, and their acceptance is optimistic. However, implementing such logical concepts frequently necessitates complex mathematical and statistical procedures. Today's computational snags have been substantially streamlined and simplified because to the availability of strong hardware that is also reasonably priced, as well as the full FbD software. Software for computers is only available to undertake data analysis using the FbD methodology (**Figure 6**).

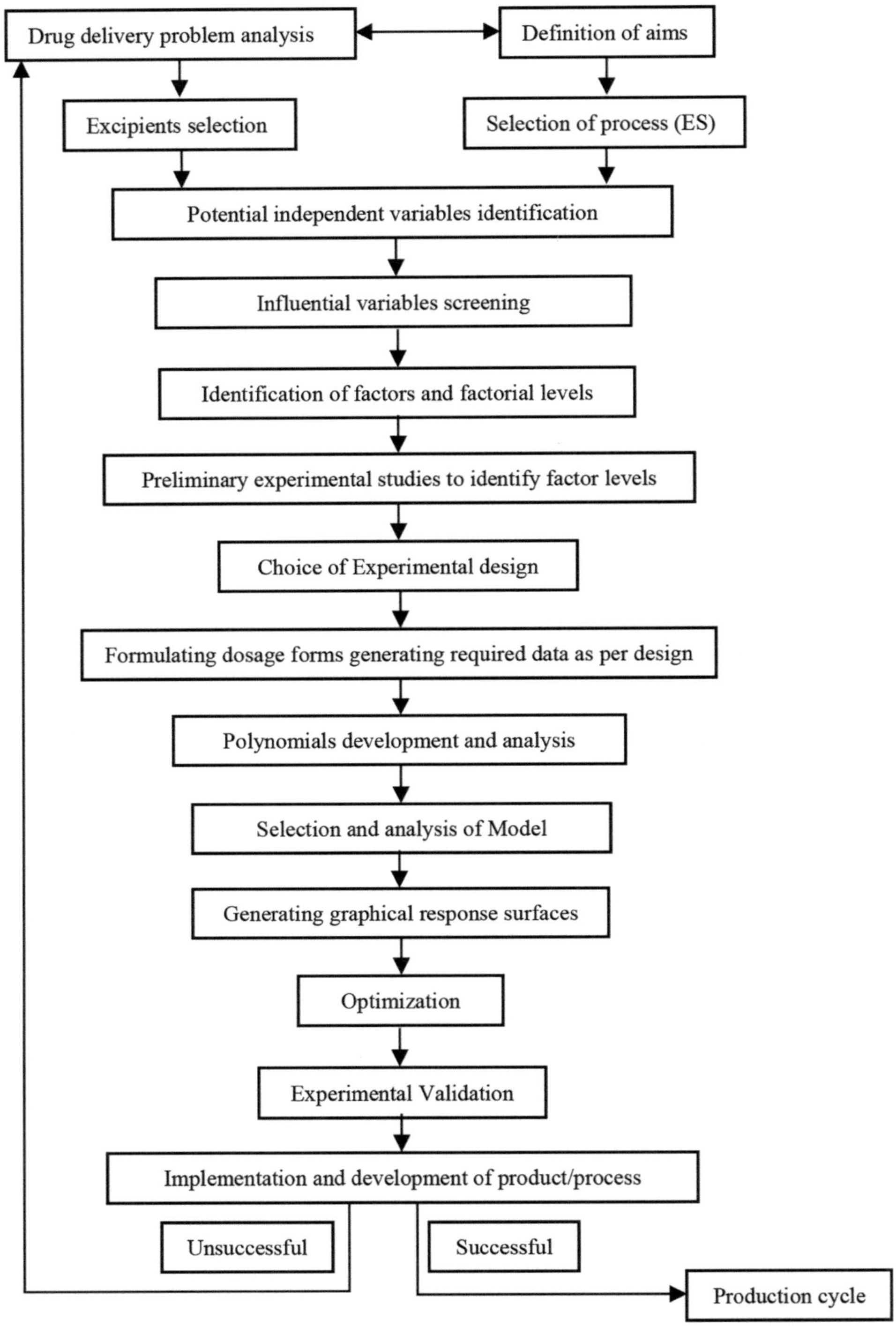

Figure 5.
Overall FbD strategy during drug delivery development.

An interface like this provides guidance at every stage of the optimization cycle, including the design selection, factor screening, use of response surface designs, generation of the design matrix, plotting of 3-D response surfaces and 2-D contour

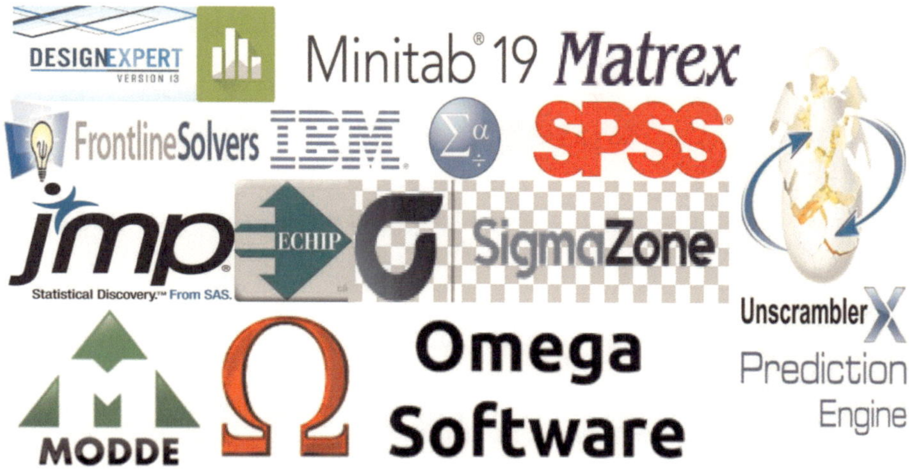

Figure 6.
Selected computer software used during FbD implementation for product and process optimization.

Software	Features
Design Expert	Pharmaceutical formulations and processes can be improved; this enables the screening and analysis of key factors for FD, FFD, BBD, CCD, PBD, and mixture designs; gives 2D contour maps and rotateable 3D plots to show the response surfaces; Optimization using numbers and graphics.
DE PRO XL and DE KISS	Software for automated data analysis employing Taguchi, FD, FFD, and PBD that is MS-Excel compatible. However, only one response variable can be used with the reasonably cheap program, DoE KISS.
Mini Tab	Powerful DoE software with practically all RSM designs, graphic and help features, and compatibility with MS-Excel.
MATREX	Software for optimization that works with Excel and has facilities for a number of experimental designs, including the Taguchi design.
OPTIMA	Constructs the experimental design, calculates the data fit to a mathematical equation, and visually displays the response surfaces.
OMEGA	Only a program that enables multi-criteria decision making using Pareto-optimality, up to six objectives, and includes numerous statistical functions is available for mixed designs.
FACTOP	Develops polynomials and grid searches to aid in the optimization of formulation utilizing various FDs and other designs; contains computer-aided-education module for optimization.
GRG2	Using a mathematical optimization program, you can find a function's maximum or minimum with or without restrictions [40].

Table 4.
List of computer Softwares available commercially for formulation by design (FbD) studies.

plots as design spaces, optimum search, partial interpretation of the results, and validation of the methodology. **Table 4** outlines the specific computer software products that are commercially available for conducting FbD studies in an industrial setting. **Tables 5** and **6** illiterates examples of several approaches of FbD in the optimization of micro and nanoformulations and a comprehensive account of the independent variables and response variables used for various DDS.

DDS	Drug	Factors	Design	Year (Ref)
Self-nanoemulsifying	Bosentan	Oil phase percentage, surfactant percentage, and co-surfactant percentage	Box-Behnken	2022 [41]
Floating Gastroretentive	Famotidine	Concentrations of Guar gum and the concentrations of Rice Bran Wax	3^2 factorial	2022 [42]
Self-microemulsifying (SMEDDS)	Teriflunomide	Concentration of oil (Sefsol 218), surfactant (Acrysol EL-135), and cosurfactant (PEG 400)	Mixture design	2022 [43]
Nanoencapsulation	Crocin component of saffron (*Crocus sativus* L.)	pH and the concentrations of CS, ALG, and calcium chloride ($CaCl_2$)	Taguchi	2022 [44]
Gastro-retentive (GRDDS)	Itopride Hydrochloride	Concentrations of Eudragit L 100, PEG, and sodium bicarbonate	Box-Behnken	2022 [45]
Magnetite Nanoparticles	Ciprofloxacin	Concentrations of CIP (35–80 mg/L), adsorbent doses (20–60 mg), and pH values (4–10) at reaction time (80 min)	Box-Behnken	2022 [46]
Nano invasomal gel	Glibenclamide (GLB) and Atenolol (ATN)	Amount of phospholipid (mg), ethanol (%), and terpene (%)	Box-Behnken	2021 [47]
Gastroretentive	Ranitidine Hydrochloride	Concentration of HPMC/ NaCMC and Concentration of $NaHCO_3$	Central Composite Design	2021 [48]
Emulsomes	Bifonazole	Phospholipid to Bifonazole ratio; Phospholipid to Tristearin ratio and Phospholipid to Stearylamine ratio	Box-Behnken	2021 [49]
Solid lipid nanoparticle	Eflornithine hydrochloride	Drug: lipid, Surfactant concentration, Stirring time	Central Composite Design	2021 [50]
Microspheres	Pentazocine	Polymer concentration, Stirring speed, Surfactant concentration	Box-Behnken	2021 [51]
Solid lipid nanoparticle	Clarithromycin	Homogenization speed (rpm), Sonication time (min), Amount of lipid (mg), Surfactant ratio, Surfactant concentration (%)	3^2 full factorial design	2021 [52]
Orodispersible films	Vitamin B12	Amount of Glycerine, Menthol and Polymer Soluplus® amount	Box-Behnken	2021 [53]
Cubosomes	Ketoconazole	Stabilizer, Surfactant amount	3^2 full factorial design	2021 [54]

DDS	Drug	Factors	Design	Year (Ref)
Nanoparticles	L-arginine	Oleic acid concentration, Poloxamer 188 concentration, Sonication rate	2^3 full factorial design	2021 [55]
Self-nanoemulsifying (SNEDDS)	Candesartan	Oil percentage (Capmul PG-8), surfactant percentage (Kolliphor EL), and a co-surfactant percentage (Transcutol P)	D-optimal mixture	2020 [56]
Self-nanoemulsifying (SNEDDS)	Andrographolide	Amount of Capryol-90 as the oil phase (20–50%), Kolliphor RH 40 as the surfactant (40–70%), and propylene glycol	Simplex lattice	2020 [57]
Solid lipid nanoparticle	Pioglitazone	Concentration of lipid (Compritol® 888 ATO), surfactant (tween80) and homogenization speed	Box-Behnken	2020 [58]
Nanoparticles	Benzylisothiocynate	Amount of polymer Concentration of surfactant	Central Composite Design	2020 [59]
Microspheres	Epichlorohydrin	Concentration of epichlorohydrin Duration of cross-linking	Two-level full factorial design	2020 [60]
Microbeads	Nitazoxanide	Percentage of chitosan, Percentage of sodium tripolyphosphate	Central Composite Design	2020 [61]
Nanoparticles	Ansamycin	Homogenization speed, Drug/ polymer ratio, PVA concentration	Central Composite Design	2020 [62]
Nanoparticles	Clonazepam	PLGA amount, Poloxamer 188 concentration	3^2 full factorial design	2020 [63]
Nanoparticles	Clarithromycin	Time of sonication, Lipid amount	3^2 full factorial design	2020 [64]
Microspheres	Theophylline	Starch:alginate ratio (X1) and polymer:drug ratio (X2)	2 factor, 2 Level CCD	2020 [65]
Polymeric nanoparticle	Zoledronic acid	Zoledronic acid content, PLGA/Pluronic F68 ratio, Organic to aqueous phase ratio	Central Composite Design	2020 [66]
Fast disintegrating oral film	Zolmitriptan	Amount of polymer and Plasticizer	2^2 factorial design	2019 [67]
Magnetic nanoparticles (MNPs)	(3-amino propyl) triethoxy silane (APTES)	Concentration of Fe_3O_4, Tragacanth Gum (TG): Chitosan (CS) ratio, nanocomposite weight, and curcumin weight on the drug loading	Taguchi	2019 [68]

DDS	Drug	Factors	Design	Year (Ref)
Nanoparticles and nanosuspension	Loratadine	Drug amount, Solvent to anti-solvent ratio, Stabilizer type, Stabilizer concentration, Sonication time, Sonication power	Central Composite Design	2019 [69]
Encapsulated nanoparticle	Sorafenib	Concentration of HPMC, PVP concentration, Poloxamer concentration	Box-Behnken	2019 [70]
Floating matrix tablets	Ciprofloxacin Hydrochloride	Amount of HPMC K100M and Xanthan gum	3^2 factorial	2018 [71]
Encapsulated Eudragit® microspheres	Vildagliptin	Eudragit RS-100 concentration, Span-80 amount, Volume of methanol, Volume of acetone, Stirring speed	Plackett-Burman design	2018 [72]
Encapsulated Chitosan nanoparticle	Cefadroxil	Polymer weight, Polymer concentration	2^2 factorial design	2018 [73]
Mucoadhesive microspheres	Quetiapine fumarate	Ethyl cellulose concentration, Chitosan concentration, Stirring speed, Type of HPMC, HPMC concentration	2^2 factorial design	2018 [74]
Mucoadhesive buccal tablets	Risperidone	Amount of Carbopol® (CP) and sodium alginate (SA)	Response surface methodology	2017 [75]
Multiparticulate pellets	Naproxen	Level of microcrystalline cellulose (MCC), polyvinylpyrrolidone K-90 (PVP K-90), croscarmellose sodium (CCS), and polacrilin potassium (PP)	Mixture design	2017 [76]
Cellulose nanofiber (CNF) aerogels	Bendamustine hydrochloride	Optimization of stirring time varied from 3 to 8 hours and the CNF ratio varied from 0.6 to 3.	Central composite design	2017 [77]
Hot Melt Extrusion Amorphous Dispersion Tablet	Compound X	Type of polymer, filler (microcrystalline cellulose (MCC), lactose, and dicalcium phosphate anhydrous (DCPA)), and disintegrant (Crospovidone, croscarmellose sodium, and sodium starch glycolate (SSG))	Full factorial	2016 [78]
Osmotic	Dicloxacillin sodium and Amoxicillin trihydrate	Screening of three categories of polymers, Optimization of osmotic tablets	Plackett-Burman and Box-Behnken	2016 [79]
Self-microemulsifying (SMEDDS)	Atorvastatin calcium	Concentrations of Capmul MCM, Tween 20, and Tetraglycol	D-optimal mixture design with response	2015 [80]

DDS	Drug	Factors	Design	Year (Ref)
			surface methodology	
Transdermal delivery	Risperidone	Amount of cholesterol, span 60, phospholipid G90, and risperidone	4^3 factorial design	2015 [81]
In situ gel	Glipizide	Concentration of gelling agent, drug release retardant polymers and concentration of drug release retardant polymers	Taguchi	2015 [82]
Sustained Release Mucoadhesive Microcapsules	Venlafaxine HCl	concentration of sodium alginate, HPMC type (i.e., K4M, K15M, HPMC K100M), amount of HPMC K100M and crosslinking time	Plackett-Burman and Box-Behnken	2014 [83]
Oro-dispersible	Clobazam	Amount of disintegrant (crospovidone) and the diluent (MCC)	Response surface methodology	2013 [84]

Table 5.
FbD optimization of various oral DDSs.

Types of drug delivery system	Factors	Response variables
Oral sustained release matrices	Drug loading, polymer type and content, polymer grades, ratio of polymers, ratio of polymer to filler, drug-polymer ratio, heating time, solvent ratio, binder, lubricant, film former, adhesive, amount of water in granulating liquid, volume of granulation solvent, granulation time, compression force, storage temperature, relative humidity, light, punch face tip geometry	Dissolution kinetics, tablet thickness, hardness, moisture uptake, friability, lag time, visual tablet quality, tensile strength, tapped density of granules, weight variation
Sustained release coated tablets	Polymer, solid content, volume of coating dispersion, plasticizer, weight gain, curing time, particle size, hardness, lubricant	Dissolution profile, in vivo plasma profile, lag time
Multiple-layered tablets	Core polymer concentration, lubricant, hardness of compressed core, compression force for complex layer	Drug release, adhesion strength in complex layer
Gastroretentive floating and bioadhesive tablets	Polymer-drug ratio, polymer grades, ratio of polymers, ratio of diluents	Dissolution kinetics, duration of buoyancy, detachment force, shear force, compression force, tablet density
Osmotic tablets	Orifice size, coating level, content of pore former, polymer content, coat weight, plasticizer type and content, cure time and cure temperature	Drug release rate, lag time, burst strength, correlation coefficient of cumulative amount of drug released and time
Buccoadhesive tablets	Amounts of polymer	Drug release, bioadhesion, and diffusion parameters

Types of drug delivery system	Factors	Response variables
Macroparticulates	Drug content, surfactant content, water content, impellar speed, mixing time, plasticizer concentration, polymer coating load, concentration of lacquer in the coating dispersion, extruder speed and screen size, spheronizer speed and load, spheronization time, extrusion rate, spray rate and temperature, curing time and temperature, agitation, osmolality and polarity of the medium	Pellet yield, dissolution time, percentage of stuck pellets, steady state extrusion force, bulk density, friability, flowability, pellet size, morphological characteristics
Microparticulates (microspheres)	Polymer type and content, polymer:drug ratio, polymer grades, molecular weight of polymer, amount of hardening agent, cross linking agent, cross linking time, emulsifier concentration, solvent, pH, phase volume ratio, stirring speed, stabilization time, surfactant, composition of internal phase, emulsifier type, deaggregating agent, dehydrating agent, precipitant, injection rate, needle gauge size	Dissolution kinetics, yield, percent drug loading, particle size, loose surface crystals, drug entrapping efficiency, surface morphology, angle of repose
Microparticulates (microcapsules)	Core-wall ratio, particle size, pH of the medium, surfactant concentration, speed of stirring, ratio of total polymer to total volume of solution	Dissolution time, stability of the capsule walls
Nanoparticulates	Monomer concentration, polymer, surfactant, volume of oily phase, stabilizer, pH, stirring speed, temperature of aqueous phase, oxygen level	Percent yield, drug loading, drug release profile, polydispersity index, particle diameter, zeta potential
Vesicular systems	Average molecular weight, surface affinity, number of additional steps, temperature, phospholipids, stabilizers, inlet pressure of homogenizer, shaking time, incubation time for annealing vesicles, lipid charge, sonication time, pH, solvent, hydration time	Percent encapsulation, average amount of polymer adsorbed per lipid, entrapment volume, size of vesicles, drug leakage, stabilization ratio
Solid dispersions, coevaporates and coprecipitates	Carrier, polymer, disintegrant, lubricant, solvent, spray feeding volume, polymer to drug ratio, diluent, compressional pressure, polymer-lubricant ratio	Release rate, dissolution time, dissolution efficiency, weight variation, hardness, friability, disintegration,
Fast release tablets	Drying time, compression force, particle size, moisture content of wet granules	Distintegration time, tensile strength, tablet porosity
Self-nanoemulsified tablet dosage forms	Amount of copolyvidone, microcrystalline cellulose and maltodextrin, surfactant, cosolvent	Weight, flowability index, tensile strength, friability, disintegration time, drug release

Table 6.
List of various independent variables and response variables chosen for various types of drug delivery system: [85].

11. Conclusions

Today, rather than relying on end-product testing, the federal agencies want assurance of QbD-centric quality that is "built-in" to the system. Therefore, understanding the formulation or process factors utilizing FbD will assist in achieving the targeted goals of product/process excellence with extraordinary ease and efficiency. Almost all types of oral DDS have successfully utilized FbD employing experimental designs to improve not only the drug formulations but also the development procedures. It has proven effective even if choosing the best formulation is not the main goal because it tends to reveal how much the product qualities improve when (any) excipient or process parameter is changed (s). By enhancing (rather than substituting) the essential formulation abilities, inventiveness, and product knowledge, FbD tends to speed up the formulation process.

Author details

Ushasi Das[1*], Dilip Kumar Panda[1] and Sanchita Mandal[2]

1 Department of Pharmacology and Toxicology, Central Drugs Laboratory, Kolkata, West Bengal, India

2 Department of Pharmaceutical Technology, Jadavpur University, Kolkata, West Bengal, India

*Address all correspondence to: ushasidas88@gmail.com

References

[1] Fukuda I, Pinto C, Moreira C, Saviano A, Lourenço F. Design of Experiments (DoE) applied to pharmaceutical and analytical quality by design (QbD). Brazilian. Journal of Pharmaceutical Sciences. 2018:54(spe). DOI: 10.1590/s2175-9790201800000 1006

[2] Singh B. QbD in pharma product development life cycle. Chronicle Pharma Biz. 2013:72-79

[3] ICH, Pharmaceutical development Q8 (R2), International Conference on Harmonisation, IFPMA, Geneva (Switzerland), 2009 [Accessed on August 3, 2022]

[4] https://www.ema.europa.eu/en/human-regulatory/research-developme nt/quality-design [Accessed: August 3, 2022]

[5] Kovács B, Péterfi O, Kovács-Deák B, Székely-Szentmiklósi I, Fülöp I, Bába L, et al. Quality-by-design in pharmaceutical development: From current perspectives to practical applications. Acta Pharmaceutica. 2021; **71**(4):497-526. DOI: 10.2478/acph-2021-0039

[6] Singh B, Sharma T, Saini S, Kaur R, Jain A, Raza K, et al. Systematic development of drug Nanocargos using formulation by design (FbD): An updated overview. Critical Reviews™ in Therapeutic Drug Carrier Systems. 2020; **37**(3):229-269. DOI: 10.1615/CritRevTherDrugCarrierSyst.2020 032040

[7] Aksu B, Beg S, Garg B, Kapil R, Singh B. Quality by design (QbD) in the development of nanostructured drug delivery systems. In: Singh B, Vyas SP, Kaur IP, editors. NanoBioMedicine. Houston, Texas, USA: Studium Press LLC; 2015. pp. 1-30

[8] Singh B. Quality by design (QbD) for holistic pharma excellence and regulatory compliance. Pharma Times. 2014;**46**(8):26-33

[9] Beg S, Rahman M, Kohli K. Quality-by-design approach as a systematic tool for the development of nanopharmaceutical products. Drug Discovery Today. 2019;**24**(3):717-725. DOI: 10.1016/j.drudis.2018.12.002

[10] Raza K, Beg S, Singh B. Developing "optimized" drug products employing "designed" experiments. Chemical Industry Digest. 2013;**12**:1-7

[11] Huang J, Goolcharran C, Ghosh K. A quality by design approach to investigate tablet dissolution shift upon accelerated stability by multivariate methods. European Journal of Pharmaceutics and Biopharmaceutics. 2011;**78**(1):141-150. DOI: 10.1016/j.ejpb.2010.12.012

[12] Shah M, Chuttani K, Mishra A, Pathak K. Oral solid compritol 888 ATO nanosuspension of simvastatin: Optimization and biodistribution studies. Drug Development and Industrial Pharmacy. 2011;**37**(5):526-537. DOI: 10.3109/03639045.2010.527983

[13] Shirsand S, Suresh S, Jodhana L, Swamy P. Formulation design and optimization of fast disintegrating lorazepam tablets by effervescent method. Indian Journal of Pharmaceutical Sciences. 2010;**72**(4):431-436. DOI: 10.4103/0250-474X.73911

[14] Nagori S, Jethwa B, Gohel M, Parikh R. Fabrication and evaluation of bi-layer tablet containing conventional

paracetamol and modified release diclofenac sodium. Indian Journal of Pharmaceutical Sciences. 2010;**72**(2): 191-196. DOI: 10.4103/0250-474X.65035

[15] Aboelwafa A, Basalious E. Optimization and In vivo pharmacokinetic study of a novel controlled release venlafaxine hydrochloride three-layer tablet. AAPS PharmSciTech. 2010;**11**(3):1026-1037. DOI: 10.1208/s12249-010-9467-z

[16] Tuntikulwattana S, Mitrevej A, Kerdcharoen T, Williams DB, Sinchaipanid N. Development and optimization of micro/nanoporous osmotic pump tablets. AAPS PharmSciTech. 2010;**11**(2):924-935. DOI: 10.1208/s12249-010-9446-4

[17] Zhang Y, Geng Y. Preparation of sinomenine hydrochloride delayed-onset sustained-release tablets. Zhongguo Zhong Yao Za Zhi. 2010;**35**(6):703-707. DOI: 10.4268/cjcmm20100609

[18] Singh B, Kapil R, Nandi M, Ahuja N. Developing oral drug delivery systems using formulation by design: Vital precepts, retrospect and prospects. Expert Opinion on Drug Delivery. 2011; **8**(10):1341-1360. DOI: 10.1517/17425247.2011.605120

[19] Malladi M, Jukanti R. Formulation development and evaluation of a novel bidependent clarithromycin gastroretentive drug delivery system using box-Behnken design. Journal of Drug Delivery Science and Technology. 2016;**35**:134-145. DOI: 10.1016/j.jddst.2016.06.003

[20] Singh B, Kumar R, Ahuja N. Optimizing drug delivery systems using "Design of Experiments" part 1: Fundamental aspects. Critical Reviews in Therapeutic Drug Carrier Systems. 2005; **22**:27-37

[21] Westerhuis JA, Coenegracht PMJ. Multivariate modeling of the pharmaceutical two step process of wet granulation and tabletting with multiblock partial least squares. Chem. 1997;**11**:372-392

[22] Bolton S, Factorial designs. Pharmaceutical Statistics: Practical and Clinical Applications. 3rd ed. New York: Marcel Dekker; 1997

[23] Kollipara S, Bende G, Movva S, et al. Application of rotatable central composite design in the preparation and optimization of poly(lactic-co-glycolic acid) nanoparticles for controlled delivery of paclitaxel. Drug Development and Industrial Pharmacy. 2010;**36**(11):1377-1387

[24] Singh B, Ahuja N. Response surface optimization of drug delivery systems. In: Jain NK, editor. Progress in Controlled and Novel Drug Delivery Systems. 1st ed. New Delhi: CBS Publishers; 2004. pp. 470-509

[25] Kincl M, Turk S, Vrecer F. Application of experimental design methodology in development and optimization of drug release method. International Journal of Pharmaceutics. 2005;**291**(1–2):39-49. DOI: 10.1016/j.ijpharm.2004.07.041

[26] Sousa JJ, Sousa A, Moura MJ, et al. The influence of core materials and film coating on the drug release from coated pellets. International Journal of Pharmaceutics. 2002;**233**(1–2):111-122. DOI: 10.1016/s0378-5173(01)00921-8

[27] Sousa JJ, Sousa A, Podczeck F, et al. Factors influencing the physical characteristics of pellets obtained by extrusion-spheronization. International Journal of Pharmaceutics. 2002; **232**(1–2):91-106. DOI: 10.1016/s0378-5173(01)00908-5

[28] Lundqvist AE, Podczeck F, Newton JM. Compaction of, and drug release from, coated drug pellets mixed with other pellets. European Journal of Pharmaceutics and Biopharmaceutics. 1998;**46**(3):369-379. DOI: 10.1016/s0939-6411(98)00039-3

[29] Hogan J, Shue PI, Podczeck F, et al. Investigations into the relationship between drug properties, filling, and the release of drugs from hard gelatin capsules using multivariate statistical analysis. Pharmaceutical Research. 1996; **13**(6):944-949. DOI: 10.1023/a:1016025817183

[30] Vaghani SS, Patel SG, Jivani RR, et al. Design and optimization of a stomach-specific drug delivery system of repaglinide: Application of simplex lattice design. Pharmaceutical Development and Technology. 2012; **17**(1):55-65. DOI: 10.3109/10837450.2010.513988

[31] Gohel MC, Parikh RK, Aghara PY, et al. Application of simplex lattice design and desirability function for the formulation development of mouth dissolving film of salbutamol sulphate. Current Drug Delivery. 2009;**6**(5): 486-494. DOI: 10.2174/156720109789941696

[32] Shah PP, Mashru RC, Rane YM, et al. Design and optimization of artemether microparticles for bitter taste masking. Acta Pharmaceutica. 2008;**58**(4): 379-392. DOI: 10.2478/v10007-008-0027-y

[33] Leonardi D, Salomon CJ, Lamas MC, et al. Development of novel formulations for Chagas' disease: Optimization of benznidazole chitosan microparticles based on artificial neural networks. International Journal of Pharmaceutics. 2009;**367**(1–2):140-147. DOI: 10.1016/j.ijpharm.2008.09.036

[34] Zhang XY, Chen DW, Jin J, et al. Artificial neural network parameters optimization software and its application in the design of sustained release tablets. Yao Xue Xue Bao. 2009;**44**(10): 1159-1164

[35] Gohel M, Nagori SA. Fabrication and evaluation of captopril modified-release oral formulation. Pharmaceutical Development and Technology. 2009; **14**(6):679-686

[36] Barmpalexis P, Kanaze FI, Kachrimanis K, et al. Artificial neural networks in the optimization of a nimodipine controlled release tablet formulation. European Journal of Pharmaceutics and Biopharmaceutics. 2010;**74**(2):316-323. DOI: 10.1016/j.ejpb.2009.09.011

[37] Miyazaki Y, Yakou S, Yanagawa F, et al. Evaluation and optimization of preparative variables for controlled-release floatable microspheres prepared by poor solvent addition method. Drug Development and Industrial Pharmacy. 2008;**34**(11):1238-1245

[38] Lewis GA, Mathieu D, Phan-Tan-Luu R. Pharmaceutical experimental design. In: Singh B, Ahuja N, editors. Book review on "pharmaceutical experimental design". 1st edition. Marcel Dekker, New York. 2000. International Journal of Pharmaceutics. 1999;**195**: 247-248

[39] Myers WR. Response surface methodology. In: Chow SC, editor. Encyclopedia of Biopharmaceutical Statistics. New York: Marcel Dekker; 2003

[40] Reha S, Chodankar DA. Optimisaton techniques: A futuristic approach for formulating and processing of pharmaceuticals. Indian Journal of

Pharmaceutical Biology Research. 2016; **4**:32-40

[41] Usta DY, Timur B, Teksin ZS. Formulation development, optimization by box-Behnken design, characterization, in vitro, ex-vivo, and in vivo evaluation of bosentan-loaded self-nanoemulsifying drug delivery system: A novel alternative dosage form for pulmonary arterial hypertension treatment. European Journal of Pharmaceutical Sciences. 2022; **174**(106159):106159. DOI: 10.1016/j.ejps.2022.106159

[42] Sabale VP, Gadge GG. Factorial design approach to fabricate and optimize floating tablets based on combination of natural polymer and rice bran wax. Beni-Suef University Journal of Basic and Applied Sciences. 2022;**11**:5. DOI: 10.1186/s43088-021-00186-9

[43] Patel AD, Shah S, Patel MS, Vyas G. Quality by design approach to the development of self-microemulsifying systems for oral delivery of teriflunomide: Design, optimization, and in vitro and in vivo evaluation. Egypt Pharmaceutical Journal. 2022;**21**(2): 167-186. DOI: 10.4103/epj.epj_84_21

[44] Nasrpour S, Yousefi G, Niakosari M, Aminlari M. Nanoencapsulation of saffron crocin into chitosan/alginate interpolyelectrolyte complexes for oral delivery: A Taguchi approach to design optimization. Journal of Food Science. 2022;**87**(3):1148-1160. DOI: 10.1111/1750-3841.16052

[45] Alaithan S, Naveen NR, Goudanavar PS, Bhavani PD, Ramesh B, Koppuravuri NP, et al. Development of novel unfolding film system of Itopride hydrochloride using box-Behnken design—A gastro retentive approach. Pharmaceuticals. 2022;**15**(8):981. DOI: 10.3390/ph15080981

[46] Salari M. Optimization by box–Behnken design and synthesis of magnetite nanoparticles for removal of the antibiotic from an aqueous phase. Adsorption Science & Technology. 2022; **2022**:13. DOI: 10.1155/2022/1267460

[47] Anitha P, Satyanarayana S. Design and optimization of nano invasomal gel of Glibenclamide and atenolol combination: in vitro and in vivo evaluation. Future. Journal of Pharmaceutical Sciences. 2021;**7**(1):92. DOI: 10.1186/s43094-021-00240-4

[48] Nigusse B, Gebre-Mariam T, Belete A. Design, development and optimization of sustained release floating, bioadhesive and swellable matrix tablet of ranitidine hydrochloride. PLoS One. 2021;**16**(6): e0253391. DOI: 10.1371/journal.pone.0253391

[49] Malviya V. Preparation and evaluation of Emulsomes as a drug delivery system for Bifonazole. Indian J of Pharmaceutical Education and Research. 2021;**55**(1):86-94. DOI: 10.5530/ijper.55.1.12

[50] Grewal IK, Singh S, Arora S, Sharma N. Application of central composite design for development and optimization of eflornithine hydrochloride-loaded sustained release solid lipid microparticles. Biointerface Research in Applied Chemistry. 2021; **112**:618-637. DOI: 10.33263/briac121.618637

[51] Jabar A, Madni A, Bashir S, Tahir N, Usman F, Rahim MA, et al. Statistically optimized pentazocine loaded microsphere for the sustained delivery application: Formulation and characterization. PLoS One. 2021;**16**(4): e0250876. DOI: 10.1371/journal.pone.0250876

[52] Nair AB, Shah J, Al-Dhubiab BE, Jacob S, Patel SS, Venugopala KN, et al. Clarithromycin solid lipid nanoparticles for topical ocular therapy: Optimization, evaluation and in vivo studies. Pharmaceutics. 2021;**13**(4):523. DOI: 10.3390/pharmaceutics13040523

[53] Suryawanshi D, Wavhule P, Shinde U, Kamble M, Amin P. Development, optimization and in vivo evaluation of cyanocobalamin loaded orodispersible films using hot-melt extrusion technology: A quality by design (QbD) approach. Journal of Drug Delivery Science Technology. 2021; **63**(102559):102559. DOI: 10.1016/j.jddst.2021.102559

[54] Rapalli VK, Banerjee S, Khan S, Jha PN, Gupta G, Dua K, et al. QbD-driven formulation development and evaluation of topical hydrogel containing ketoconazole loaded cubosomes. Materials Science and Engineering: C. 2021;**119**(111548):111548. DOI: 10.1016/j.msec.2020.111548

[55] Patel D, Patel M, Soni T, Suhagia B. Topical arigine solid lipid nanoparticles: Development and characterization by QbD approach. Journal of Drug Delivery Science Technology. 2021;**61**(102329): 102329. DOI: 10.1016/j.jddst.2021.102329

[56] Verma R, Kaushik D. Design and optimization of candesartan loaded self-nanoemulsifying drug delivery system for improving its dissolution rate and pharmacodynamic potential. Drug Delivery. 2020;**27**(1):756-771. DOI: 10.1080/10717544.2020.1760961

[57] Indrati O, Martien R, Rohman A, Nugroho AK. Application of simplex lattice design on the optimization of Andrographolide self nanoemulsifying drug delivery system (SNEDDS). Indonesian Journal of Pharmacy. 2020; **31**(2):124. DOI: 10.14499/indonesianjpharm31iss2pp124

[58] Shaveta S, Singh J, Afzal M, Kaur R, Imam SS, Alruwaili NK, et al. Development of solid lipid nanoparticle as carrier of pioglitazone for amplification of oral efficacy: Formulation design optimization, in-vitro characterization and in-vivo biological evaluation. Journal of Drug Delivery Science and Technology. 2020;**57**(101674):101674. DOI: 10.1016/j.jddst.2020.101674

[59] Parmar A, Kaur G, Kapil S, Sharma V, Sharma S. Central composite design-based optimization and fabrication of benzylisothiocynate-loaded PLGA nanoparticles for enhanced antimicrobial attributes. Applied Nanoscience. 2020;**10**(2):379-389. DOI: 10.1007/s13204-019-01185-0

[60] Tesfay D, Abrha S, Yilma Z, Woldu G, Molla F. Preparation, optimization, and evaluation of epichlorohydrin cross-linked enset (Enseteventricosum (Welw.) Cheeseman) starch as drug release sustaining excipient in microsphere formulation. BioMed Research International. 2020;**2147971**:1-19. DOI: 10.1155/2020/2147971

[61] Bharti C, Nagaich U, Pandey J, Jain S, Jain N. Development of nitazoxanide-loaded colon-targeted formulation for intestinal parasitic infections: Centre composite design-based optimization and characterization. Future Journal of Pharmaceutical Science. 2020;**6**(1):1-17. DOI: 10.1186/s43094-020-00130-1

[62] Gusai T, Dhavalkumar M, Soniwala M, Dudhat K, Vasoya J, Chavda J. Formulation and optimization of microsponge-loaded emulgel to improve the transdermal application of acyclovir-a DOE based approach. Drug Delivery and Translational Research. 2021;**11**(5):2009-2029. DOI: 10.1007/s13346-020-00862-w

[63] Nair KG, Velmurugan R, Sukumaran SK. Formulation and optimization of ansamycin-loaded polymeric nanoparticles using response surface methodology for bacterial meningitis. Bio NanoScience. 2020; **10**(1):279-291. DOI: 10.1007/s12668-019-00713-0

[64] Shah P, Sarolia J, Vyas B, Wagh P, Ankur K, Kumar MA. PLGA nanoparticles for nose to brain delivery of clonazepam: Formulation, optimization by 32 Factorial design, in vitro and in vivo evaluation. Current Drug Delivery. 2021; **18**(6):805-824. DOI: 10.2174/1567201817666200708115627

[65] Okunlola A, Akaeze DI. Formulation design and optimization of theophylline microspheres containing Akidi beans (Vigna Unguiculate) starch as polymer using central composite design. East and Central African Journal of Pharmaceutical Sciences. 2020;**23**:16-27

[66] Saka OM, Öz UC, Küçüktürkmen B, Devrim B, Bozkır A. Central composite design for optimization of zoledronic acid loaded PLGA nanoparticles. Journal of Pharmaceutical Innovation. 2020; **15**(1):3-14. DOI: 10.1007/s12247-018-9365-6

[67] Chauhan I, Yasir M, Verma M. Oral delivery of zolmitriptan loaded fast disintegrating film: Formulation development, statistical optimization, in-vitro and in-vivo evaluation. Journal of Applied Pharmaceutical Sciences and Research. 2019;**2**(1):13-22. DOI: 10.31069/japsr.v2i1.3

[68] Shafiee S. Hossein Abbastabar Ahangar, Ali Saffar, Taguchi method optimization for synthesis of Fe3O4 @chitosan/Tragacanth gum nanocomposite as a drug delivery system. Carbohydrate Polymers. 2019; **222**(114982):114982. DOI: 10.1016/j.carbpol.2019.114982

[69] Alshweiat A, Ambrus R, Katona G, Csóka I. QbD based control strategy of loratadine nanosuspensions and dry nanoparticles stabilized by soluplus. Farm. 2019;**67**(4):729-735. DOI: 10.31925/farmacia.2019.4.23

[70] Park SY, Kang Z, Thapa P, Jin YS, Park JW, Lim HJ, et al. Development of sorafenib loaded nanoparticles to improve oral bioavailability using a quality by design approach. International Journal of Pharmaceutics. 2019;**566**: 229-238. DOI: 10.1016/j.ijpharm.2019.05.064

[71] Pasa G, Choudhury P, Panigrahi G. Formulation design and optimization of oral floating matrix tablets of ciprofloxacin hcl by using hpmc and xanthan gum with experimental design. Asian Journal of Pharmaceutical Research and Development. 2018;**6**(6): 23-35. DOI: 10.22270/ajprd.v6i6.430

[72] Naik J, Waghulde M. Development of vildagliptin loaded Eudragit® microspheres by screening design: in vitro evaluation. International Journal of Pharmaceutical Investigation. 2018; **48**(6):627-637. DOI: 10.1007/s40005-017-0355-3

[73] Basha M, AbouSamra MM, Awad GA, Mansy SS. A potential antibacterial wound dressing of cefadroxil chitosan nanoparticles in situ gel: Fabrication, in vitro optimization and in vivo evaluation. International Journal of Pharmaceutics. 2018;**544**(1): 129-140. DOI: 10.1016/j.ijpharm.2018.04.021

[74] Komati S, Swain S, Rao MEB, Jena BR, Unnam S, Dasi V. QbD-based design and characterization of

mucoadhesive microspheres of quetiapine fumarate with improved oral bioavailability and brain biodistribution potential. Bulletin of Faculty Pharmacy Cairo University. 2018;**56**(2):129-145. DOI: 10.1016/j.bfopcu.2018.09.002

[75] Çelik B. Risperidone mucoadhesive buccal tablets: Formulation design, optimization and evaluation. Drug Design, Development and Therapy. 2017;**11**:3355-3365. DOI: 10.2147/dddt.s150774

[76] Shah N, Mehta T, Gohel M. Formulation and optimization of multiparticulate drug delivery system approach for high drug loading. AAPS PharmSciTech. 2017;**18**(6):2157-2167. DOI: 10.1208/s12249-016-0689-6

[77] Bhandari J, Mishra H, Mishra PK, Wimmer R, Ahmad FJ, Talegaonkar S. Cellulose nanofiber aerogel as a promising biomaterial for customized oral drug delivery. International Journal of Nanomedicine. 2017;**12**:2021-2031. DOI: 10.2147/ijn.s124318

[78] Agrawal A, Dudhedia M, Deng W, Shepard K, Zhong L, Povilaitis E, et al. Development of tablet formulation of amorphous solid dispersions prepared by hot melt extrusion using quality by design approach. AAPS PharmSciTech. 2016;**17**(1):214-232. DOI: 10.1208/s12249-015-0472-0

[79] Patel A, Dodiya H, Shelate P, Shastri D, Dave D. Design, characterization, and optimization of controlled drug delivery system containing antibiotic drug/s. Journal of Drug Delivery. 2016;**2016**:1-15. DOI: 10.1155/2016/9024173

[80] Yeom DW, Son HY, Kim JH, Kim SR, Lee SG, Song SH, et al. Development of a solidified self-microemulsifying drug delivery system (S-SMEDDS) for atorvastatin calcium with improved dissolution and bioavailability. International Journal of Pharmaceutics. 2016;**506**(1–2):302-311. DOI: 10.1016/j.ijpharm.2016.04.059

[81] Imam SS, Aqil M, Akhtar M, Sultana Y, Ali A. Formulation by design-based proniosome for accentuated transdermal delivery of risperidone: in vitro characterization and in vivo pharmacokinetic study. Drug Delivery. 2015;**22**(8):1059-1070. DOI: 10.3109/10717544.2013.870260

[82] Swathi G, Lakshmi PK. Design and optimization of Hydrodynamically balanced Oral In situ gel of glipizide. Journal of Applied Pharmaceutical Science. 2015;**5**(Suppl. 1):031-038. DOI: 10.7324/japs.2015.54.s6

[83] Swain S, Behera A, Dinda SC, Patra CN, Jammula S, Beg S, et al. Formulation design, optimization and Pharmacodynamic evaluation of sustained release Mucoadhesive microcapsules of venlafaxine HCl. Indian Journal of Pharmaceutical Sciences. 2014;**76**(4):354-363

[84] Bala R, Khanna S, Pawar PK. Formulation and optimization of fast dissolving intraoral drug delivery system for clobazam using response surface methodology. Journal of Advanced Pharmaceutical Technology & Research. 2013;**4**(3):151-159. DOI: 10.4103/2231-4040.116785

[85] Singh B, Dahiya M, Saharan V, Ahuja N. Optimizing drug delivery systems using systematic "Design of Experiments." part II: Retrospect and prospects. Critical Reviews in Therapeutic Drug Carrier Systems. 2005;**22**(3):215-294. DOI: 10.1615/CritRevTherDrugCarrierSyst.v22.i3.10

Chapter 3

Metal-Based Nanomaterials Photodynamic Action with a Focus on Au and Ag Nanomaterials

Atiyeh Nomani, Anvarsadat Kianmehr, Shahriyar Abdoli and Siamak Javani

Abstract

Photodynamic action is the interaction between cells and oxygen, light, and chemical reagent (photosensitizers). Photodynamic techniques include photodynamic diagnosis (PDD), fluorescence-guided tumor resection, and photodynamic therapy (PDT). PDD and PDT have the exact mechanism. They are based on light and tissue interaction with a difference. PDT is along with the destruction of the lesion against PDD that the diagnosis is made without destruction. Photosensitizers (PSs) could be organic and inorganic. Metal-based PSs were considered, due to the disadvantages of organic PSs such as low quantum yield and small stock shift, and high toxicity. We have examined the metal-based nanomaterials PDT in recent years. The titles considered are including the introduction that consists of explanations about photodynamic action, PDD, PDT and history of PDT, PDT mechanism, PDT effects on the immune system, photosensitizers, and metal-based nanomaterials in the photodynamic application, which this section addresses along with the application of metal nanomaterials (with a focus on gold and silver nanomaterials) in photodynamic techniques.

Keywords: photodynamic, metal nanomaterials, photosensitizers, gold nanoparticles, silver nanoparticles

1. Introduction

Photodynamic is defined as the effect of light on living systems in combination with oxygen and chemical reagents. Photodynamic diagnosis (PDD), fluorescence-guided tumor surgery (FGS), and photodynamic therapy (PDT) are most recent types of photodynamic technology. FGS is the use of fluorescence imaging in surgery for defining tumor location and its margins. PDT and PDD are non- or minimally invasive therapeutic and diagnosis techniques. PDD is an effective diagnosis method with a wide application in medical diagnosis including dermatology, gastroenterology, urology, and oncology. Similar to PDT, the mechanism of PDD is based on light and tissue interaction but does not along with the destruction of the lesion. When a specific wavelength of light is irradiated to a tissue, endogenous or exogenous fluorophores absorb the light energy leading to electrons being raised to an excited state, and subsequent relaxation and returning to the ground state lead to emission fluorescence of a specific wavelength [1–7].

Photodynamic therapy (PDT) is a form of phototherapy and the joint action of nontoxic photosensitizer (PS), a light source, and molecular form of oxygen. The PS, in the presence of oxygen, is activated by a suitable wavelength of light to generate reactive oxygen species (ROS) (**Figure 1**). This phototoxicity leads to oxidative stress and cytotoxicity to elicit cell injury and cell death [5, 8–10]. PDT has been used clinically to treat a wide range of neoplastic and non-malignant diseases with minimal side effects on the surrounding normal cells. PDT was approved by the US Food and Drug Administration as the first drug-device combination for cancer therapy [3, 11]. In addition to oncological diseases, PDT is a very efficient therapeutic modality for non-oncological diseases. Recently, PTD was used as a new approach for elimination of human pathogens too. Microbial infections continue to be an outstanding cause of morbidity and mortality worldwide. The wide utilization of antibiotics and vaccination strategies cannot avert the prevalence of microbial infections. Frequent and immeasurable utilization of antimicrobial drugs may be associated with side effects such as gastrointestinal disorders, liver toxicity, and secondary fungal infections. These factors sternly diminish the therapeutic effect of antimicrobials and develop drug resistance in microbes. By broad monitoring commissioned by the UK Government and Wellcome Trust in 2016, it has been estimated that mortality of antimicrobial resistance will rise to over 10 million worldwide by 2050. Some clinical trial studies have demonstrated that microbial infection could be diminished using PDT techniques. To this, PS as a photodynamic agent suitably is engineered to target the structural elements of microbial cells selectively. Despite PDT advantages, there are some limitations such as effective PS with properties of an ideal PS, leading to reduce the efficacy of PDT. Nanotechnology-based PDT and combination therapy including chemotherapy, radiotherapy (RT), immunotherapy and anti-angiogenesis therapy, hypothermia, and employment of antioxidants and receptor inhibition strategies

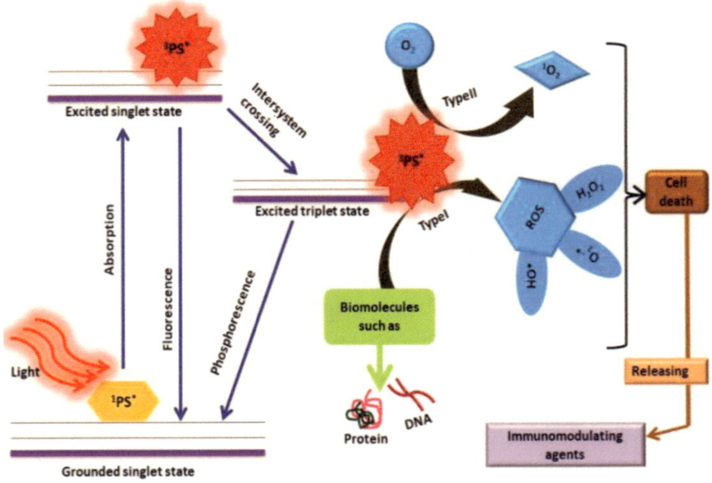

Figure 1.
Schematic illustration of PDT mechanism. PS reaches to $^1PS^*$ through absorption of light with specific wavelength. The $^1PS^*$ undergoes intersystem crossing to an $^3PS^*$ (an electronically different excited state lower in energy). $^3PS^*$ generates ROS through interaction with the surrounding biomolecules.

during PDT are methods to overcome these obstacles. Nanotechnology has garnered a great deal of attention in PDT, due to targeting potential and selective accumulation at the desired site and reduced toxicity to normal cells and tissues, improving the solubility of hydrophobic PSs and controlling the released rate of PSs. Nanoparticles have been used as PSs, conjugating agents, and carriers for PSs, followed by the creation of the fourth generation of PSs [8, 12–15]. This review article addresses the metal nanomaterial-based photodynamic applications in recent years. The main focus of this paper is on the application of silver and gold nanomaterial-based photodynamic therapy in recent years.

2. Photosensitizers

PSs are agents that absorb light of a specific wavelength, triggering the activation processes leading to the selective demolition of the improper cells [9]. Several PSs have already received FDA approval for use in photodynamic treatment for various types of cancer [2]. The physicochemical and biological characteristics of a PS could be summarized as the following: (1) composition uniformity, purity, and negligible of dark toxicity; (2) high clearance from the body patients [12]; (3) excellent solubility in body tissues; (4) stability at room temperature [9]; (5) potent absorption with a high extinction coefficient at near-infrared (NIR) wavelength range (700–1300 nm), where tissue penetration is increased, and the auto-absorption is reduced by other endogenous molecules (such as the hemoglobin); (6) inexpensive, affordable, and easy to synthesize; (7) the capability of high tumor selectivity and subcellular targeting [16].

There are different categorizations for PSs. PSs can be categorized based on their response to NIR light: direct NIR-responsive PSs and indirect NIR-responsive PSs. The direct PSs can directly convert light energy into the production of radical agents, and they are composed of NIR-responsive organic and inorganic PSs. The indirect PSs include UV- or visible light responsive PSs and an up-conversion nanomaterial.

Based on the time of application, PSs are classified into four distinct generation categories. The first generations are based on hematoporphyrin and its derivatives (e.g., Photofrin, Photosan, and Photocan), acridine dyes, and eosin solution. Photofrin (the trade name of sodium porfimer) is a mixture of purified porphyrin dimers and oligomers from hematoporphyrin derivatives. The limitations of the first-generation PSs include low penetration into tissues due to short wavelength of maximum absorption, low chemical purity, long half-life, and high accumulation in the skin that lead to skin hypersensitivity to light leading to investigate the next generation of PSs. The second generation of PSs, which have better chemical purity, consist of hematoporphyrin derivatives, synthetic PSs such as 5-aminolevulinic acid, and pure synthetic compounds of an aromatic macrocycle such as porphyrins, benzoporphyrins, and chlorins. Moreover, PSs of this generation show higher quantum yield of $^1O_2$ production, better tissue penetration due to maximum absorption in the wavelength of 650–800 nm, improved selectivity for target tissue, and fewer side effects, extended extinction coefficient. Despite such mentioned benefits of second-generation PSs, they have poor solubility in water, which limits their intravenous administration.

Third-generation PSs are developed by altering existing PSs from earlier generations and combining them with nanomaterials or substances that have a higher affinity for tumor tissue. These modifications can include combination with target receptor ligand molecules and LDL lipoprotein, conjugation with a monoclonal antibody specific for cancer cell antigen, and the use of tumor surface markers. Increased selectivity, greater accumulation in the target site, better bioavailability, and reduced therapeutic doses to produce satisfactory therapeutic effects are among the benefits of third-generation photosensitizers [9, 11, 17].

Next generation of PSs are nanomaterial-based PSs and living-organism-derived, protein in the name of genetically encoded photosensitizers (GEPSs) has been developed. GEPSs are more beneficial than synthetic PSs due to their facility intracellular localization, spatiotemporal protein expression, and ROS generation through designing with genetic engineering methods as following selective and controlled expression by using particular promotors, efficient PSs owning to high speeding of intersystem crossing and excited triplet state generation, the study of the mechanisms that occur in living cells by recruitment chromophore-assisted light inactivation (CALI), PDT, correlative light-electron microscopy (CLEM) and photoablation, widely high-specific targeting capability, reducing toxicity by proteolysis and spatiotemporal inactivation of cellular proteins. Due to the mentioned features, GEPS is an effective tool in biomedical applications such as PDT, immune PDT, antimicrobial PDT

FPPS	Features	Source	Ref.
KillerRed	Red fluorescent protein and the first GEPS, ROS generation through the type-I mechanism of PDT	Arised from non-fluorescent hydrozoan jellyfish-derived chromoprotein	[18]
KillerOrange	A dimeric orange variant, mechanism of ROS generation is similar to KillerRed	Developed from KillerRed	[18]
SuperNova Red (SNR)	Monomeric variant, expression of SNR in the cell as a fusion partner with various cellular proteins	Developed from KillerRed	[18]
SuperNova Green(SNG)	A monomeric variant and a green emitting PS protein	Developed from KillerRed	[18]

Table 1.
Fluorescent protein photosensitizers.

FBPS	Features	Source	Ref.
Mini singlet oxygen generator (MiniSOG)	A green-emitting and monomeric PS protein, surrounded by binding positions to flavin mononucleotide(FMN) chromophore as a required cofactor for ROS generation	Generated from an *Arabidopsis thaliana*-derived light-oxygen-voltage-sensing (LOV) domain of phototropin-2	[18]
Singlet oxygen protein PSs (SOPP)	Generated from site-directed mutagenesis, mutation of FMN-binding glutamine in SOPP to leucine (Q102L), improved photosensitizing performance	Developed from of MiniSOG	[18]
Pp2FbFP	A monomeric flavin binding PS with variants such as Pp2FbFP Y112L, Pp2FbFP Q116V, and Pp2FbFP L30M	Arised from *Pseudomonas putida*	[18]

Table 2.
Flavin-binding photosensitizers.

(aPDT), and CALI. Oligomeric and monomeric types of GEPS have been utilized in cellular applications with photophysical features. GEPS-based photosensitizers could be categorized into fluorescent protein photosensitizers (FPPSs) (**Table 1**) and flavin-binding photosensitizers (FBPSs) (**Table 2**) [18].

2.1 PDT mechanism

After light irradiation, PS absorbs a quantum of light and will reach its excited singlet state ($^1PS^*$). The single excited PS undergoes intersystem crossing to an excited triplet state ($^3PS^*$). During this transfer, part of the energy is irradiated in the form of a quantum of fluorescence.$^3PS^*$ produces ROS through interaction with the surrounding biomolecules via type I and type II mechanisms. In the type I reaction, excited triplet state $^3PS^*$reacts directly with biomolecules such as cell membrane, then transferring hydrogen or electron between PS and substrate, leading to the formation of highly reactive products of the PS and the substrate including hydroxyl radicals ($HO^•$), superoxide anion ($O_2^{-•}$), and hydrogen peroxide (H_2O_2). After the start of the radical chain reactions, cell components will begin to be destroyed, which will cause the signaling pathways for autophagy or apoptosis to be triggered. In the type II mechanism, $^3PS^*$ transfers directly energy to the molecular oxygen in the ground triplet state to form excited singlet oxygen ($^1O_2$) having high quantum yields. On the other hands, $^1O_2$ produced by type II reaction increases the level of ROS that causes damages to proteins, nucleic acids, lipids, membranes, and organelles, which can lead to activation of cell death processes such as apoptosis or necrosis [9, 10, 15].

3. Metal-based nanomaterials in photodynamic application

Nanomaterials usually refer to materials that possess at least one dimension in sizes ranging from 1 to 100 nm. They can be used alone as a PS or conjugated with PS and GEPS, in various types of PDT such as antimicrobial PDT and immune-PDT. Lipid PS nanoparticles (LPNs), polymer PS nanoparticles (PPNs), inorganic PS nanoparticles (IPNs), and self-assembled PS nanoparticles (SAPNs) are four groups of nanoparticles-based PSs in which IPNs are addressed in this review [18].

Due to the limitations of organic PSs, which include small stoke shift in porphyrin derivatives and low quantum yield due to aggregated form of porphyrin derivatives by steady p–p stacking in concentrated solutions, high toxicity, non-selectivity for tumor, and poor light absorption such as suboptimal tumor selectivity and poor light penetration into the tumor in second-generation PS, the interest of metal-based nanomaterial for PDT has been growing. Metal-based nanomaterials have been utilized as PSs and delivery vehicles because of properties that include: (1) relatively narrow size of metal nanoparticles, which can affect circulation time in the bloodstream and accumulation rate in tumors. Longer circulation time could be observed in therapeutic nanoparticles with a size of lower than 100 nm and higher accumulation in therapeutic nanoparticles with 20–200 nm size. (2) Shape distribution of metal nanoparticles that play a critical role in their internalization into the targeted cell. (3) Metal nanoparticles show surface plasmon resonance (SPR), which is associated with the surface plasmon resonance of the nanoparticles with a size smaller than the resonant absorption wavelength, used in PTT. According to this, the light wavelength used in PDT should be longer than the wavelength range of surface plasmon resonance. (4) Stability in water dispersion and long-term activity [11, 12, 19]. (5) Lower

PS leaching and higher loading efficiency of PSs. (6) High ability to interact with many compounds and generate both active and passive PS adsorption via the EPR effect [20]. Integration of PSs to nanoparticles is done via electrostatic or covalent interactions [21]. Subsequently, we discuss about various metal-based nanomaterials such as copper, O_2 self-enriched metal-based nanoplatforms, transition metal oxides (TMOs), and transition metal dichalcogenides (TMD), upconversion (UCNPs) and metal organic frameworks. After that, we concentrate on photodynamic therapy based on gold and silver nanomaterials.

Copper ions have a vital role in biosystems including proliferation and differentiation of cells, promoting angiogenesis by stabilizing the expression of hypoxia-inducible factor (HIF-1α) and secretion of vascular endothelial growth factor (VEGF), cell migration, accelerating wound healing by collagen deposition, keeping the immune system functioning in such a way that copper ion deficiency causes immunodeficiency through reducing the phagocytic activity of granulocytes and the immunoglobulins synthesis, copper-composed nanomaterials have biomedical applications including antibacterial applications such as anti-multidrug-resistant bacteria and Cu-based enzymes, drug delivery, bioimaging, bioeffect and biosafety, catalytic nanotherapeutics, and nanotherapy. Due to photonic properties, Cu-based nanomaterials are used in PTT and PDT [12, 22]. In 2020, tumor microenvironment (TME) stimuli-responsive theranostic nanoplatform via assembling PS (chlorine e6, Ce6) modified carbon-dots (CDs-Ce6) and Cu_2^+ is designed. The existence Cu_2^+ in this nanoplatform creates extra chemodynamic therapy (CDT) via $^{\bullet}OH$ generation through reaction with endogenous H_2O_2. Also, it enhances therapeutic efficiency by supernormal intracellular glutathione (GSH) depletion via a redox reaction This nanoplatform shows important features of FL imaging, synergistic treatment by PTT, PDT, and CDT [23].

Metal–organic frameworks (MOFs) are a kind of coordination polymers, which are usually composed of a metal oxide center and organic linkers. MOFs formed by self-assembly of metal ions clusters and organic ligands through the coordination bonds. MOFs have shown characteristics such as tunable sizes/shapes, high porosity, versatility, intrinsic biodegradability, well-defined biocompatibility, designable and ease of synthesis, and great drug delivery. They are multifunctional composites that enhance the PDT effect with other therapeutic modalities synergistically. PS molecules incorporate in MOF pores, therefore self-quenching and aggregation of PS molecules don't occur, and the distribution of ROS throughout the porous and rigid structure of MOF is easily accomplished [12, 24–27]. Nanoscale metal–organic frameworks (nMOFs) have potential characteristics, which lead to great biomedical applications. These properties include synthetic tunability in structures and compositions of nMOFs, high molecular payloads without self-quenching in photosensitizers, and facilitated diffusion of ROS through nMOFs pores to enhance the efficacy of PDT, radiotherapy (RT), radiotherapy-radiodynamic therapy (RT-RDT), and CDT, also reduce the adverse effect of hypoxia in aggressive tumors, which is based on evidence, hypoxia-inducible factor 1 (HIF-1) pathway activation triggers survival signaling in cancer cells. nMOFs could be used as immunoadjuvants, which leads to adaptive immunity boosting and PDT efficiency improvement. Passive and active targeting, regulation of singlet oxygen generation, innate biodegradability, prohibition of ROS neutralization, the capability of theranostic function, pH-responsive treatment of cancer [13, 26, 28, 29].

Transition metal oxides (TMOs) exhibit semiconductors such as properties including adjustable and different bandgaps, conductivity, absorption of light at certain wavelengths, various proportions of oxygen's and metals, consequently creating various structures, photocatalytic efficiency, and possible wide usage of them in the PDT/PTT fields. The process of photo-catalysis is as follows: photons with energy equal to or greater than the TMO bandgap energy cause the excitation of electrons from the valence band to the conduction band (CB) and create electronic holes. These electrons and created holes during redox reactions, and adsorption of molecules to the surface of TMOs causes the creation of free radicals such as hydrogen peroxide (H_2O_2), superoxide ion ($O_2^{\bullet -}$), and hydroxyl radicals ($OH^{\bullet}$). ZnO, TiO_2, MoO_3, and WO_3 are among the TMOs that have great photo-induced antibacterial activity. Doping metal ions in TMOs, which maintains charge balance due to the presence of oxygen vacancies, is one method for increasing photocatalytic activity. TMOs have improved photocatalytic efficiency. There can be polymorphism due to the possibility of their synthesis manipulation that nanofibers, nanorods, nanobelts, and nanowires are instances of their diverse forms [2]. For example, the tubular structure of TiO_2 can perform as photocatalysis-propelled micro/nanomotors, and in an environment containing H_2O_2 (1%), O_2 bubbles are produced due to the decomposition of H_2O_2. Titanium dioxide (TiO_2), iron oxide, and cerium oxide are among the TMOs that can induce the lysosome-autophagy system through different pathways. TiO_2 is one of the common TMOs that has attracted a lot of attention in biomedicine due to its low cost, chemical stability, and biocompatibility, including as PSs in PDT, anticancer, and surface coating, and substrates for stem cell expansion. TiO_2 is usually an n-type semiconductor that has four polymorphisms. Anatase and rutile forms have efficient photocatalytic applications due to their broader band gap [14].

Transition metal dichalcogenides (TMDs) are semiconductors with stacking configurations and several structural phases. TMDs' structural phases are the coordination of the three atomic planes of transition metal (group IV, V, VI, VII, IX, or X) and two chalcogenides (S, Se, and Te). TMDs have bandgap energies within the range of 1.6–2.4 eV, which are suitable for visible light catalysis. TMDs act as co-catalysts and link to other photocatalysts. TMDs have electron sinks so they could retard photogenerated electron–hole recombination, which causes it widely used in photodynamic therapy and biosensing. Molybdenum disulfide (MoS_2) is one of the TMDs with poor cytotoxicity and higher NIR absorption. MoS_2 as a member of graphene-analog materials has graphene-derived features such as superior surface-to-volume ratios and hydrophobic surface nature leading to absorbing biomolecules, hydrophobic drugs, and genes, so it could be a drug delivery vehicle. According to studies, MoS_2 has PDT ability without adding other PSs. For example, MoS_2 nanoflowers have high NIR absorption and peroxidase-like activity, leading to decomposition of a low concentration of H_2O_2 and hydroxyl radical generation. Also, MoS_2 QDs could generate $^1O_2$ with radiation of 630 nm laser light [2, 30].

Upconversion NPs (UCNPs) and quantum dots are two major groups of transducing nanoparticles. The limited penetration depth of UV and visible light is a challenge for PDT, so transducing nanoparticles are a solution for this challenge so that they could transfer energy with wavelength out of PSs' absorption range to conjugated PS molecules Quantum dots (QDs) as semiconductor nanocrystals are constructed of different elements such as silicon, cadmium, selenide, and graphene, and they have optical and emission properties – dependent size (1–10 nm). QDs with larger sizes after that are excited by a specific wavelength of light, emitting light with low energy in the red spectrum range while the emission wavelength of smaller QDs is in the blue spectrum range. QDs could generate ROS by transferring energy to triplet oxygen, but their $^1O_2$ yield is low so it is necessary to design QDs conjugated with PSs that have enhanced energy transfer for increasing $^1O_2$ yield [2, 15]. Other groups of nano-transducer are UCNPs, constructed of a crystalline host lattice that may possess transition metals, lanthanide, or actinide ions, such as ytterbium (Yb^{3+}), erbium (Er^{3+}), and thulium (Tm^{3+}) [15, 31]. UCNPs provide anti-stoke luminescent because they could generate short-wavelength light (visible or UV light) from short-wavelength incident light (NIR). Up-conversion luminescence (UCL) efficiency depends on dopant ion ratio and up-conversion luminescence mechanisms.

Excited state absorption (ESA), photon avalanche (PA), and energy transfer up-conversion (ETU) are three main mechanisms that are observed in UCNPs either alone or in combination, for a luminescent generation. Energy transfer is the dominant mechanism that is existence in UCNPs such as $NaYF_4$ doped with Yb^{3+} (sensitizer), Er^{3+}, or Tm^{3+} (activator). ETU mechanism occurs in a two-ion-involved system, in which one of them donates energy is named sensitizer (S) ion and the other is activator (A) with the ability of visible or UV light emission. Each of the two neighboring ions absorbs the same energy, when the excited state of S and A is near enough, non-radiative energy transferring occurs from S to A, then the activator is excited to the upper energy state and emits higher-energy photons, while sensitizer comes back to ground state [2, 31, 32]. UCNPs could act as PSs, drug delivery systems, and bioconjugated, so they have wide applications in PDT including deep tumors PDT, antimicrobial PDT, and the PDT of viral infections. UCNPs such as lanthanides-doped platforms could incorporate into the design of MOF-based hybrid nanomaterials and act as a wavelength-shifting platform to broaden the light-harvesting properties of MOFs, which could absorb NIR light [2, 31, 33].

3.1 O_2 self-enriched metal-based nanoplatform for PDT improving

Due to requiring a high concentration of O_2 for PDT, one of the obstacles in PDT of solid tumors is the lack of enough oxygen because of the hypoxic microenvironment existence. The hypoxic microenvironment is a marking of solid tumors (50~60% of malignant solid tumors are recognized by hypoxia), which creates through imbalance between the oxygen consumption caused by tumor cell reproduction and insufficient oxygen supply created by tumor vascular systems abnormally. In addition to creating tumor resistance to PDT, hypoxia causes tumorigenesis and tumor progression, which can result from the production of hypoxia-inducible factors (HIFs), DNA methylation, and also the production of unwanted metabolites such as hydrogen peroxide (H_2O_2), which promotes tumor cell metastasis and invasion. Strategies for hypoxia relieving and PDT efficacy improvement, including: (1) hyperbaric oxygen therapy; (2) direct transport to tumor sites by oxygen-carrying agents (e.g., hemoglobin and perfluorocarbon); (3) in situ production of oxygen by degradation of chemicals (such as C_3N_4 and CaO_2), which is delivered by nanomaterials into tumor sites; (4) O_2 generation by catalytic conversion of some common appearances of ROSs such as $O_2^{\bullet-}$ and H_2O_2 into the tumor microenvironment. Pathophysiologic mechanisms (e.g., NADPH oxidase (NOX) enzymes overexpression), in tumors, lead to the production of elevated H_2O_2 that has a generation rate of 5 nmol per 105 cells h^{-1}.

Catalysis of endogenous H_2O_2 and conversion to O_2 are carried out by natural catalase and catalyze-like oxygen generators or artificial enzymes such as manganese dioxide (MnO_2), copper oxide (CuO), nanozymes, and biocatalytic cascades. Due to high sensitivity to TME and fast decomposition in an acidic environment, MnO_2 nanostructures were considered a TME-responsive drug carrier. MnO_2 and its various forms (e.g., MnO_2 nanosheets, MnO_2 nanoshell, and MnO_2 nanozymes) enhance

PDT efficacy through interaction with tumoral H_2O_2, as a result, O_2 generation and ameliorating tumor hypoxia. Also, MnO_2 moderates intratumoral GSH, as follows after MnO_2 interaction with GSH, Mn^{4+} converts to Mn^{2+}, which can form hydroxyl radical($^{\bullet}OH$), through Mn^{2+} interaction with H_2O_2 by Fenton-like catalytic reaction. Tumor overexpressed GSH as a scavenger of ROS, causing tumor cells to become resistant to PDT-induced oxidative stress, thus reducing the efficiency of photodynamic therapy with intratumoral GSH. Nanozymes have enzyme mimetic activity. Nobel metal nanomaterials (such as platinum (Pt), palladium (Pd) nanoparticles, rhodium (Rh)-based nanomaterials), and cerium oxide nanoparticles have served as nanozymes and generate oxygen to promote ROS production for PDT of tumor cells. Rh decomposes H_2O_2 into O_2 through its catalase-like activity, and Rh alloys have a more catalytic effect. Cerium oxide (ceria, CeO_2) nanoparticles have the dual performance of superoxide dismutase (SOD) and catalase-like activity and could generate oxygen via the $O_2^{\bullet-}$and H_2O_2 catalysis. The bifunctional activity of ceria is the result of electron shuttle between Ce^{3+} and Ce^{4+}, which are mixed valence states, as follows Ce^{3+} decompose superoxide anion ($O_2^{\bullet-}$) and Ce^{4+} catalysis hydrogen peroxide (H_2O_2). Natural catalase's poor stability and nonporous properties of artificial enzymes reduce $^1O_2$ yield and their effect on the tumor environment hypoxia. Also, the amount of H_2O_2 produced by tumor cells is not large enough that artificial enzymes have a good catalytic function and generate a high amount of O_2. For this reason, smart biocatalytic cascade systems designed such as well-assembled multicatalytic nanoreactors have been interested. These systems can supply a large amount of molecular oxygen as a substrate for PDT and also provide more effective communication between catalyst and substrate in these systems [27, 34–36].

3.2 Gold-based nanomaterials

Gold nanomaterials (AuNMs) have different biomedical applications such as PTT and PDT, due to their physicochemical properties (**Figure 2**).

AuNMs features are including ease and the possibility of achieving different sizes of synthesis, flexibility in surface modification, great nanocarriers for transporting a wide range of components such as small molecules, nucleic acids, proteins, and antibodies, controlled-release, site-specific triggering, low toxicity, high conductivity, and localized surface plasmon resonance (LSPR). LSPR is one of the optical properties of AuNMs, which refers to the total oscillations of the conduction band electrons of metal nanoparticles. The absorption band of LSPR in AuNMs is affected by shape and aspect ratio, so that with tuning the shape and aspect ratio due to the surface photon confinement effect, the absorption spectrum reaches to NIR range. AuNMs are one of the NIR-responsive materials that have an absorption spectrum with a longer wavelength in the range of NIR (750–1000 nm), where the depth of light penetration into the target tissue is greater in this range. Therefore, they overcome the organic PSs' limitations, whose absorption spectrum has a shorter wavelength (300–700 nm) and a lower penetration depth (less than 1 mm) and can create a novel generation of PSs [2, 3, 37–40]. Gold nanoparticles' (Au NPs) appropriate wavelength for PDT is between 800 and 900 nm [12].

Au NPs can exist in different shapes, such as spheres, rods, shells, stars, cages, and gold nanoflowers (**Figure 2**). Au NPs can be isotropic and anisotropic based on their shapes and characteristics. Just as the size alterations affect the plasmon absorption band, the geometry alterations of the nanoparticles also affect the SPR band, so according to Mie's theory, the particle's electric surface charge density changes with

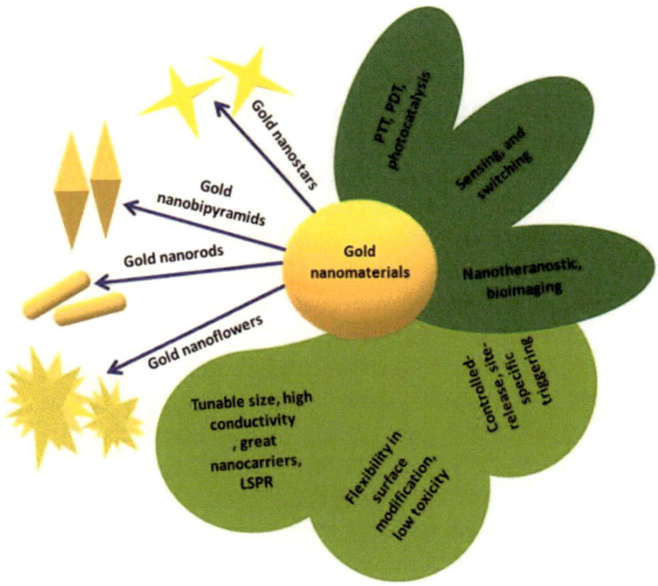

Figure 2.
Au NMs: shapes, features, and applications.

the alteration of the particle diameter. Therefore, with the increase in size, a shift in the location of the SPR absorption band toward longer wavelengths is observed. In addition, a small change in the particle geometry causes significant changes in the characteristics of the SPR absorption band. These alterations are also observed in anisotropic AuNPs, which are even higher than the changes caused by the increase in size in isotropic AuNPs. Anisotropic AuNPs have multiple SPR absorption bands contrary to the isotropic morphology, which has only one SPR absorption band. Therefore, the wavelength of the SPR absorption band shifts from the visible region to the near-infrared region (NIR), by changing the shape of the gold nanoparticle. Among the anisotropic morphologies of AuNPs, we can mention gold nanoflowers (AuNFs), gold nanostars (GNSs), gold nanorods (AuNRs), gold nanoplates, etc. Due to their anisotropic shape and symmetric structure with branches, GNSs possess tunable localized surface plasmon resonance (LSPR) in the near-infrared (NIR) region of the electromagnetic spectrum, and they are appropriate nanoplatforms for theranostic applications [3, 37, 41, 42].

The GNS@ICG-Ab-CIK nanoplatform designed by Shujing Liang et al. in 2020 is a nano-theranostics system that has the potential for cancer theranostics. In this nanoplatform, GNS (gold nanostars) was combined with anti-HER2 (trastuzumab) and targeted. Anti-HER2 (trastuzumab) is a monoclonal antibody that acts against HER2-overexpressing human breast cancer cells. This monoclonal antibody prevents cell cycle progression and inhibits angiogenesis and antibody-dependent cytotoxicity. GNS combined with trastuzumab was loaded with Indocyanine green (ICG) through electrostatic adsorption, and a new nanoprobe was formed that has the ability of tri-model imaging (photoacoustic (PA), computed tomography (CT), and fluorescence imaging) and also creates effective synergistic PTT/PDT of HER-2-positive breast cancer. GNSs protect ICG from photo-thermal damage and improve $^1O_2$ production, as well as increase their stability in the bloodstream and reduce blood clearance. To improve targeting efficiency, cytokine-induced killer (CIK) cells, which have the tumor-homing ability, were used. These cells activate the immune system after intravenous administration, so the constructed nanoplatform acts against cancer through immunotherapy in addition to PDT and PTT [37, 43].

AuNFs possess branch structures and flower-like shapes along with absorbing light in the red deep region (600—900 nm). AuNFs have a high surface-to-volume ratio and tissue penetration compared with other forms of AuNPs such as spherical and rod-shaped and are used as an agent for imaging, nano-vehicle, and therapy [3, 44]. PDA-Ce6-GSH-AuNF is a multifunctional system capable of cancer synergistic therapy through PDT and PTT treatments, in which AuNFs with a diameter of about 80 nm and an absorption band in the vis-near infrared (Vis–NIR) range of 800–900 nm are used. AuNFs were synthesized using HAuCl4 salt at 0°C, through the template-free method, which has two steps. In the first step, HAuCl4 was reduced by ascorbic acid (AA) and Au seeds were formed. In the second step, through the seed-mediated approach, and using $NH_2OH{\cdot}HCl$ as a reducing agent, gold ions (Au^{3+}) were converted into gold nanoparticles. These nanoparticles are deposited on Au seeds (crystal nucleus) and branch structures of AuNFs are constructed. Then glutathione (GSH) molecules are anchored to the gold surface by their thiol group, and it is utilized as a linker for connecting chlorin e6 (Ce6) to AuNFs through the activated carboxyl group of GSH. Then Ce6-modified AuNFs were coated with polydopamine (PDA). PDAs are surface modification agents with high chemical and thermal stability and containing catecholamine functional groups with great adhesion properties, which create thin nanoscale layers on the surface of organic materials. Thin PDA layers increase cellular absorption of nanoparticles and their mucopenetration and also play a role in hydrophobic drug delivery, which is due to the hydrophilicity and zwitterionic properties they give to the material. PDA has an elevated absorption capability in the NIR region and high efficiency of energy conversion and creates red-shift adsorption, so as a photothermal agent, it can increase the PTT efficiency of the nanoplatforms. The nanoplatform was examined in vitro and in vivo, through a near-infrared (NIR) laser with a wavelength of 660 nm for PDT and 808 nm for PTT. Based on the results, the amount of Ce6 loaded in Au NFs was 14.0 wt.%, the singlet oxygen production efficiency by the designed nanoplatform was approximately 91.0% of free Ce6, and the photothermal conversion efficiency was 23.6% (7.0% more than free Au NFs). As regards that the antitumor efficiency was increased by combining PDT and PTT treatments, PDA-Ce6-GSH-AuNFs were considered as dual phototherapy agents [3].

Au NRs are one-dimensional anisotropic nanoparticles. Contrary to spherical gold nanoparticles, which have one LSPR band in the range of 520 nm, AuNRs have two LSPR bands; transverse LSPR (t-LSPR) with a wavelength in the range of 520 nm and longitudinal-LSPR (l-LSPR) with higher wavelengths in the range of the biological window (560–950 nm) and (1000–1350 nm). l-LSPR can be adjusted by changing the aspect ratio of AuNRs, and compared with the LSPR of spherical nanoparticles, AuNRs are more sensitive to environmental variations resulting from dielectrics. These features make AuNRs possess wide applications in biomedical, including LSPR-biosensing. AuNRs are one of the metal nanoparticles that are used in non-aggregation plasmonic colorimetric sensors as a mediator in the etching/growth process. This process alters the shape, size, and environmental dielectrics of metal nanoparticles, which follows the plasmon band changes. Based on the studies on Au NRs, gold nanoshells (nanocages, nanorod-in-shell, and nanoparticle-in-shell) and gold nanobipyramids (Au NBPs) (**Figure 2**), have been used as PS in PDT and can produce singlet oxygen ($^1O_2$) [45–47]. Au NBPs are, like the Au NRs, one of the novel plasmonic nanoparticles, which have longitudinal dipolar plasmon with a tunable wavelength from the visible region to the near-infrared. Au NBPs have higher shape and size uniformity and against Au NRs, which have curved or flat ends, Au NBPs contain two sharp end apexes, so Au NBPs could create higher regional electric field enhancements with more slender peak width. Au NBPs possess broad plasmonic usage in the areas of photocatalysis, sensing, and switching (such as plasmonic index-change-based sensing method, colorimetric and selective immunoassay, and electrochemical plasmonic switching), biomedical applications (PTT, PDT, real-time bioassays, as thermocycling-creating nanoreactors for rapid and quantitative real-time PCR, plasmon-enhanced fluorescence bioimaging agents, etc.), and plasmon-enhanced spectroscopies (PL), surface-enhanced Raman spectroscopy (SERS), etc.) [48].

Au NP creates antimicrobial effects through mechanisms, which include interaction with bacterial cell barriers, interaction with biomolecules such as enzyme activity inhibiting, DNA binding or interference in protein synthesis, bacteria-killing by photothermal effect, the redox imbalance, and increasing the effectiveness of antimicrobial photodynamic therapy (aPDT). According to studies, AuNPs do not cause the redox imbalance by making changes in the ROS level, but they affect the level of glutathione (GSH) [49]. According to reports, the mechanisms through which gold nanoparticles can increase the effect of aPDT are as follows: improving the relative distribution and production of ROS, and also, it can increase the amount of PS excitation and improving the efficiency of aPDT through conjugation with PS such as AuNPs-conjugated methylene blue (MB) against bacteria such as the mature methicillin-resistant *Staphylococcus aureus* (MRSA) biofilm [50–52]. By reducing photobleaching, AuNPs also increase the efficiency of photodynamic therapy. In a study in 2021, the effect of biosynthetic AuNPs-mediated mycelium of *Mucor plumbeus* on aPDT efficiency was investigated. Based on the observations of this study, biogenic AuNPs in combination with (Mb) methylene blue as PS can cause effective aPDT of both Gram-negative (*Escherichia coli*) and Gram-positive (*S. aureus*) bacteria. Biogenic AuNPs reduce the photobleaching speed of methylene blue by changing the kinetics of the photofading process [50]. In 2017, phototheranostic nanoagents (PTNAs) were designed, which possess biosynthesized AuNPs using *Syzygium cumini*'s fruit extract (ScAuNPs). In this study, the effects of ScAuNPs have been compared with chitosan-mediated AuNPs (ChAuNPs). According to the results, antioxidant efficacy, drug loading, fluorescence quantum yield (Q), singlet oxygen quantum yield, and antimicrobial PDT of ScAuNPs and their conjugated probes/nanoprobes were better than those of ChAuNPs [53].

Other forms of AuNMs are nanoclusters (**Figure 3**). Generally, metal nanoclusters (Au, Ag, Cu, etc.) have a different structure from metal nanoparticles, and subsequently, their characteristics, including their optical characteristics, change, too. These nanomaterials have several to 100 atoms and their size is less than 2 nm, which is comparable with the Fermi wavelength of electrons, which is usually less than 1 nm because as the size decreases, the continuous energy band of metals changes to a discrete energy level, which is associated with molecular-like electronic transitions (i.e., HOMO – LUMO transitions) in valence states. Metal nanoclusters (MNCs) could be categorized as water-soluble MNCs stabilized by biomolecules (proteins, peptides, DNA, etc.), and oil-soluble MNCs with easy crystallization, such as $Au_{25}(PET)_{18}$ (PET is phenethyl mercaptan), that is, oil-soluble mono-metallic NCs nobel metal nanoclusters (MNCs) have capping agents such as protein, DNA, and small organic molecules, good biocompatibility, and the ability to easily modify the surface characteristics. Also, they are good fluorescent labels, due to large stock

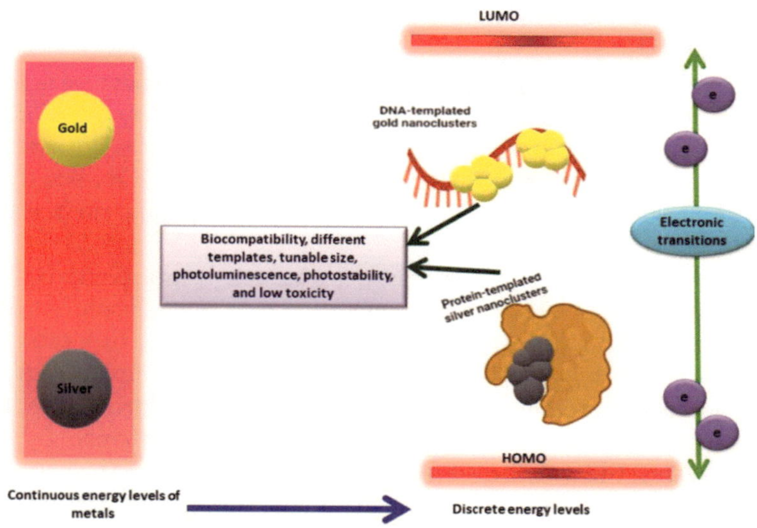

Figure 3.
Properties of AuNCs and AgNCs.

shift, size-dependent excitation and emission wavelength, and high optical stability [54–57]. Gold nanoclusters (AuNCs) consist of less than 100 gold atoms and have a size smaller than 2 nm, which is comparable with the Fermi wavelength of electrons (< 1 nm). AuNCs do not have localized surface plasmon resonance like gold nanoparticles because the electrons of the valence layer of AuNCs cannot move freely. AuNCs do not absorb plasma resonance in the visible region. The maximum fluorescence of gold nanoclusters is in the visible to NIR region, which is the appropriate wavelength for tissue penetration. Also, high photostability and great fluorescence lifetime in vivo conditions are other characteristics of AuNCs. Therefore, they have biomedical applications such as biosensing, bio-imaging, and therapy. AuNCs are used as inorganic PS in PDT. In 2014, in a study, a nanoprobe was designed in which Doxorubicin (DOX) was loaded in a nanocomposite consisting of AuNCs encapsulated in Zeolitic imidazolate framework-8 (ZIF-8). Due to their small size, AuNCs have limitations such as low enhanced permeability and retention (EPR) effect, short duration in blood circulation, and low accumulation in tumor sites due to fast clearance. To solve these limitations in this study, AuNCs were encapsulated in the inner of ZIF-8 and DOX in the channel of ZIF-8. This nanocomposite is pH-responsive and bifunctional so that it uses synergistic PDT/chemotherapy to treat breast cancer. And due to being pH-responsive, it is not released in neutral environments and normal cells are not affected. Their release occurs in acidic tumor sites, so the performance of PDT and chemotherapy is enhanced [29, 38, 54].

3.3 Silver-based nanomaterials

Due to the innate antibacterial properties of silver ions, it has been used by humans for many years and recently has been noticed in cancer therapeutics. According to studies, mechanism of Ag-based agents for therapy is irreversible apoptosis along with contacting Ag^+ to a thiol-rich protein that is located on the cell, and bacterial membrane leads to decrease of these proteins. So superficial contact is a factor that regulates antimicrobial effects. Ag^+ is restricted by a lack of stability in the physiological body environment and target ability for tumors. So synthesis of nanoplatforms for Ag^+ accumulation in the diseased region and making synergistic therapeutic effects is vital [58]. Silver nanoparticles usually possess a size between 20 and 25 nm due to their high surface-to-volume ratio [12]. They have wide contact areas with viruses and bacteria, which subsequently improves the bactericidal performance. Therefore, the effects of silver nanoparticles on Gram-positive and Gram-negative bacteria depend on the size, dose, shape, and total surface area of the nanoparticle.

According to the studies, silver nanoparticles have high antibacterial effects on *Streptococcus mutans* in low concentrations, so their toxicity is reduced. Silver nanoparticles affect the morphology of *E. coli* and *S. aureus*, also they can alter the expression of some coating proteins such as (OmpA, OmpC, OmpF, OppA, and MetQ) and heat shock proteins (IbpA and IbpB). Ions released from silver nanoparticles can also have a biocidal effect [59]. Silver nanoparticles enhance photodynamic performance against the wide-broad spectrum of microorganisms bacterial and fungal species and including antibiotic-resistant strains, which is a public health threat all over the world. They can be used as carriers for PSs or as hybrids, composites, and conjugates with PSs [12, 60]. Silver core-mesoporous silica shell nanoparticles-containing HPIX (Hematoporphyrin IX dihydrochloride) is a hybrid PS that was synthesized in 2016 by Tevhide Ozkaya Ahmadov et al. [61] which exhibited significant photodynamic inactivation ability against MRSA (a multidrug-resistant strain of *S.aureus*) in such a way that its lethal efficiency increased up to six times [62]. As the size of silver nanoparticles decreases, their antimicrobial effect will be greater due to the increase of surface-to-volume, such that silver nanoclusters (AgNCs) with a size smaller than 2 nm exhibit stronger antimicrobial effects. Similar to AuNCs, AgNCs participate in photodynamic therapy. AgNCs have remarkable luminescence properties, biocompatibility, tunable size and photoluminescence, photostability, and low toxicity. Ag NCs have more antimicrobial capability than AuNCs, but their stability is lower than AuNCs, in a way that they don't preserve for a long time such as a few months while some AuNCs could preserve for more than a few months [63, 64].

The optical features of AgNCs are attributed to factors such as the quantum confinement effect, surface ligand effect, and the electronic transition between the highest occupied molecular orbital (HOMO) and the lowest unoccupied molecular orbital (LUMO) (**Figure 3**) [65]. Surface ligand affects the intramolecular and intermolecular control of nanoclusters, which are two kinds of continuous systems of nanoclusters control and both together adjust nanocluster systems. Intramolecular control points out the manipulation of metal–ligand compositions and bonding environment at the single-molecule level. Intermolecular control refers to changes in the aggregation pattern in amorphous or crystallographic forms. Ligand exchange and heteroatom alloying are methods for intramolecular control. Among the methods used for intermolecular control, we can mention cluster-based metal–organic framework, aggregation-induced emission, and intercluster metallophilic reaction. Based on the studies, manipulation of nanocluster crystallographic networks at the supramolecular level and the adjustment of intramolecular and intermolecular interactions make the nanoclusters become CIEE (crystallization-induced emission enhancement)-active or -inactive nanomaterials [62].

There are various methods for metal nanoclusters synthesis, among these approaches, the template-based method is suitable for the generation of metal nanoclusters, and they involve improving the stability, shape, and size-controlled and fluorescence tunability of metal nanoclusters. Templates or capping agents can be dendrimers, proteins, peptides, and DNAs [50]. Bovine serum albumin (BSA) and human serum albumin (HSA) are the common proteins used as capping agents in the synthesis of nanoclusters (NCs). BSA has various functional groups such as -OH, -NH_2, -COOH, and -SH, which are involved in the synthesis of metal nanoclusters (MNCs) by creating steric stabilization. BSA has disulfide bonds that establish a covalent bond with the MNCs core through the sulfur. Also, the pH of the environment participates in the formation of nanomaterials and MNCs. For instance, BSA converts silver ions into silver nanoparticles at pH (6–8) and generates silver nanoclusters at pH higher than 11. Of course, the protein itself can also reduce the silver ions (Ag^+) without adding external reducing agents and turning them into silver nanoparticles and nanoclusters. BSA obtains various conformations, including -N (native), B (basic), A (aged), and U (unfolded), along with alterations of environment pH from neutral to alkaline that different nanomaterials are stable in some of these conformations [65].

AgNCs are also constructed with DNA templates in the way that this nanocluster has a high affinity to N_3 cytosine. The number of single-stranded cytosines installed in the primary and secondary structures of DNA (such as hairpin loops, i-motifs, and G-quadruplexes) controls the size and shape of AgNCs. Another feature of DNA-AgNCs is their resistance to photobleaching, which makes them have applications in nanophotonics and biosensing. One of the advantages of using oligonucleotides for the synthesis of AgNCs is the possibility of their synthesis with different sequences. AgNCs can exert antimicrobial effect through DNA intercalation and inactivation of type II topoisomerases. In 2016, Siamak Javani et al. investigated the antibacterial performance of fluorescent DNA-AgNCs, which has an inhibitory effect on the growth of Gram-positive and -negative bacteria in sub-micromolar concentrations. These DNA-AgNCs were synthesized with three types of oligonucleotide sequences named Seq1, Seq2, Seq3, and the absorption wavelengths of the resulting nanoclusters are 370 nm, 480 nm, and 560 nm, respectively, and their emission wavelengths are 475 nm, 572 nm, and 630 nm, respectively. The result of the antibacterial test for *E.coli* showed that Seq3 had more inhibitory effect than Seq2 and Seq1 showed the least inhibitory activity. Based on the results of this study, the factors that regulate the antibacterial performance of DNA-AgNCs are the amount of silver and factors such as sequence, structure, and Ag arrangement [66, 67].

4. PDT effects on immune system

PDT can lead to cell death through apoptosis, necrosis, autophagy, or proptosis. The type of cell death induced by PDT depends on the location of the PS and the amount of photodamage. Each of these cell death leads to the release of molecules such as alarmins or damage-associated molecular patterns (DAMPs), cytokines, growth factors, and other immunomodulating agents. Alarmins as immunostimulators are released after photooxidative damage that triggers innate immunity, which leads to the activation of adaptive immunity. They are detected by pattern recognition receptors (PRRs) that are expressed on immune cells, and subsequently, activate immune cells after DAMPs are attached to the PRRs. Similar to the lesion from infection and other tissue damage, PDT- mediated damage of tumor and endothelial cells is caused by release of inflammatory factors including arachidonic acid-derived metabolites arising from membrane lipids peroxidation (such as thromboxanes, prostaglandin, and leukotriene), high amount of cytokines such as the interleukin

(IL)-6, IL-1β, IL-2, IL-1β (possess a prominent role in PDT efficiency), MIP2 (CXCL2), tumor necrosis factorα (TNFα), acute phase proteins, pro-aggregatory and vasoactive mediator releasing (result in platelets activation and clotting cascade initiation). These factors lead to the migration of innate immune cells toward the tumor site for tumor cell elimination. The PDT immune cells from PDT-mediated damage include neutrophils, macrophages, natural killers (NK), and dendritic cells (DCs). Previous studies demonstrated that systemic neutrophilia is incorporated in immune-PDT interaction of tumor cells through various factors resulting from PDT-mediated damage, which can be mentioned in some cases, including: (1) Complement activation upon PDT is caused to release tumor tissue anaphylatoxins (such as C3a and C5a), subsequently, vascular permeability increasing and neutrophil infiltration. (2) Adhesion molecules such as E-selectin and ICAM1 for neutrophil adherence on tumor tissue and micro vessels, also adhesion to the subendothelial matrix by the β2 integrin receptors (3) Acute-phase proteins (APPs), which facilitate neutrophils migrate, mature neutrophil progenitors more quickly, and help them leave the bone marrow [68].

Macrophages as effector cells participate in immune-PDT of cancer cells. The release of HSP70 from tumor cells damaged by PTD will activate macrophages. Hsp70 is bound to PRRs (which are expressed on macrophages such as the toll-like receptors (TLRs) and as a result of this binding, TLR2/4 of macrophages is activated, followed by TNFα releasing. TNFα as a cytolytic cytokine leads to indirect tumor cell elimination. C3 and MBLs (mannose-binding lectins) opsonization of tumor cells provides their phagocytose possibility by macrophages, due to complement receptors expressed by macrophages could recognize opsonized agents. NK cells have also been interested in cancer PDT. According to reports, major histocompatibility (MHC) class I-related molecule (MICA) and Natural Killer Group 2D (NKG2D) ligands from photodamage are recognized by NKG2D receptors on NK cells and lead to activation of these receptors, consequently enhancing PDT-induced immunity. Dendritic cells (DCs) as antigen-presenting cells communicate between innate and adaptive immune systems. PRRs of DCs detect DAMPs, released by PDT-damage, following it to activate/mature dendritic cells leading to augment MHC class II and co-stimulatory factors expression, which will be associated with the presenting of antigens to T lymphocytes and activation of type 1, 2, and 3 of adaptive immunity. In type 1 immunity cytokines such as IL-12 and IFN-γ are expressed by $CD4^+$ T cells leading to the activation of the cytotoxic function of $CD8^+$ T cells. In type 2 immunity, $CD4^+$ T cells deviate to the Th2 phenotype, which is associated with cytokines expression such as IL-4 and antibody generation from B cells. According to studies demonstrated, $CD8^+$ T cells have a pivotal role in immune-PDT, in a way defects in these cells reduce the efficacy of PDT. Type 3 immunity induced by PDT arises from the increasing of T helper (Th17) cell numbers in the tumor-draining lymph nodes (TDLNs). Th17 cells are a subset of $CD4^+$ T cells that generate IL-17 cytokine that according to studies, this molecule has a significant role in neutrophils recruitment in TDLNs upon PDT and also neutrophils are effective in activated $CD8^+$T cells accumulation into tumor cells [68, 69].

5. Conclusions and perspectives

In the first parts of the paper, PDT as one of the applications of photodynamic function is addressed, then gold and silver nanomaterials-based PDT and finally, the challenges of metal nanomaterial-based PDT. Photodynamic is determined as an action in which cells react with oxygen, light, and PS. Utilizin effective PS is an important agents in improving of PDT efficacy. There are different generations of PSs. Due to limitations of organic PSs, the attention toward metal-based nanomaterials for PDT has been increasing, due to their unique properties such as relatively narrow size, shape distribution, simplified functionalization, and consequently, active absorption, stability, and SPR. Metal nanomaterial-based PDT has challenges, including accumulation and long retention time of PSs, hypoxia and low PDT efficiency, low therapeutic penetration of light, brief half-life of $^1O_2$ and shorter diffusion amplitude in comparison with cell and organelles size, and metal nanomaterials toxicity. These challenges, especially nanotechnology risks, must be addressed in future studies. However, photodynamic techniques are frontier approaches for diagnosis and treatment of disease such as cancer and microbial resistances. Photodynamic applications and nanomedicine are the multidisciplinary fields that could design improved novel PSs with usage of different areas such as biology, physics, engineering, electronic, chemistry, informatics, pharmaceutic, and medicine. Therefore, PDT, especially along with other therapies (combination therapy), deserves attention in future research studies and clinical applications.

Acknowledgements

This work was supported by the Golestan University of Medical Sciences financial support (Grant number, 31-111679).

Conflict of interest

The authors of this project have no conflict of interest.

Author details

Atiyeh Nomani[1], Anvarsadat Kianmehr[2], Shahriyar Abdoli[2*] and Siamak Javani[2*]

1 School of Advanced Technologies in Medicine, Golestan University of Medical Sciences, Gorgan, Iran

2 Medical Cellular and Molecular Research Center, Golestan University of Medical Sciences, Gorgan, Iran

*Address all correspondence to: drabdoli@goums.ac.ir; siamak.javani@imdea.org and siamackjavani@yahoo.com

References

[1] Wu J, Niu S, Bremner DH, Nie W, Fu Z, Li D, et al. A tumor microenvironment-responsive biodegradable mesoporous nanosystem for anti-inflammation and cancer theranostics. Advanced Healthcare Materials. 2020;**9**(2):1-12. DOI: 10.1002/adhm.201901307

[2] Lee HP, Gaharwar AK. Light-responsive inorganic biomaterials for biomedical applications. Advancement of Science. 17 Jul 2020;**7**(17):2000863. DOI: 10.1002/advs.202000863

[3] Wu F, Liu Y, Wu Y, Song D, Qian J, Zhu B. Chlorin e6 and polydopamine modified gold nanoflowers for combined photothermal and photodynamic therapy. Journal of Materials Chemistry B. 2020;**8**(10):2128-2138. DOI: 10.1039/c9tb02646k

[4] Bochenek K, Aebisher D, Międzybrodzka A, Cieślar G, Kawczyk-Krupka A. Methods for bladder cancer diagnosis – The role of autofluorescence and photodynamic diagnosis. Photodiagnosis and Photodynamic Therapy. 2019;**27**:141-148. DOI: 10.1016/j.pdpdt.2019.05.036

[5] Gomez S, Tsung A, Hu Z. Current targets and bioconjugation strategies in photodynamic diagnosis and therapy of cancer. Molecules. 27 Oct 2020;**25**(21):4964. DOI: 10.3390/molecules25214964

[6] Endlicher E, Messmann H. Photodynamic diagnosis in the gastrointestinal tract. Gastrointestinal Endoscopy Clinics of North America. 2004;**14**(3):475-485. DOI: 10.1016/j.giec.2004.03.009

[7] Nagaya T, Nakamura YA, Choyke PL, Kobayashi H. Fluorescence-guided surgery. Front Oncologia. 22 Dec 2017;**7**:314. DOI: 10.3389/fonc.2017.00314

[8] Abdel-kader MH. Chapter 1 the journey of PDT throughout history: PDT from pharos to present. In: Photodynamic Medicine: From Bench to Clinic. The Royal Society of Chemistry; 2016. pp. 1-21. DOI: 10.1039/9781782626824-00001

[9] Kwiatkowski S, Knap B, Przystupski D, Saczko J, Kędzierska E, Knap-Czop K, et al. Photodynamic therapy – Mechanisms, photosensitizers and combinations. Biomedicine and Pharmacotherapy. 2018;**106**:1098-1107. DOI: 10.1016/j.biopha.2018.07.049

[10] Warrier A, Mazumder N, Prabhu S, Satyamoorthy K, Murali TS. Photodynamic therapy to control microbial biofilms. Photodiagnosis and Photodynamic Therapy. 2021;**33**:102090. DOI: 10.1016/j.pdpdt.2020.102090

[11] Dhanalekshmi KI, Sangeetha K, Magesan P, Johnson J, Zhang X, Jayamoorthy K. Photodynamic cancer therapy: Role of Ag- and Au-based hybrid nano-photosensitizers. Journal of Biomolecular Structure & Dynamics. Jul 2022;**40**(10):4766-4773. DOI: 10.1080/07391102.2020.1858965

[12] Sun J, Kormakov S, Liu Y, Huang Y, Wu D, Yang Z. Molecules recent progress in metal-based nanoparticles mediated photodynamic therapy. Molecules. 12 Jul 2018;**23**(7):1704. DOI: 10.3390/molecules23071704

[13] Sakamaki Y, Ozdemir J, Heidrick Z, Watson O, Shahsavari HR, Fereidoonnezhad M, et al. Metal–organic

frameworks and covalent organic frameworks as platforms for photodynamic therapy. Comments on Inorganic Chemistry. 2018;**38**:238-293. DOI: 10.1080/02603594.2018.1542597

[14] Mohammadalipour Z, Rahmati M, Khataee A, Moosavi MA. Differential effects of N-TiO_2 nanoparticle and its photo-activated form on autophagy and necroptosis in human melanoma A375 cells. Journal of Cellular Physiology. 2020;**235**(11):8246-8259. DOI: 10.1002/jcp.29479

[15] Bekmukhametova A, Ruprai H, Hook JM, Mawad D, Houang J, Lauto A. Photodynamic therapy with nanoparticles to combat microbial infection and resistance. Nanoscale. 2020;**12**(41):21034-21059. DOI: 10.1039/d0nr04540c

[16] Diaz-Diestra D, Gholipour HM, Bazian M, Thapa B, Beltran-Huarac J. Photodynamic therapeutic effect of nanostructured metal sulfide photosensitizers on cancer treatment. Nanoscale Research Letters. 8 Mar 2022;**17**(1):33. DOI: 10.1186/s11671-022-03674-8

[17] Kim MM, Darafsheh A. Light sources and dosimetry techniques for photodynamic therapy. Photochemistry and Photobiology. 2020;**96**(2):280-294. DOI: 10.1111/php.13219

[18] Das S, Tiwari M, Mondal D, Sahoo BR, Tiwari DK. Growing tool-kit of photosensitizers for clinical and non-clinical applications. Journal of Materials Chemistry B. 2020;**8**(48):10897-10940. DOI: 10.1039/d0tb02085k

[19] Yetisgin AA, Cetinel S, Zuvin M, Kosar A, Kutlu O. Therapeutic Nanoparticles and Their Targeted Delivery Applications. Molecules. 8 May 2020;**25**(9):2193. DOI: 10.3390/molecules25092193

[20] Shang L, Zhou X, Zhang J, Shi Y, Zhong L. Metal nanoparticles for photodynamic therapy: A potential treatment for breast cancer. Molecules. 2021;**26**(21):6532. DOI: 10.3390/molecules26216532

[21] Kadkhoda J, Tarighatnia A, Barar J, Aghanejad A, Davaran S. Recent advances and trends in nanoparticles based photothermal and photodynamic therapy. Photodiagnosis and Photodynamic Therapy 2022;**37**(December 2021):102697. DOI: doi:10.1016/j.pdpdt.2021.102697

[22] Dong C, Feng W, Xu W, Yu L, Xiang H, Chen Y, et al. The coppery age: Copper (Cu)-involved nanotheranostics. Advancement of Science. 2020;**7**(21): 1-38. DOI: 10.1002/advs.202001549

[23] Sun S, Chen Q, Tang Z, Liu C, Li Z, Wu A, et al. Tumor microenvironment stimuli-responsive fluorescence imaging and synergistic cancer therapy by carbon-Dot–Cu2+ nanoassemblies. Angewandte Chemie International Edition. 2020;**59**(47):21041-21048. DOI: 10.1002/anie.202007786

[24] Chen M, Long Z, Dong R, Wang L, Zhang J, Li S, et al. Titanium incorporation into Zr-porphyrinic metal–organic frameworks with enhanced antibacterial activity against multidrug-resistant pathogens. Small. 2020;**16**(7): 1-11. DOI: 10.1002/smll.201906240

[25] Yu W, Zhen W, Zhang Q, Li Y, Luo H, He J, et al. Porphyrin-based metal–organic framework compounds as promising nanomedicines in photodynamic therapy. ChemMedChem. 2020;**15**(19):1766-1775. DOI: 10.1002/cmdc.202000353

[26] Cai Z, Xin F, Wei Z, Wu M, Lin X, Du X, et al. Photodynamic therapy combined with antihypoxic signaling

and CpG adjuvant as an in situ tumor vaccine based on metal–organic framework nanoparticles to boost cancer immunotherapy. Advanced Healthcare Materials. 2020;**9**(1):1-12. DOI: 10.1002/adhm.201900996

[27] You Q, Zhang K, Liu J, Liu C, Wang H, Wang M, et al. Persistent regulation of tumor hypoxia microenvironment via a bioinspired Pt-based oxygen nanogenerator for multimodal imaging-guided synergistic phototherapy. Advancement of Science. 29 Jul 2020;**7**(17):1903341. DOI: 10.1002/advs.201903341

[28] Ni K, Luo T, Nash GT, Lin W. Nanoscale metal-organic frameworks for cancer immunotherapy. Accounts of Chemical Research. 2020;**53**(9):1739-1748. DOI: 10.1021/acs.accounts.0c00313

[29] Zhang L, Gao Y, Sun S, Li Z, Wu A, Zeng L. PH-Responsive metal-organic framework encapsulated gold nanoclusters with modulated release to enhance photodynamic therapy/chemotherapy in breast cancer. Journal of Materials Chemistry B. 2020;**8**(8):1739-1747. DOI: 10.1039/C9TB02621E

[30] Vankayala R, Kuo CL, Sagadevan A, Chen PH, Chiang CS, Hwang KC. Morphology dependent photosensitization and formation of singlet oxygen (1Δg) by gold and silver nanoparticles and its application in cancer treatment. Journal of Materials Chemistry B. 2013;**1**(35):4379-4387. DOI: 10.1039/c3tb20806k

[31] Liang G, Wang H, Shi H, Wang H, Zhu M, Jing A, et al. Recent progress in the development of upconversion nanomaterials in bioimaging and disease treatment. Journal of Nanobiotechnology. 2020;**18**(1):1-22. DOI: 10.1186/s12951-020-00713-3

[32] Chen J, Zhao JX. Upconversion nanomaterials: Synthesis, mechanism, and applications in sensing. Sensors. 2012;**12**(3):2414-2435. DOI: 10.3390/s120302414

[33] He L, Ni Q, Mu J, Fan W, Liu L, Wang Z, et al. Solvent-assisted self-assembly of a metal-organic framework based biocatalyst for cascade reaction driven photodynamic therapy. Journal of the American Chemical Society. 2020;**142**(14):6822-6832. DOI: 10.1021/jacs.0c02497

[34] Wang J, Sun J, Hu W, Wang Y, Chou T, Zhang B, et al. A porous Au@Rh bimetallic core–shell nanostructure as an H_2O_2-driven oxygenerator to alleviate tumor hypoxia for simultaneous bimodal imaging and enhanced photodynamic therapy. Advanced Materials. 2020;**32**(22):1-14. DOI: 10.1002/adma.202001862

[35] Liu X, Liu J, Chen S, Xie Y, Fan Q, Zhou J, et al. Dual-path modulation of hydrogen peroxide to ameliorate hypoxia for enhancing photodynamic/starvation synergistic therapy. Journal of Materials Chemistry B. 2020;**8**(43):9933-9942. DOI: 10.1039/D0TB01556C

[36] Zhu D, Zhu XH, Ren SZ, Lu YD, Zhu HL. Manganese dioxide (MnO_2) based nanomaterials for cancer therapies and theranostics. Journal of Drug Targeting. 2021;**29**(9):911-924. DOI: 10.1080/1061186X.2020.1815209

[37] Liang S, Sun M, Lu Y, Shi S, Yang Y, Lin Y, et al. Cytokine-induced killer cells-assisted tumor-targeting delivery of Her-2 monoclonal antibody-conjugated gold nanostars with NIR photosensitizer for enhanced therapy of cancer. Journal of Materials Chemistry B. 2020;**8**(36):8368-8382. DOI: 10.1039/d0tb01391a

[38] Yang J, Wang F, Yuan H, Zhang L, Jiang Y, Zhang X, et al. Recent advances in ultra-small fluorescent Au nanoclusters toward oncological research. Nanoscale. 2019;**11**(39):17967-17980. DOI: 10.1039/C9NR04301B

[39] Yang D, Deng F, Liu D, He B, He B, Tang X, et al. The appliances and prospects of aurum nanomaterials in biodiagnostics, imaging, drug delivery and combination therapy. Asian Journal of Pharmaceutical Sciences. 2019;**14**(4):349-364. DOI: 10.1016/j.ajps.2018.06.002

[40] Hu X, Zhang Y, Ding T, Liu J, Zhao H. Multifunctional gold nanoparticles: A novel nanomaterial for various medical applications and biological activities. Frontiers in Bioengineering and Biotechnology. 2020;**8**:1-17. DOI: 10.3389/fbioe.2020.00990

[41] Fabris L. Gold nanostars in biology and medicine: Understanding physicochemical properties to broaden applicability. Journal of Physical Chemistry C. 10 Dec 2020;**124**(49):26540-26553. DOI: 10.1021/acs.jpcc.0c08460

[42] Ortiz-Castillo JE, Gallo-Villanueva RC, Madou MJ, Perez-Gonzalez VH. Anisotropic gold nanoparticles: A survey of recent synthetic methodologies. Coordination Chemistry Reviews. 2020;**425**:213489. DOI: 10.1016/j.ccr.2020.213489

[43] Albanell J, Codony J, Rovira A, Mellado B, Gascón P. Mechanism of action of anti-HER2 monoclonal antibodies: Scientific update on trastuzumab and 2C4. Advances in Experimental Medicine and Biology. 2003;**532**:253-268. DOI: 10.1007/978-1-4615-0081-0_21

[44] Pacaud M, Hervé-Aubert K, Soucé M, Makki AA, Bonnier F, Fahmi A, et al. One-step synthesis of gold nanoflowers of tunable size and absorption wavelength in the red & deep red range for SERS spectroscopy. Spectrochimica Acta Part A: Molecular and Biomolecular Spectroscopy. 2020;**225**:117502. DOI: 10.1016/j.saa.2019.117502

[45] Chen J, Fan T, Xie Z, Zeng Q, Xue P, Zheng T, et al. Advances in nanomaterials for photodynamic therapy applications: Status and challenges. Biomaterials. Apr 2020;**237**:119827. DOI: 10.1016/j.biomaterials.2020.119827

[46] Pellas V, Hu D, Mazouzi Y, Mimoun Y, Blanchard J, Guibert C, et al. Gold nanorods for LSPR biosensing: Synthesis, coating by silica, and bioanalytical applications. Biosensors (Basel). 17 Oct 2020;**10**(10):146. DOI: 10.3390/bios10100146

[47] Zhang Z, Wang H, Chen Z, Wang X, Choo J, Chen L. Plasmonic colorimetric sensors based on etching and growth of noble metal nanoparticles: Strategies and applications. Biosensors & Bioelectronics. 2018;**114**:52-65. DOI: 10.1016/j.bios.2018.05.015

[48] Chow TH, Li N, Bai X, Zhuo X, Shao L, Wang J. Gold nanobipyramids: An emerging and versatile type of plasmonic nanoparticles. Accounts of Chemical Research. 2019;**52**(8):2136-2146. DOI: 10.3390/ijms222111411

[49] Tian EK, Wang Y, Ren R, Zheng W, Liao W. Gold nanoparticle: Recent progress on its antibacterial applications and mechanisms. Journal of Nanomaterials. 2021;**2021**:2501345. DOI: 10.1155/2021/2501345

[50] Maliszewska I, Wanarska E, Thompson AC, Samuel IDW, Matczyszyn K. Biogenic gold nanoparticles decrease methylene

blue photobleaching and enhance antimicrobial photodynamic therapy. Molecules. 2021;**26**(3):623. DOI: 10.3390/molecules26030623

[51] Silvestre ALP, Di Filippo LD, Besegato JF, de Annunzio SR, Furquim A, de Camargo B, et al. Current applications of drug delivery nanosystems associated with antimicrobial photodynamic therapy for oral infections. International Journal of Pharmaceutics. 2021;**592**:120078. DOI: 10.1016/j.ijpharm.2020.120078

[52] Mesquita MQ, Dias CJ, Neves MGPMS, Almeida A, Faustino MAF. Revisiting current photoactive materials for antimicrobial photodynamic therapy. Molecules. 21 Sep 2018;**23**(10):2424. DOI: 10.3390/molecules23102424

[53] Thakur NS, Bhaumik J, Kirar S, Banerjee UC. Development of gold-based phototheranostic nanoagents through a bioinspired route and their applications in photodynamic therapy. ACS Sustainable Chemistry & Engineering. 2017;**5**(9):7950-7960. DOI: 10.1021/acssuschemeng.7b01501

[54] Zhang Y, Zhang C, Xu C, Wang X, Liu C, Waterhouse GIN, et al. Ultrasmall Au nanoclusters for biomedical and biosensing applications: A mini-review. Talanta. 2019;**200**:432-442. DOI: 10.1016/j.talanta.2019.03.068

[55] Yang TQ, Peng B, Shan BQ, Zong YX, Jiang JG, Wu P, et al. Origin of the photoluminescence of metal nanoclusters: From metal-centered emission to ligand-centered emission. Nanomaterials. 2020;**10**(2). DOI: 10.3390/nano10020261

[56] Zare I, Chevrier DM, Cifuentes-Rius A, Moradi N, Xianyu Y, Ghosh S, et al. Protein-protected metal nanoclusters as diagnostic and therapeutic platforms for biomedical applications. Materials Today. 19 Feb 2021;**35**:1-35. DOI: 10.1016/j.mattod.2020.10.027

[57] Yang Y, Zhou Y, Wang S, Wang X, Liu X, Xie A, et al. A structurally precise Ag: XAu25-xnanocluster based cancer theranostic platform with tri-targeting/in situ O2-generation/aggregation enhanced fluorescence imaging/photothermal-photodynamic therapies. Chemical Communications. 2020;**56**(68):9842-9845. DOI: 10.1039/x0xx00000x

[58] Li Z, Fu Q, Ye J, Ge X, Wang J, Song J, et al. Ag+-coupled black phosphorus vesicles with emerging NIR-II photoacoustic imaging performance for cancer immune-dynamic therapy and fast wound healing. Angewandte Chemie International Edition. 2020;**59**(49):22202-22209. DOI: 10.1002/anie.202009609

[59] Yin R, Agrawal T, Khan U, Gupta GK, Rai V, Huang YY, et al. Antimicrobial photodynamic inactivation in nanomedicine: Small light strides against bad bugs. Nanomedicine. 2015;**10**(15):2379404. DOI: 10.2217/nnm.15.67

[60] Chen J, Yang L, Chen J, Liu W, Zhang D, Xu P, et al. Composite of silver nanoparticles and photosensitizer leads to mutual enhancement of antimicrobial efficacy and promotes wound healing. Chemical Engineering Journal. 2019;**374**:1373-1381. DOI: 10.1016/j.cej.2019.05.184

[61] Ahmadov TO, Ding R, Zhang J, Wang P, Tang H, Zhang P. Silver nanoparticle-enhanced hybrid photosensitizer for photoinactivation of multidrug-resistant: *Staphylococcus aureus* (MRSA). RSC Advances. 2016;**6**(59):54318-54321. DOI: 10.1039/c6ra11072j

[62] Wu S, Wei X, Li H, Shen H, Han J, Kang X, et al. Ligand effects on intramolecular configuration, intermolecular packing, and optical properties of metal nanoclusters. Nanomaterials (Basel). 9 Oct 2021;**11**(10):2655. DOI: 10.3390/nano11102655

[63] Yang J, Jin R. Advances in enhancing luminescence of atomically precise Ag nanoclusters. Journal of Physical Chemistry C. 2021;**125**(4):2619-2625. DOI: 10.1021/acs.jpcc.0c08693

[64] Tang J, Shi H, Ma G, Luo L, Tang Z. Ultrasmall Au and Ag nanoclusters for biomedical applications: A review. Frontiers in Bioengineering and Biotechnology. 2020;**8**:1-12. DOI: 10.3389/fbioe.2020.01019

[65] Sahu DK, Sarkar P, Singha D, Sahu K. Protein-activated transformation of silver nanoparticles into blue and red-emitting nanoclusters. RSC Advances. 2019;**9**(67):39405-39409. DOI: 10.1039/c9ra06774d

[66] Javani S, Lorca R, Latorre A, Flors C, Cortajarena AL, Somoza Á. Antibacterial activity of DNA-stabilized silver nanoclusters tuned by oligonucleotide sequence. ACS Applied Materials & Interfaces. 2016;**8**(16):10147-10154. DOI: 10.1021/acsami.6b00670

[67] Rolband L, Yourston L, Chandler M, Beasock D, Danai L, Kozlov S, et al. DNA-templated fluorescent silver nanoclusters inhibit bacterial growth while being non-toxic to mammalian cells. Molecules. 2021;**26**(13):1-14. DOI: 10.3390/molecules26134045

[68] Falk-Mahapatra R, Gollnick SO. Photodynamic Therapy and Immunity: An Update. Photochem Photobiol. May 2020;**96**(3):550-559. DOI: 10.1111/php.13253

[69] Wachowska M, Muchowicz A, Demkow U. Immunological aspects of antitumor photodynamic therapy outcome. Central-European Journal of Immunology. 2015;**40**(4):481-485. DOI: 10.5114/ceji.2015.56974

Chapter 4

Development of Liquisolid Compacts: An Approach for Dissolution Enhancement of Poorly Aqueous Soluble Drugs

Madhavi Kasturi

Abstract

Solubility plays a key role to achieve desired concentration of drug in systemic circulation and show its pharmacological action. An approach of liquisolid technique, developed by Spireas, was employed for the dissolution enhancement of poorly aqueous soluble drugs. Initially, liquid medication (liquid drug or drug solution or suspension in hydrophilic liquid vehicle) is transformed to free-flowing, non-sticky, compressible powder by the addition of suitable carrier material and coating materials for the development of liquisolid compacts. The postulated mechanism for enhanced solubility was improved wettability of drug and enhanced surface area of molecularly dispersed drug in the liquid environment. Pre- and post-the compression tests were performed for the developed liquisolid compacts to obtain optimized formulation. For the optimized compacts, FTIR and DSC studies were performed for determining drug-excipient compatibility; SEM and PXRD studies were performed to study the solid-state characterization. Furthermore, accelerated stability studies were performed for optimized liquisolid compacts for 6 months according to ICH guidelines and the results were compared with freshly prepared formulations. In conclusion, liquisolid compact formulation was proved to be safe, economic and alternative approach to formulate solid oral dosage forms of poorly aqueous soluble drugs.

Keywords: solubility enhancement, carrier material, coating material, flowable liquid retention potential, liquisolid compacts

1. Introduction

Oral route is considered as the easiest, convenient and most frequently preferred route for the administration of pharmaceutical dosage forms. Drug solubility is the most important key factor to achieve desired concentration of drug in the systemic circulation and show its pharmaceutical action. The poor dissolution properties of non-aqueous soluble drugs possess major challenge for researchers in pharmaceutical field in the course of development of solid dosage forms intended for oral administration. The development of several methods during the past few years includes the application of pro-drug and drug derivatization processes, micronization, co-precipitation, salt formation, solid dispersions, inclusion complex formation, lyophilization, micro-encapsulation, incorporation of drug solutions into soft gelatin capsules, self-emulsifying drug delivery systems, etc. In order to increase drug dissolution rate profiles, powder solutions are also designed that contain liquid medications in powdered form.

The rate of oral absorption is frequently regulated by the rate of dissolution in the GIT, in case of Biopharmaceutical Classification Class II drugs (low soluble and high permeable drugs). Therefore, solubility and dissolution rate characteristics of drugs are most important determinants of their oral bioavailability, together with permeation [1]. Hence, the notion of powdered solutions enables the creation of moderately flowing powders from liquid medications or drug solutions obtained by admixing drug solutions or liquid pharmaceuticals with selected powder excipient. Similar methods have been employed by certain researchers to improve the drug release patterns of numerous water-insoluble medicines.

The most recent, modern solubility enhancement approach known as liquisolid (LS) technique or "Powder Solution Technology" introduced by Spireas and Bolton, has been employed to develop rapid release solid dosage forms for water-insoluble or poorly water-soluble drugs [2]. The powdered forms of liquid medications produced via liquisolid process are thought to flow smoothly and also possess compressible nature. The liquid medication can be turned into dry (moistureless), non-sticky powder that can be easily flowable and compressible by simple mixing with chosen carriers, coating excipients [3]. In this method, the medication is dissolved in solvent followed by admixing with powder excipients and administered as solid dosage form. In this instance, the medication has been entirely molecularly distributed. As a result, insoluble or poorly water-soluble pharmaceuticals are anticipated to have improved dissolution rate characteristics and, consequently, higher bioavailability due to notably improved wetting capabilities and increased drug surface area accessible for dissolution.

2. Liquisolid technology

In order to create a "liquisolid powder system," a non-volatile solvent is first used to prepare either a lipophilic liquid medication or a drug solution/suspension of a water-insoluble or poorly aqueous soluble drug. This substance is referred to as "liquid medication." Additionally, it is transformed into easily compressible and freely flowing powders by mixing with excipients such carrier and coating ingredients. Liquid medication is combined with a carrier material (Avicel PH 102) having good absorption properties and coating material (Aerosil 200) having high adsorptive properties to obtain non-sticky, free-flowing readily compressible powder. It is further mixed with disintegrants to form immediate release compacts. The liquisolid (LS) powder can be further transformed to conventional solid dosage forms in which they can be compressed to compacts or encapsulated into hard gelatin capsules. The compacts so obtained are termed as liquisolid compacts (LSCs). Increased solubility, wettability, and drug surface area accessible for dissolution from the LSCs are thought to be the causes of the increased drug release rates [4]. However, the features of the medication and the different excipients employed in the formulation play a major role in determining the drug release profile. Therefore, using the LS approach, formulations that may either accelerate or delay the release of the medicine can be created by changing any one of these excipients. The novelty of the current study is application of liquisolid technique for the preparation of drug loaded tablets known as liquisolid compacts, which showed higher drug release profiles compared to that of directly compressed tablets, especially in case of poorly aqueous soluble drugs.

2.1 Constitution of LS formulation

The LS formulations contain some key constituents such as

i. Lipid liquid drug, solution or suspension of drug in hydrophilic vehicle,

ii. carrier excipient, and

iii. coating excipient

2.1.1 Non-volatile solvent

The non-volatile solvents should be able to solubilize the lipidic drug to the greatest extent, be inert, have a high boiling point, be water-miscible by nature, and not be excessively viscous. In the LS formulation, these hydrophilic solvents serve as a binding agent. Propylene glycol (PG), polysorbate 80, and polyethylene glycol (PEG) are a few examples of hydrophilic non-volatile solvents that are employed in LS formulations [5].

2.1.2 Carrier materials

The majority of liquid absorption is facilitated by carrier materials, which are typically porous materials with great absorption capabilities. These can maintain appropriate flow and compression properties while containing only a limited or fixed volume of solvent. However, an excessive rise in the carrier material's moisture content causes a deterioration in the powder flow properties. Various MCC grades, such as Avicel PH 101, PH 102, and PH 200, are examples of carrier materials [6].

2.1.3 Coating materials

The coating materials should have tiny, highly adsorbent particles that help to cover the wet surface of the carrier particles and retain the powder's flowability. Finally, complete adsorption of surplus liquid results in non-adherent, dry-looking powder. It is necessary to coat the surface with coating ingredients such as lactose, starch, syloid, aerosil 200, and silica (Cab-O-Sil M520) [2]. In addition to these, new coating materials with high adsorbent qualities as Sylysia (amorphous silica gel) and Neusilin (magnesium aluminum metasilicate) can also be employed.

2.1.4 Additives

It appears that the release of the drug is influenced by the process of disintegration of solid dosage forms. Therefore, disintegrants are typically added to LSCs to enable rapid disintegration. Examples of super disintegrants are low substituted hydroxypropyl cellulose (HPC), cross carmellose sodium, starch glycolate sodium, and crosspovidone [7]. In some instances, LS systems that typically function as a release retarding agent are supplemented with an additive called HPMC in order to

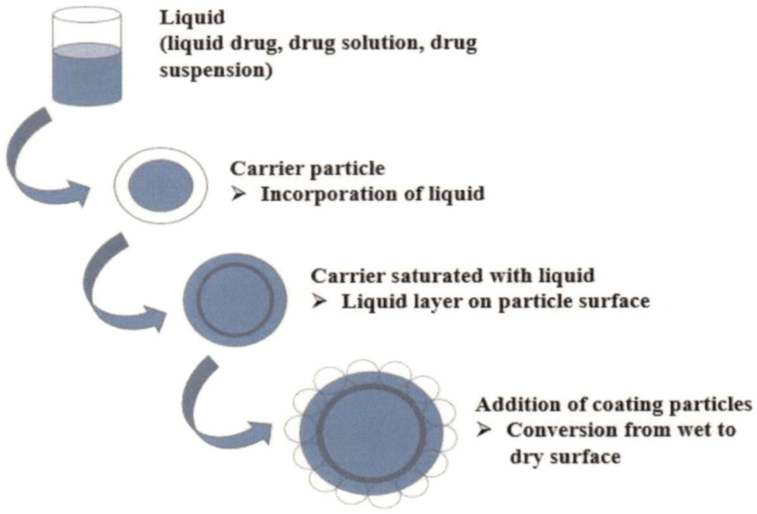

Figure 1.
Diagrammatic representation of formation of LS system.

prolong medication release [8]. **Figure 1** depicts the diagrammatic picture of the creation of the LS system.

2.2 Various forms of LS systems

1. Based on the type of liquid medication, the LS systems are divided into four categories.

    a. Powdered liquid drugs

    b. Powdered drug solutions

    c. Powdered drug emulsions

    d. Powdered drug suspensions

2. Based on the formulation technique used, two different types of LS systems are identified.

    a. LS compacts

    b. LS microsystems

The two main formulation elements of LSCs are liquid medicine and powder substrate. The major components of the powder substrate are: (a) carrier particles that are preferably big and porous to improve compression; (b) coating material particles that are ideally very fine and highly adsorptive to improve flow.

The schematic representation of various steps involved in preparation of LS formulations is shown in **Figure 2**.

DOI: http://dx.doi.org/10.5772/intechopen.108706

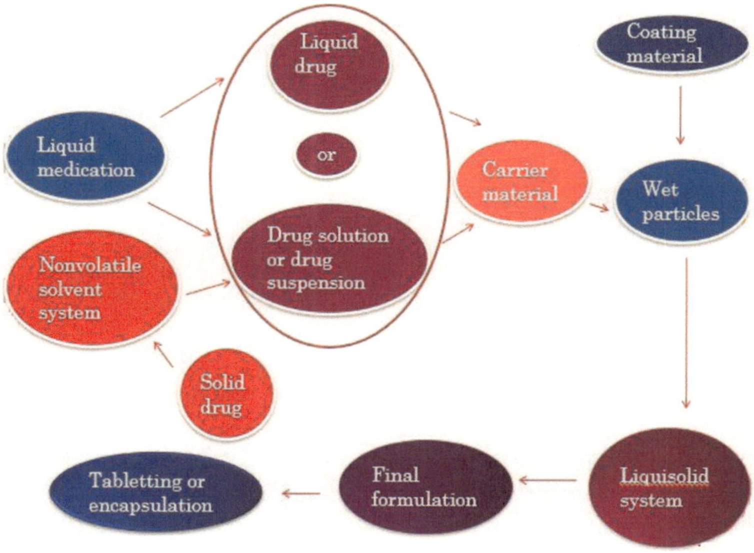

Figure 2.
Representation of several stages involved in development of LS formulations.

The amounts of various excipients required for the formulation of powder solutions are predicted using a novel mathematical model expression [9]. The absorbate molecules diffuse through the absorbent until they are eventually consumed by the powder particles inside their bulk, which causes the liquid to be absorbed. Adsorption is the phenomena where liquid is not really absorbed and the molecules merely cling to the solid's accessible surface, both internal and external, rather than being disseminated throughout the solid's interior. However, sorption is a mechanism where simultaneous occurrence of both of these processes occur which majorly depends on powder characteristics.

2.3 Mechanisms for enhanced drug release in LS systems

The mechanisms for enhanced drug release in LS systems include.

a. enhanced drug surface area

b. enhanced aqueous solubility

c. enhanced wettability

2.3.1 Enhanced drug surface area

Even if the drug particles are totally dissolved in the preferred hydrophilic non-volatile solvent in the LS system, the drug is still present in the powder substrate, either in molecularly distributed or completely solubilized state. As a result, when compared to directly compacted tablets (DCTs), the surface area of the drug in LS systems is substantially higher. However, when the drug content rises, the solubility limit rises with it. Hence, as the amount of undissolved drug in the liquid carrier increased, the rate of drug release decreased. Furthermore, the rate of drug release increases along with the proportion of molecularly dispersed drug (FM). Spireas' percentage of the molecularly dispersed drug is the ratio of drug solubility (Sd) in the liquid vehicle to the genuine drug concentration (Cd) in the liquid vehicle transported by each system (FM). It can be calculated using Eq. (1).

$$\mathrm{FM} = \frac{\mathrm{Sd}}{\mathrm{Cd}} \tag{1}$$

where, FM is equal to 1, in case if $S_d \geq C_d$.

2.3.2 Enhanced aqueous/water solubility of drug

A small volume of liquid vehicle in the LS formulation may not be sufficient in the case of the LS system to entirely solubilize the medication and increase drug solubility in dissolution medium. The solvent diffusing out of an LS particle is sufficient to increase the solubility of poorly aqueous soluble drugs in the dissolution medium at the interface microenvironment of the solid particle and liquid carrier, which is the most likely explanation for the increase in aqueous solubility of poorly aqueous soluble drugs [2]. It's also feasible that a small amount of the liquid carrier diffuses with the medication from the total amount, acting as a co-solvent to boost the drug's solubility in water.

2.3.3 Enhanced wetting properties

In the instance of the LS system, the wetting property is explained by measuring the contact angles as well as the water rising times. By lowering the interfacial tension between the powder/tablet surface and the dissolution medium, a non-volatile liquid vehicle aids in the wetting of drug particles in the system. The low contact angle of LSCs compared to conventional tablets proves improved wettability. The wettability of the LS system is improved by lowering the interfacial tension when the liquid vehicle acts as a surfactant. Water growing times and contact angles were used to demonstrate the wettability of the LS system.

By measuring the contact angles and the water rising times in the case of the LS system, the wetting property is described. A non-volatile liquid vehicle facilitates the wetting of drug particles in the system by reducing the interfacial tension between the surface of the powder or tablet and the dissolving media. The superior wettable quality of LSCs is demonstrated by their low contact angle when compared to traditional tablets. When the liquid vehicle functions as a surfactant, the interfacial tension is reduced, which enhances the wettability of the LS system. Water growth times and contact angles were employed to demonstrate the wettability of the LS system.

2.4 Parameters affecting LS formulations

2.4.1 Basis of selection of excipients in LS technology

The LS technology majorly deals with the selection of suitable carrier and coating materials that are mainly responsible for loading of drug in the liquid medication. This may be liquid drug or suspension of drug in a solvent or a solution of drug in suitable liquid (non-volatile) vehicle. This is further adsorbed on the porous carrier material.

A liquid layer starts forming on the surface of the particles, when once the carrier material is saturated with liquid, a moist or sticky blend is formed [10]. Dry and free flowing and compressible powder is obtained upon addition of dry coating material that physically exists in a very fine powder, instantly adsorbs fine layer of drug solution over the carrier material. Various forms of microcrystalline cellulose (such as MCC, Avicel PH101, Avicel PH102) are used as carrier materials and mostly amorphous silicon dioxide is used as coating material. Application of LS technique to poorly aqueous soluble drug enhances the drug release due to increased surface area of the drug, that in turn lead to increased solubility and improved wettability of the drug particles. The LS technology may also be applied to prolong the drug release. According to the principle, sustained release or extended release dosage forms provide desirable therapeutic plasma levels which are maintained throughout the therapy. It has been stated that usage of hydrophobic carriers like Eudragit® RL and RS instead of hydrophilic carriers or by addition of a matrix forming polymers like HPMC, sustained release formulations are developed. It was observed that the enhancement in solubility or release characteristics has been successfully improved in case of low dose poorly water-soluble drugs by the application of LS technology. The drug release rate is exactly proportional to the percentage of molecularly (FM) dispersed drug in the liquid vehicle, according to the main concept of LS technology [11].

It is obvious that only a definite amount of powder can absorb or absorb a limited volume of non-volatile solvent to preserve acceptable flow and compression properties. Hence, high amounts of carrier and coating materials are required in case of large volume of liquid medication if high dose drug is used. This result in increase in weight of the tablet eventually leads to formation of bulky tablet. Hence it is required to minimize tablet weight and increase the liquid adsorption capacity. By adding carrier and coating materials or binding agents to the liquid medication with a high specific surface area (SSA) liquid adsorption capacity is obtained. Therefore, higher the SSA of the carrier material, higher will be the liquid load factor. It has been stated that the liquid adsorption capacity of the granular cellulose that is experimental grade exhibits SSA of 24.22 m^2/g which is higher than that of microcrystalline cellulose (MCC). Similarly, carrier materials such as Avicel PH102(SSA = 1.10 m^2/g) and Avicel PH 101 (SSA = 1.07 m^2/g) have been frequently used in the studies due to their higher SSA values. Moreover, it has to be highlighted that the physicochemical characteristics such as viscosity, polarity, lipophilicity and chemical structure of the liquid used for solubilizing or suspending the drug cannot be ignored which could also affect the adsorption capacity of both the carrier and coating materials. Subsequently, the liquid adsorption capacity of a blend of carrier and coating material not only depends on their SSA, but also depends on the liquid vehicle involved.

2.4.2 Ratio of carrier and coating material (R) importance

The pre-compression properties and drug release characteristics of LS systems increase from 5 to 1 to 50 to 1 for excipient ratios denoted by R. The reciprocal of the powder excipient ratios (1/R) and the liquid load factors (Lf) have a linear connection. The powder excipients ratio R affects the dissolving rate profiles of LS systems, with results visible within 5 minutes of the dissolution process against R values in the 5 to 20 range. At powder excipients ratios >20, the dissolving rates have risen proportionally to R until they reached an obvious maximum plateau. Lower R values should indicate medication dissolution patterns that are less than ideal. Increases in R excipient ratios cause a modest drop-in dissolution rate until the maximum degree of dissolution is attained at R values of 35 to 45. The R values greater than 50 indicate that the drug solution was embedded during the formulation process.

Carrier agents are usually able to absorb the solvent in their interiors of matrices. The production of dry-looking, non-sticky liquid pharmaceuticals necessitates large quantities of these carriers. Due to its huge specific area in comparison to other carriers such as lactose and starch, Avicel PH 102 outperformed the others [12]. As a result, the unit size of LS tablets may vary depending on the composition of the carrier material. The more uniformly the drug is adsorbed on the coated material or absorbed into the carrier material, the higher the concentration of Avicel PH 102. The strength and cohesiveness of the LSCs are provided by the H-bonds on the cellulose molecules in Avicel PH 102. Compression transforms them plastically, creating a potent compact [13].

A surface-active substance called polysorbate 80 aids in drug particle wetting by lowering the interfacial tension between the LSC surface and the dissolving solution. As a result, it has been discovered that one of the primary explanations for an increase in dissolving rate is an increase in the wetting qualities of LSCs created by the dissolution media. More uniform drug distribution in the carrier medium was indicated by higher R values, which ranged from 30 to 60 [14].

2.5 Advantages and limitations of LS technique

2.5.1 Advantages of LS technique

1. Maximum drugs belonging to BCS class II can be formulated into LS systems.

2. Improved dissolution profiles (in vitro and in vivo drug release) and enhanced bioavailability for LS formulations can be achieved when compared to conventional dosage forms.

3. Cost-effective method, since the production costs are lower than those of soft gelatin capsules.

4. Formulation of drug either in a tablet dosage form or encapsulated dosage form is possible.

5. Greater surface area of drug will come in contact with the dissolution medium.

6. The LS systems can be developed as immediate release or sustained release dosage forms.

7. In case of optimized sustained release for water insoluble drugs, LS tablets and capsules show constant dissolution rates with zero order release kinetics equivalent to osmotic pump technology and laser-drilled tablets.

8. It is also used in the development of controlled drug delivery systems.

9. The release of drug can be altered using suitable excipients or additives in the LS formulation.

10. The drug is available in molecularly dispersed state in the formulation.

11. The LS formulations can also be produced in industrial scale.

12. Color can be added into liquid vehicle for achieving uniqueness of final product.

13. Lesser excipients can be used in LS formulations when compared to other formulations like solid dispersions.

14. This technique omits the process approaches such as nanonisation, micronization techniques.

15. A number of poorly water-soluble and nearly water-insoluble drugs (ex-Digitoxin, Hydrocortisone, Prednisolone) are formed into LS systems using the new formulation-mathematical model.

16. Because the drug is present in solution form, better availability is attained when a poorly water- soluble agent is orally delivered.

17. The LS powder system available in solubilized liquid state causes increase in wetting nature of drug which further increases dissolution of drug.

2.5.2 Limitations of LS technique

1. One of the major problems with this technique is formulation of high dose lipophilic drugs into LS tablets and hence it is not applicable for the formulation of insoluble drugs with high dose. The technology has been shown successful and employed for low dose water-insoluble medications.

2. High amounts of carrier and coating materials are required to maintain acceptable flowability and compatibility for LS powder formulation. Since these drugs require large quantities of liquid vehicle which increases tablet weight above 1gm which makes them difficult to swallow. On the other hand, using traditional tablet procedures, it is difficult to convert a high dose tablet to a low-dose tablet with a weight of less than 50 mg. Several techniques have been proposed to overcome the problem mentioned above.

For example, adding some of the additives like PVP and PEG 35000, to the liquid medications ultimately increase the viscosity of liquid medication and further may decrease the quantity of carrier and coating material used in formulation development. Modern carrier and coating materials like Neusilin and Fujicalin also have greater specific surface areas (SSA), which results in increased absorption capacities.

1. This technique is only applicable for water insoluble, poorly water soluble and lipophilic drugs.

2. These LS systems require maximum solubility of drug in the hydrophilic non-volatile solvents. It was obvious that acceptable compression properties may not be achieved since during the compression process, there may be chance that liquid drug squeeze out of the LS tablet consequential in tablets of unsatisfactory hardness.

3. It needs more efficient excipients with higher adsorption capacities a smaller tablet size to improve LS formulations.

4. High solubility of the drug in liquid vehicle is prerequisite to prepare liquid solid systems [15].

5. This method of dispersing large amounts of carrier material with small amounts of viscous liquid solutions may not be feasible on large industrial scale.

2.6 Applications of LS technique

2.6.1 Dissolution and solubility enhancement

To overcome the limited solubility of drugs in pharmaceutical area, these are formulated as LS tablets. Basically, the method of preparation of LS tablets and the effect of various formulation and processing variables on the preparation and release properties of LS tablets are studied. This technique is proved and successfully applied for low dose drugs up to 50 mg only. In case of LS tablet, formulation of high dose water insoluble drugs is a limitation. Furthermore, by adding materials like PVP to liquid medications, only a small amount of carrier is needed to generate a dry powder with good flow ability and compatibility.

2.6.2 Flowability and compressibility

LSCs possess acceptable flowability as well as compressibility properties. They are prepared by mixing or simple blending with selected powder excipients such as the carrier material (ex. cellulose, lactose, starch) and the coating materials (ex. silica). In such LS powder systems, the drug exists in form of molecular state of subdivision. These LS systems were also free flowing, non-adherent and dry looking powders. Microcrystalline cellulose (compression enhancer) can be used in the LS problem of 'Liquid Squeezing Out' phenomenon whenever observed. Hence, in this system liquid medication is admixed with the excipients and then compressed into tablets. It was also showed that, lesser the drug concentration in the liquid medication, rapid is the release rates. If the drugs are present in high concentration in LS system, they tend to precipitate within the polymers pores.

2.6.3 Designing of sustained release tablet

Several ways have been explored to achieve this goal, including coating with specific materials, preparing a salt variant of the drug, and incorporating drugs into hydrophobic carriers. Hydrophobic carriers like Eudragit RL and RS are used to develop sustained release LS systems. The LS formulations can give both rapid release and sustained release of drugs. Sustained release propranolol hydrochloride (water soluble) by the use of LSC technique was developed [6]. LS method can also be employed to design controlled release of tablets.

2.6.4 Bioavailability improvement

In the solid powdered solution and LS systems drug is present in solution form or almost molecularly dispersed state. As a result of the large increase in wetting properties, the surface area of drug accessible for dissolution, the LSCs of non-aqueous soluble substances are expected to have better drug release properties. As a result, bioavailability is enhanced.

2.7 LSCs formulation development

LSCs are the compressible pulverized forms of the liquid medications containing drugs. These are prepared as a result of compression of LS powder systems containing lipophilic drug, carrier and coating materials.

2.7.1 Formulation design for LSCs

While developing the LSC formulations the following components should be incorporated.

Non-Volatile solvents: Poly Ethylene Glycol (PEG)-200. PEG- 400, PEG- 6000, PEG- 4000, Propylene Glycol (PG), Polysorbate80, Tween–80 etc. Addition of PVP to liquid medication, may lead to production of dry powder formulations comprising liquid with a high drug concentration.

Carriers: Avicel RTM 105, Avicel PH 102 granular Microcrystalline cellulose (MCC) grade, Avicel PH 200 coarse granular MCC grade, lactose and starch. MCC has granular grades with fine particle sizes, which results in good compression capabilities for tablet manufacture.

Super Disintegrates: Sodium starch glycolate (SSG), Crospovidone, croscarmellose sodium (CCS).

Coating Materials: Aerosil PH 200, Colloidal silica, Cab-O-sil RTM M5, Sylysia (amorphous silica gel) and Neusilin (magnesium aluminum metasilicate).

Initially, the saturation solubility studies for drug will be performed in various hydrophilic solvents such as polyethylene glycols (PEG 200, PEG 400, PEG 600); propylene glycol (PG); Span 80; glycerine; Tween 80; Span 20; Tween 20; etc. Saturated drug solutions were obtained by addition of excess drug to each 5 ml solvent taken in screw cap vials. After sealing, the vials were kept on rotary shaker under constant vibration at 25°C and shaken for about 72 hrs. Afterwards, sample aliquots were taken and further filtered. Later, filtrate was diluted appropriately with distilled water and drug content was analyzed using UV–VIS spectrophotometer. The liquid vehicle showing maximum solubility for drug was finally selected as solvent to prepare liquid medication which is further transformed to liquisolid compacts by the addition of excipients.

2.7.2 New mathematical paradigm for LS system design

Spireas [2] developed a novel mathematical model to formulate LSCs with good flow and compressibility properties. The basic building blocks for creating this formulation are a suitable drug, a non-volatile solvent of choice with the highest solubility for the drug, a suitable carrier material with acceptable absorption, and a coating material with good adsorption properties. The new fundamental features of powder systems known as flowable liquid retention potential and compressible liquid retention potential of the powdered excipients included in the formulation serve as the foundation for this model.

The ϕ value can be explained as the extreme amount of liquid that can be held in unit volume of carrier material while still maintaining acceptable flow characteristics following admixing.

The ψ value can be explained as the extreme amount of liquid that can be held in unit volume of carrier material while still maintaining compression property following admixture [16].

The excipients ratio (R) or the ratio of carrier: coating material is given by the Eq. (2)

$$R = Q/q \tag{2}$$

where,

R is ratio of carrier material to coating material, Q is carrier material and q is coating material.

For successful LS formulation design, the ratio R should be properly selected.

Liquid load factor (Lf) is defined as the ratio of amount of liquid medication to that of carrier in the LS powder system having acceptable appropriate properties and is given by the Eq. (3).

$$Lf = W/Q \tag{3}$$

Where, W is the amount of liquid medication and Q is amount of carrier material.

The Lf value was calculated from the below Eq. (4).

$$Lf = \phi + \phi(1/R) \tag{4}$$

Where, ϕ is flowable liquid retention potential value for carrier material and ϕ is flowable liquid retention potential value coating materials, respectively.

As a result, Lf value was initially derived using Eq. (4) for the purpose of developing LS system, using R value as a predetermined fixed value. Then, W can be calculated further as it is the weight of liquid medication (combined weight of drug and non-volatile solvent). Given that W and Lf values are known, Q (quantity of carrier) can be computed using Eq. (3). So, using the Eq. (2), it is possible to calculate the amount of q (amount of coating material) after knowing the values of Q and W.

2.7.3 Determination of angle of slide

The flowable nature of prepared LS powder can be assessed by specific parameter known as Angle of slide (θ). Powder flowability is considered an important factor as it plays a crucial role in pharmaceutical industries.

Uniformly prepared powder/solvent blends containing 10 grams of carrier or coating material with increasing amounts of solvent were prepared. Further, it is placed at one edge of metal plate containing smooth surface and tilted slowly till the admixture starts to slide. The angle of slide (θ) was defined as the angle produced between the plate and the horizontal surface. The angle matching to 33° is regarded as optimal flow behavior for LS powder system [17].

2.7.4 Flowable liquid retention potential determination

The Φ value indicating flowable liquid retention potential can be determined from the angle of slide (θ) values. To 10 grams of carrier or coating powder gradually increasing quantity of liquid vehicle was added; then mixed using a mortar and pestle to attain powder admixtures. On one end of a smooth polished metal plate, the powder-solvent admixtures were positioned individually. Later, the plate was gradually raised until it made an angle with the horizontal planet, at which point the mixture began to slide. This obtained angle (θ) gives the angle of slide [18].

Using Eq. (5), the flowable liquid retention potentials for each solvent-powder admixtures can be calculated

$$\Phi \text{ value} = \text{weight of liquid vehicle/weight of carrier or coating material} \quad (5)$$

2.7.5 Compressible liquid retention potential (Ψ value)

The Compressible liquid retention potential (Ψ value) for each solid powder excipient with solvent is carried out by gradually adding liquid vehicle to 1 gm powder material till uniform admixture is obtained. Then this admixture was compressed in the rotary tablet machine to prepare a tablet. The crushing strength value obtained between 5 and 7 Kgf was considered as an acceptable one. During compression, leakage of liquid medicament from the powder admixture must not be observed [2].

2.7.6 Load factor calculation (Lf)

The quantity of liquid retained by the carrier agent and coating agent depends on the excipient ratio (R) to maintain adequate flowable and compressible properties. As per the LS powder system preparation, the maximum amount of solvent retained within carrier material should not be exceed a limit. This characteristic amount of liquid is named as liquid Lf. The weight of the liquid medicine (W) divided by the weight of the carrier powder (Q) in an LS powder system yields the liquid load factor, or Lf.

$$\text{Lf} = \text{W/Q}$$

Liquid load factor can be calculated by using Eq. (6) after determining Φ–values of carrier and coating agents.

$$\text{Lf } \Phi = \Phi_{\text{CA}} + \Phi_{\text{CO}}(1/\text{R}) \quad (6)$$

where, Φ_{CA} represents flowable liquid retention potential value for carrier agent and Φ_{CO} represents flowable liquid retention potential value for coating material.

R is the ratio of carrier (Q) weight to coating (q) weight present in the formulation. Eq. (6) is used to calculate load factor in LS formulations for obtaining acceptable flowability.

$$\text{Lf } \Psi = \Psi_{\text{CA}} + \Psi_{\text{CO}}(1/\text{R}) \quad (7)$$

Where, Ψ_{CA} and Ψ_{CO} represents compressible liquid retention potential values for carrier agent and coating agent respectively.

Eq. (7) is used to calculate load factor in LS formulations for obtaining acceptable compressibility [19].

Finally, suitable amounts of carrier and coating materials can be calculated using the above equations to produce acceptable flowing and compactible powders.

2.7.7 Preparation of drug loaded LSCs

LSCs were prepared according to the method described by Spireas and Bolton [2]. They were prepared by dispersing accurately weighed quantity of drug (50 mg) in non- volatile liquid vehicle showing maximum solubility for the drug. In a 20 mL glass beaker, a calculated quantity of drug equivalent to the dose is added to a calculated amount of vehicle and thoroughly mixed to generate liquid medication. Then a binary mixture was formulated comprising calculated amounts of carrier agent and coating agent; and continuously mixed for about 10 minutes in a mortar. The resulting liquid medication was mixed with binary mixture and blended in a porcelain mortar avoiding excessive trituration and particle size reduction.

The mixing process comprises of three stages as follows

1. Mixing the LS powder at a speed of 1 rotation/min for uniform distribution of liquid medication in powder blend containing carrier and coating material (binary mixture).

2. The LS powder should be applied in a homogeneous coating to the inner surface of mortar and left for 5 minutes to allow powder particles to absorb liquid medication.

3. Scrapping off LS powder off the surface of mortar using aluminum spatula.

Finally, super disintegrant was added to each batch and mixed for 30 sec, followed by addition of lubricant and mixed for 2 min. This resultant final LS powder formulation was compressed into LSCs using suitable punch in rotary tablet compression machine [20].

2.8 Characterization of drug loaded LSCs

The drug loaded LSCs are characterized in terms of both pre compression and post compression evaluation tests. The precompression evaluation tests include determination of powder flow properties for prepared LS powder systems. The flow properties of the LS powder system were characterized in terms of Tapped and Bulk density, Compressibility Index, Angle of repose and Hausner's ratio.

2.8.1 Angle of repose (θ) (funnel method)

It is measured by fixed funnel method. The powder blend is passed through funnel until apex of powder pile touches tip of the funnel. A rough circle is drawn around the base of the pile. The angle of repose is measured using Eq. (8)

$$\text{Tan}\ (\theta) = \text{height of powder (h) in cm/radius of powder (r) in cm} \qquad (8)$$

2.8.2 Bulk density

The bulk density is obtained by dividing mass of powder with its bulk volume. It was calculated using Eq. (9) in gm/ml.

$$\text{Bulk density} = \frac{\text{Weight of powder}}{\text{Bulk volume of powder}} \qquad (9)$$

2.8.3 Tapped density

It is measured by taking accurately weighed 10 g of powder blend into a 100 ml graduated measuring cylinder. The initial volume was determined. The cylinder was initially tapped for 200 times from a distance of 14 ± 2 mm. The tapping process was again repeated additionally for 200 times. Finally, the tapped volume was noted [12]. The tapped density was calculated using Eq. (10) the following formula in gm/ml.

$$\text{Tapped density} = \frac{\text{Weight of powder}}{\text{Tapped volume}} \tag{10}$$

2.8.4 Carr's index or compressibility index

Compressibility Index is calculated using Eq. (11) based on tapped and bulk densities which determines the ease of powder flow property.

$$\text{Compressibility index (\%)} = \frac{\text{Tapped Density–Bulk Density}}{\text{Tapped Density}} \times 100 \tag{11}$$

2.8.5 Hausner's ratio

The Hausner's ratio is the proportion of a powder tapped density to its bulk density. It is calculated using Eq. (12).

$$\text{Hausner's ratio} = \text{Tapped density/Bulk density} \tag{12}$$

Powders with Hausner's ratio 1 to 1.11, 1.12 to 1.18, 1.19 to 1.25, 1.26 to 1.34, 1.35 to 1.60 indicate free flowing, good, fair, passable, poor flow of powder respectively.

The post compression tests for the prepared LSC formulations were performed similar to that of tablets according to IP specifications [21].

2.8.6 Weight variation test

The weight of tablet is determined to ensure that tablet contains exact amount of drug. Around 20 LSCs from each formulation were selected randomly. They were weighed individually and the average weight was calculated using digital balance. The individual weights were then compared with that of average weight for each formulation batch. It is calculated using Eq. (13) the below formula,

$$\text{\%Deviation} = \frac{\text{(Individual weight of tablet–Average weight tablets)}}{\text{Average weight of tablets}} \times 100 \tag{13}$$

2.8.7 Hardness

It is also termed as crushing strength of tablet. It is measured using Monsanto hardness tester and was expressed in kg/cm^2. The LSC whose hardness to be tested was placed between the spindle and anvil of Monsanto hardness tester. The screw knob is moved clockwise and then pressure is applied that holds the tablet in position. The scale is moved in order that the indicator is fixed at zero. The pressure is applied continuously until tablet breaks. The reading is noted, that indicates the pressure required to break the tablet. The test is performed thrice and the mean value was determined.

2.8.8 Friability

It is used to measure the mechanical strength of tablets. The friability of prepared LSCs can be determined using Roche friabilator (Mumbai, India). Around, 10 LSCs from each batch were weighed and placed in the chamber of friabilator. The chamber is rotated at speed of 25 rpm for a period of 4 min (100 rotations). At the end of test, the tablets were then dusted, re-weighed collectively and the percentage weight loss (friability) was calculated [22]. It is measured using Eq. (14)

$$\%\text{friability} = \frac{\text{Initial weight} - \text{final weight}}{\text{Initial weight}} \text{x } 100 \quad (14)$$

2.8.9 Drug content uniformity

About 10 LSCs were randomly selected and crushed to powder in a mortar. The powder was weighed equivalent to unit dose of drug which was taken into 100 ml volumetric flask. Initially, 10 ml volume of methanol was added, followed by addition of buffer to make up final volume. The resulting solution was diluted, filtered and analyzed using spectrophotometer to determine the drug content [19].

2.8.10 Disintegration time

Disintegration time for LSC was performed by placing one tablet in each of the six tubes of the basket of USP Disintegration Tester (Electrolab, India) apparatus. Disc was placed above each tube and the apparatus was run using buffer solution as immersion medium. The apparatus is maintained at temperature of $37 \pm 2°C$. The assembly will be lifted up and down between 30 cycles/min. The time required for all the six tablets to disintegrate completely was noted as DT. The process is repeated thrice and the average disintegration time is determined [19].

2.8.11 In vitro drug release studies

The *in vitro* drug release profiles for LSCs were determined by means of Rotating Paddle, USP Type II dissolution test apparatus (Electrolab, Mumbai, India). The dissolution was performed in 900 ml of selected dissolution media (SGF or SIF) with paddle speed of 50 rpm. Aliquots of 5 ml samples were collected at predefined time intervals. To maintain constant volume and sink conditions, the dissolution medium was replaced with 5 ml of fresh medium. These samples were analyzed using UV–VIS spectrophotometer at λ_{max} of prepared drug. It is carried out in triplicates for each LSC batch and also compared with conventionally prepared directly compressed compacts containing an equivalent amount of drug for comparison [23].

2.9 Analysis of optimized LSCs

Based on the results of evaluation tests, one LSC formulation was optimized from the prepared batch and selected for further analytical characterization. This optimized drug loaded LSC was subjected to FTIR and DSC studies to determine presence of any possible interaction between drug and excipients. SEM studies were also performed to study surface morphology and XRD studies for determining the solid-state characterization.

2.9.1 Fourier-transform infrared spectroscopy (FTIR)

Drug-excipient interactions play crucial role in release of drug from the formulation and hence the compatibility studies were performed using FT-IR spectrophotometer. IR spectrum was determined for samples by FTIR-8400S spectrophotometer (Shimadzu, Japan) using KBr pellet method. In this method, 100 mg of dry KBr IR powder is carefully mixed with 5 mg of sample (drug or formulation). It is further compressed to transparent discs at a pressure of 12,000 psi under vacuum for about 3 min. The obtained disc was mounted in holder and the sample was scanned over a wave range of 4000 to 400 cm^{-1}, at a resolution of 4 cm^{-1} using FTIR spectrophotometer. FTIR was executed for both the pure drug and LS powders [24].

2.9.2 Differential scanning calorimetry (DSC)

DSC Thermograms of pure drug and the optimized LSC formulation for drug were recorded using the calibrated Shimadzu DSC-60 (Shimadzu, Kyoto, Japan) [19]. Samples of weight around 3 to 5 mg were weighed. They were placed in aluminum pans whose lids were crimped taking Shimadzu crimper. The samples were investigated over a scanning rate of 10°C/min to determine their thermal behavior, covering a wide temperature range of 30–200°C under nitrogen atmosphere. The DSC was calibrated using indium standard [25].

2.9.3 Powder X-ray diffraction (PXRD)

The crystalline nature pure drug as well as samples can be determined by Philips Analytical XRD using copper target. At room temperature, the operating voltage was 40 kV and current used was around 55 mA [26].

2.9.4 Scanning electron microscopy (SEM)

The surface morphology characteristics of pure drug as well as the drug–carrier systems or formulations were assessed using scanning electron microscopy. The external surface morphology of the LSCs were studied using a scanning electron microscope (Hitachi TM 1000, Tokyo, Japan). The samples were first adhered to aluminum stubs, gold-coated sputter with double sided conductive tape of 12 mm diameter, and examined in the scanning microscope [27].

2.10 Stability studies

Stability can be explained as the extent to which a product will retain its specified limits throughout the shelf life. The accelerated stability studies for optimized LSC formulation were performed according to ICH guidelines at temperature of 40 ± 2°C and relative humidity (RH) of 75% RH ± 5% for duration of 6 months in a stability chamber. USP Type I flint vials are used to place the selected optimized formulations. They are then hermetically closed using bromo butyl rubber plugs and further sealed with aluminum caps. The samples were taken at specific time periods and evaluated for post compression tests. These results of aged samples were compared with fresh (initial) samples kept at room temperature and similarity factor was determined [28].

3. Conclusion

The purpose of the present study was to investigate the effect of liquisolid technique in improving the dissolution profile of poorly aqueous soluble drugs mostly that belong to BCS Class II and Class IV. In this investigation, preformulation study i.e. saturation solubility was performed for drug in order to determine extent of its solubility in liquid vehicle, which forms basis for preparation of LSCs. However, solvent showing highest solubility for drug was selected as liquid vehicle for preparing liquid medication.

Further, liquisolid systems were formulated by the technique described and patented by Spireas et al. The liquisolid compacts were formulated with addition of carrier material (such as Avicel PH102) and coating material (such as Cab-O-Sil M5). During formulations the chemical compatibility between drug and excipients was checked and confirmed by FTIR study. The liquisolid preparations were initially characterized by precompression study for flowability and compressibility. The liquisolid powder systems were compressed to obtain liquisolid compacts which were further characterized for post compression tests such as hardness, content uniformity, disintegration and dissolution profiles. The stability studies were also conducted and the tablet properties like hardness, drug content, disintegration and dissolution profiles were compared for freshly prepared and aged tablets.

The drug loaded liquisolid formulations showed higher drug release profiles when compared with the conventional dosage forms for the same drug. Hence, this technique proved a substitute method to develop solid oral dosage forms for poorly water-soluble drugs. The method uses appropriate excipient ratios of biodegradable polymers which not only improve drug release but also sustain the drug release characteristics of the water-soluble drugs. Finally, it can be concluded that LS technology was effective for enhancing the dissolution behavior as well as the bioavailability of poorly water soluble or practically water insoluble drugs in presence of non-volatile solvents. Thus, liquisolid approach has potential application for formulation research in improvement of dissolution rate and hence proved to be a promising tool as well an alternative technique to enhance the dissolution profiles of very low aqueous soluble drugs.

Abbreviations

BCS	biopharmaceutics classification system
LS	liquisolid
LSC	liquidolid compacts
PEG	polyethylene glycols
PG	propylene glycol
MCC	microcrystalline cellulose
HPC	hydroxypropyl cellulose
PVP	polyvinylpyrrolidone
HPMC	hydroxypropyl methyl cellulose
SSA	specific surface area
FM	fraction of molecularly dispersed drug
Sd	drug solubility
Cd	drug concentration

Author details

Madhavi Kasturi
Department of Pharmaceutics, Smt. S.M. Shah Pharmacy College, Ahmedabad, Gujarat, India

*Address all correspondence to: madhavi2386@gmail.com

References

[1] Jamakandi VG. Formulation and evaluation of immediate release tablet of carvedilol using liquisolid compacts technique for solubility enhancement. Asian Journal of Pharmaceutics. 2016; **10**(03):S324-S332. DOI: 10.22377/ajp.v10i03.772

[2] Spireas SS, Jarowski CI, Rohera BD. Powdered solution technology: Principles and mechanism. Pharmaceutical Research. 1992;**9**(10):1351-1358. DOI: 10.1023/a:1015877905988

[3] Chandel P, Kumari R, Kapoor A. Liquisolid technique: An approach for enhancement of solubility. Journal of Drug Delivery and Therapeutics. 2013; **3**(4):131-137. DOI: 10.22270/jddt.v3i4.556

[4] Shinkar DM, Khatik AS, Saudagar RB. Liquisolid technology: A review. Asian Journal of Research in Pharmaceutical Science. 2016;**6**(3):161-166. DOI: 10.5958/2231-5659.2016.00022.9

[5] Kapure VJ, Pande VV, Deshmukh PK. Dissolution enhancement of rosuvastatin calcium by liquisolid compact technique. Journal of Pharmaceutics. 2013;**1**(1):1-9. DOI: 10.1155/2013/315902

[6] Jassim ZE. Formulation and evaluation of furosemide liquisolid compact. International Journal of Applied Pharmaceutics. 2017;**9**(6):39-48. DOI: 10.22159/ijap.2017v9i6.21458

[7] Javadzadeh Y, Siahi-Shadbad MR, Barzegar-Jalali M, Nokhodchi A. Enhancement of dissolution rate of piroxicam using liquisolid compacts. Il Farmaco. 2005;**60**(4):361-365. DOI: 10.1016/j.farmac.2004.09.005

[8] Lu M, Xing H, Jiang J, Chen X, Yang T, Wang D, et al. Liquisolid technique and its applications in pharmaceutics. Asian Journal of Pharmaceutical Sciences. 2017;**12**(2): 115-123. DOI: 10.1016/j.ajps.2016.09.007

[9] Liao CC, Jarowski CI. Dissolution rates of corticoid solutions dispersed on silicas. Journal of Pharmaceutical Sciences. 1984;**73**(3):401-403. DOI: 10.1002/jps.2600730330

[10] Sharma V, Pathak K. Attempts and outcomes of liquisolid technology: An updated chronological compilation of innovative ideas and adjuvants in the field. Pharmaceutical and Biomedical Research. 2016;**2**(4):1-21. DOI: 10.18869/acadpub.pbr.2.4.1

[11] Schlack H, Bauer-Brandl A, Schubert R, Becker D. Properties of Fujicalin, a new modified anhydrous dibasic calcium phosphate for direct compression: Comparison with dicalcium phosphate dihydrate. Drug Development and Industrial Pharmacy. 2001;**27**(8): 789-801. DOI: 10.1081/ddc-100107242

[12] Javadzadeh Y, Jafari-Navimipour B, Nokhodchi A. Liquisolid technique for dissolution rate enhancement of a high dose water-insoluble drug (carbamazepine). International Journal of Pharmaceutics. 2007;**341**(1–2):26-34. DOI: 10.1016/j.ijpharm.2007.03.034

[13] Fahmy RH, Kassem MA. Enhancement of famotidine dissolution rate through liquisolid tablets formulation: In vitro and in vivo evaluation. European Journal of Pharmaceutics and Biopharmaceutics. 2008;**69**(3):993-1003. DOI: 10.1016/j.ejpb.2008.02.017

[14] Tayel SA, Soliman II, Louis D. Improvement of dissolution properties of carbamazepine through application of

the liquisolid tablet technique. European Journal of Pharmaceutics and Biopharmaceutics. 2008;**69**(1):342-347. DOI: 10.1016/j.ejpb.2007.09.003

[15] Singh SK, Srinivasan KK, Gowthamarajan K, Prakash D, Gaikwad NB, Singare DS. Influence of formulation parameters on dissolution rate enhancement of glyburide using liquisolid technique. Drug Development and Industrial Pharmacy. 2012;**38**(8): 961-970. DOI: 10.3109/ 03639045.2011.634810

[16] Arun RR, Ahammed SAK, Jyoti H. Formulation and evaluation of liquisolid tablets of nifedipine. Rajiv Gandhi University of Health Sciences Journal of Pharmaceutical Sciences. 2013;**3**(4): 43-50. DOI: 10.5530/rjps.2013.4.6

[17] Karmarkar AB, Gonjari ID, Hosmani AH. Liquisolid technology for dissolution rate enhancement or sustained release. Expert Opinion on Drug Delivery. 2010;**7**(10): 1227-1234. DOI: 10.1517/ 17425247.2010.511173

[18] Akinlade B, Elkordy AA, Essa EA, Elhagar S. Liquisolid systems to improve the dissolution of furosemide. Scientia Pharmaceutica. 2010;**78**(2):325-344. DOI: 10.3797/scipharm.0912-23

[19] Jaydip B, Dhaval M, Soniwala MM, Chavda J. Formulation and optimization of liquisolid compact for enhancing dissolution properties of efavirenz by using DoE approach. Saudi Pharmaceutical Journal. 2020;**28**(6): 737-745. DOI: 10.1016/j.jsps.2020.04.016

[20] Tiong N, Elkordy AA. Effects of liquisolid formulations on dissolution of naproxen. European Journal of Pharmaceutics and Biopharmaceutics. 2009;**73**(3):373-384. DOI: 10.1016/ j.ejpb.2009.08.002

[21] Bi YX, Sunada H, Yonezawa Y, Danjo K. Evaluation of rapidly disintegrating tablets prepared by a direct compression method. Drug Development and Industrial Pharmacy. 1999;**25**(5):571-581. DOI: 10.1081/ ddc-100102211

[22] Srivastava S, Srivastava D, Nimisha PV. Liquisolid technique for enhancement of dissolution properties of lornoxicam. Indo Global Journal of Pharmaceutical Sciences. 2014;**4**(2): 81-90. DOI: 10.35652/IGJPS.2014.111

[23] Anil A, Thomas L, Sudheer P. Liquisolid compacts: An innovative approach for dissolution enhancement. International Journal of Pharmacy and Pharmaceutical Sciences. 2018;**10**(6): 11-17. DOI: 10.22159/ijpps.2018v10i6. 25500

[24] Kasturi M, Malviya N. Formulation and evaluation of liquisolid compacts of BCS Class II drug ketoprofen. Journal of Pharmaceutical Research International. 2021;**33**(45B):322-334. DOI: 10.9734/ JPRI/2021/v33i45B32811

[25] Kasturi M, Malviya N. A successful attempt to enhance solubility of BCS Class II drug using liquisolid compact technique. International Journal of Pharmaceutical Sciences and Research. 2021;**12**(5):2641-2650. DOI: 10.13040/ IJPSR.0975-8232.12(5).2641-50

[26] Naureen F, Shah Y, Shah SI, Abbas M, Rehman IU, Muhammad S, et al. Formulation development of mirtazapine liquisolid compacts: Optimization using central composite design. Molecules. 2022;**27**(13):4005. DOI: 10.3390/molecules27134005

[27] Pathak BK, Raghav M, Thakkar AR, Vyas BA, Shah PJ. Enhanced oral bioavailability of etodolac by the liquisolid compact technique:

Optimisation, in-vitro and in-vivo evaluation. Current Drug Delivery. 2021; **18**(4):471-486. DOI: 10.2174/1567201817666201026111559

[28] Thakkar HP, Vasava D, Patel AA, Dhande RD. Formulation and evaluation of liquisolid compacts of itraconazole to enhance its oral bioavailability. Therapeutic Delivery. 2020;**11**(2):83-96. DOI: 10.4155/tde-2019-0050

Chapter 5

Lipid as a Vehicle/Carrier for Oral Drug Delivery

Jagruti Desai, Tapan Desai and Ashwini Patel

Abstract

The drug administered by an oral route has to withstand a harsh environment of gastrointestinal media, absorb through intestinal epithelium and circumvent first-pass metabolism in liver before reaching portal blood circulation. Moreover, hydrophobic drug molecules offer challenges for formulation with respect to their solubility and hence bioavailability. Various approaches have been developed to overcome this barrier. One of them is the use of lipids in formulation. Incorporation of the drug in lipids can result in increased solubility, absorption and thereby enhanced bioavailability. Intestinal lymphatic route of absorption has also been explored for increasing bioavailability of hydrophobic drug moieties. In this chapter, we have discussed the pathway of lipid digestion in the human body as well as the mechanism of lipid particles upon oral administration. The various lipid formulations developed and the excipients used in the formulations have also been described. The importance of lipid chain length and the effect of food in increasing the bioavailability of drug is discussed. The lymphatic pathway of lipid carriers has also been discussed.

Keywords: oral drug delivery, M-cell uptake, drug absorption, lymphatic transport, lipid chain length

1. Introduction

Although many advancements occur in other routes, the oral route pathway of drug administration still remains the most preferred route. It is because of its cost-effectiveness, safety and convenience of administration, ease of production, suitability for long-term or life-long use and does not require sterilization and flexibility in dose adjustment [1, 2]. Intravenous administration delivers the drug directly to blood circulation, but there is the possibility of extravasation of blood or drug, thrombosis and catheter infections [3]. So, oral route has always remained the first preference for drug administration. However, there are certain limitations of this route which need to be circumvented. It includes poor solubility of drug, poor permeability, instability, first-pass metabolism, intestinal metabolism and slow commencement of action compared to intravenous route. Additionally, drug absorption starts from stomach, but it has short residence time of 2 h. So, only weakly acidic and neutral drugs are absorbed efficiently from stomach lining. Thus, major drug absorption after oral administration, thus occurs from intestine as it imparts a high absorptive surface area and greater residence time [1, 4, 5]. The common mechanism of absorption includes passive diffusion and enterocyte-mediated active transport through stomach and intestine [6, 7]. BCS Class I drugs, having high solubility and permeability are absorbed efficiently by oral route. However, the drug molecules that are being discovered belong to BCS Class II having poor aqueous solubility and good permeability [8]. This leads to their poor oral bioavailability. Many advancements to increase bioavailability have been made including size reduction, recrystallization, complexation, solid dispersion and use of solubility enhancers [9].

Use of lipid as an excipient to enhance oral bioavailability has been widely explored. They are majorly derived from dietary oils and/or fats and are biocompatible, biodegradable in nature and non-toxic [10]. Further, they not only help in increasing the solubility of drug in gastrointestinal media but various lipids have been shown to decrease proteolytic degradation [11], increase lymphatic absorption [12] and modulate various mechanisms including P-gp activity [13]. It has also been shown to enhance transcellular absorption of drug molecules [14]. The various lipid-based formulations have been developed so far are described in this chapter. Since the lipids have varied properties, their appropriate selection and design of formulation affect the success of the formulation [15]. Moreover, absorption of drug through the lymphatic system greatly affects the bioavailability of formulation and its efficacy. In general, the drug upon oral administration is either absorbed via intestinal epithelium to portal blood circulation, or is taken up by lymphatic vessels to the lymphatic system. The drug entering portal blood circulation has to pass through liver before reaching heart thus chances of metabolism are high. While the drug entering into the lymphatic system is directly get drained to heart avoiding first-pass metabolism. Hence, the lymphatic system can be an alternate and a safe route to enhance drug delivery [16]. Since this system mainly transports lipids and fats, the lipidic drug delivery systems have greater chances of absorption through this route [17]. In particular, for selective lymphatic uptake, high lipophilicity (log P > 5) and the presence of triglycerides having long carbon chains are desired [18]. The possible parameters of lipid-based drug delivery system to enhance lymphatic absorption are described in this chapter. Moreover, the in vivo lysis lipid in the human body has also been discussed. Another pathway of absorption exclusively to the lymphatic system is through Microfold cells (M-cells) present in intestinal epithelium [19, 20]. It uptakes lipid nanoparticles as well. Hence, this route becomes important for nanosized lipid drug delivery system. The mechanism of absorption of nanoparticles through this route has been described in this chapter.

2. In vivo lysis of lipid in human body

Lipid digestion begins in the gastrointestinal tract from oral cavity in the presence of lingual lipase enzymes secreted by Ebner's gland present on the tongue [21]. Further physical breakdown occurs due to gastric emptying, antral contraction and retropulsion. Stomach acts as the core site for the emulsification of fat molecules into coarse emulsion droplets of size approximately 0.5 μm [22, 23] followed by the enzymatic degradation of triglyceride to form a mixture of fatty acids and monoglycerides [24]. The coarse emulsion droplets when entering the small intestine stimulate the secretion of bile salts and bile lipids from the gallbladder which stabilizes the surface of droplets leading to the formation of fine droplets upon entering the intestine and further gets homogenized with bile and pancreatic juice. In general, the chain length of triglycerides determines its absorption pathway. The short- and medium-chain length fatty acids (having carbon chain length of less than 12) are able to diffuse through enterocytes, taken up by blood vessels, enter liver and then to blood circulation. On the other hand, long-chain fatty acids (having chain length greater than 12) undergoes re-esterification and are converted back to triglyceride form. These triglycerides are taken up by the chylomicrons which are absorbed by lymph vessels and drained to the blood circulation via the thoracic duct. When these chylomicrons reach any tissue, they activate the lipoprotein lipase present on the surface of BCECs to generate fatty acids. The fatty acids so formed enter muscles and adipose tissues for use or otherwise get stored. The lipids are transported in the body through lipoprotein vehicles like chylomicrons. These vehicles remain in the circulatory system until their triglycerides are consumed. They are also taken up by liver and digested. Among lipoproteins, the chylomicrons are the largest produced by intestinal wall. Other lipoproteins include high-density lipoproteins (HDL), low-density lipoproteins (LDL) and very low-density lipoproteins (VLDL). The HDL is synthesized by liver and intestinal wall (enterocytes), VLDL by the liver and LDL partly through the metabolism of VLDL in plasma and partly by liver [25].

3. Various lipid-based formulations

Lipid nanocarriers comprise of solid lipid matrix which exists in solid form at room temperature and leads to phase transition upon physiological temperature. They are of two categories: solid lipid nanocarriers (SLNs) and nanostructures lipid carriers (NLCs). They have possessed low toxicity, a solvent-free system, inexpensive, stable during sterilization and manufacturing, can entrap both hydrophilic and lipophilic drug candidates, can prolong the drug release and easy industrial scale-up. Due to the presence of these properties, they are gaining the researchers attention. Various lipid-based systems for oral drug delivery as listed in **Table 1**.

Type of carriers	Merits	Demerits
SLN	Unique structure with nano size, protect drug from harsh gastric environment, by achieving effective concentration at the receptor location and bypassing the apical transporter protein improves drug absorption	Low drug loading as drug might undergo partition or expulsion while stored.
NLC	Use of liquid lipids tends to form a less ordered structure which improve drug loading and stability compared to SLNs	Excipient-based cytotoxicity, irritation and sensitization
Lipid drug conjugates (LDCs)	Alteration in physicochemical properties of drug molecules, minimizing toxicity	Drug expulsion, particle growth, unpredictive gelation
Liposomes	improved stability, a faster absorption rate due to increment in aqueous solubility	Elasticity and leaching of drug during transport, degradation of phospholipid during storage, reproducibility in the quality of final preparation
Phytosomes	High drug loading due to enhancement of complexation rate, improve stability, inhibit drug expulsion, improve absorption and bioavailability.	Rapid elimination of phytoconstituents from the formulation

Type of carriers	Merits	Demerits
NLCs	high drug encapsulation compared to conventional nanoparticles, no drug partition in oily compartments, two or more drugs can be encapsulated, inhibit degradation, non-toxic to healthy cells	Surfactant dependent toxicity
SEDDS	Improves permeation, ideal carrier for lipophilic and sensitive drug delivery, simplicity of manufacturing at industrial scale also.	In vitro models available are not reliable. Concentration of surfactant used is high (up to 60%)
Emulsion	Minimize non-selective spread, more affinity for tumor cells, shows controlled payload drug release behavior, minimize irritation of gut wall, ease of manufacturing	Costly due to the use of micronization and reproducibility in droplet.

Table 1.
Comparison of various lipid carrier systems.

3.1 Solid lipid nanoparticles (SLNs) and nanostructured lipid nanocarriers (NLCs)

SLNs are the first generation of lipid nanocarrier introduced in 1991. The main solid lipids used in the development of nanocarriers are fatty acids, steroids, triglycerides, partial glycerides and waxes. Physically, SLNs are colloidal dispersion having different size of particles like smaller (<100 nm), medium (100–300 nm) and larger (300–1000 nm). Structurally, they comprise of APIs and solid lipid (0.1–30%) with coating of emulsifiers in the concentration limit of 0.5–5% [26, 27]. The method of preparation is opted based on physical parameters like particle size, shape, charges, stability of formulation, drug loading and drug release manner. The different solid lipids like tripalmitin, stearic acid, tristearin, glyceryl behenate, cetyl palmitate and glyceryl monostearate are generally used to form core-shell and surfactant like tyloxapol, poloxamer 188, soybean lecithin and tween 80 are used to form monolayer coating for the stabilization of lipid particles [28]. Structurally, SLNs possess highly organized crystal lattices with small space for the entrapment of the therapeutic molecules. On the basis of the spatial arrangement of the therapeutics in the SLNs, they have been classified into three different types: API is (i) homogeneously distributed throughout the SLN—homogeneous matrix arrangement; (ii) dispersed in the periphery of the core-shell-drug enrich core model and (iii) concentrated at the centre of the core-shell-drug enrich core model.

Aziz Unnisa et al. developed dapagliflozin solid lipid nanoparticles for controlling hyperglycaemia. SLNs were formulated by hot homogenization followed by probe-sonication. They utilized lipid-compritol 888 ATO; tween 80 as an emulsifier and poloxamer 188 as a co-surfactant. Prepared SLNs were of spherical shape and nano-size in range. The in vivo pharmacokinetic studies in diabetes-induced rat model showed a rise in C_{max} (1258.37 ± 1.21 mcg/mL), AUC (5247.04 mcg/mL) and oral absorption (twofold) of the dapagliflozin compared to its marketed formulation [29]. Huma Rao et al. formulated compritol-based alprazolam solid lipid nanoparticles. Prepared formulation shows quick onset of action and sustained release of drug. Hence alprazolam SLNs would relieve early symptoms of anxiety and depression, along with long-lasting control of symptoms in patients. They optimized the formulation and optimized formulation has 92.9 nm with narrow size distribution which demonstrate desired level of homogeneity and stability. Entrapment efficiency and drug loading capacity were found to be about 89% and 77% with smooth spherical morphology. In vitro drug release data demonstrates the 24 h sustained release of alprazolam from the SLNs. Based on their finding, they have made conclusion for promising sustained release formulation of short-acting alprazolam with decreasing dosing frequency and improves patient compliance [30].

NLCs are advanced lipid nanoparticles comprised blend of solid and liquid lipids in particle form stabilized by water base surfactants. Appropriate blend of these produces unorganized or poor crystalline lipid matrix. These provide high drug loading and prevent leaking of APIs throughout their storage. SLNs have low loading capacity because of their crystalline behavior and there is always possibility of drug expulsion during storage since solid lipids might undergo phase transition. This problem is overcome in NLCs as liquid lipid is present in it that does not allow drug to expulse [31].

Jittakan Lertpairod and Waree Tiyaboonchai prepared curcumin-loaded NLCs for targeting colon. First, NLCs were prepared using micro-emulsion method. Prepared NLCs entangled in EudragitS100, a pH-sensitive polymer, by ionotropic gelation method. The formulated MLCs are of 227 nm size, negative surface charge with high drug loading (>90%). NLCs embedded in polymeric matrix inhibit the drug release in stomach. They followed sustained released behavior in the intestine and colon [32].

3.2 Lipid drug conjugates (LDCs)

As lipids are derived from the natural sources like dietary supplements or oil/fat, they show excellent biodegradability and biocompatibility. These lipids are conjugated with the drug molecules via chemical bonds like esters, amides, disulphides, etc., and form lipid drug conjugates. LCDs have potential to alter physicochemical properties like improving the lipophilic performance, improving the drug permeation through biological membrane and brain, improving bioavailability, minimizing the toxicity, improving drug loading and altering the drug release patterns [33]. Atiđa Selman et al. formulated hybrid oral liposomes for selenium nanoparticles (Lip-SeNPs) using thiolated chitosan. Lip-SeNPs liposomes were prepared by microfluidics-assisted chemical reduction and assembling process followed by covalent conjugation with chitosan-N-acetylcysteine. Thiolated Lip-SeNPs were of 250 nm size and possessed positive charge improving adhesion to mucus layer without penetrating the enterocytes [34].

3.3 Liposomes

Liposomes are spherical vesicular systems mimic the cell plasma membrane structure. The main lipid used is phospholipid like eggs or soybean phosphatidylcholine, which for the bilayer with amphiphilic nature comprising a head (hydrophilic in nature) and a tail (hydrophobic in nature). For minimizing the fluidity in the bilayer, cholesterol is added for enhancing its in vitro and in vivo stability. Both hydrophilic and lipophilic drugs can be entrapped in the vesicles. Lipophilic drugs get entrapped in the lipid portion while hydrophilic drugs get entrapped in the aqueous portion. Based on the size of the vesicles and layers, they have been classified as (i) multilaminar vesicles that are composed of around 5–20 concentric bilayers of lipid and (ii) unilamellar liposome vesicles.

Oral administration is challenging for the liposomes due to degradation by acids, enzymes like lipase and bile salts present in gastric media. To overcome this problem, new technologies including engineering of polymers or ligands have been developed [5]. The strategies that are performed to improve the stabilization and disruption in the gastric environment are as follows:

i. Bilosomes: Incorporation of bile slats like sodium taurocholate, sodium glycocholate and sodium deoxycholate. They act as a permeation enhancer, enhance absorption, prevent premature release of drug and protect liposomes against the bile salts of the intestinal media [35].

ii. Surface modification by polymer coating: Use of enteric coating polymers for the protection from the gastric environment due to stearic hindrance; mucoadhesive polymers for enhancing the drug absorption by prolonged retention in the intestinal mucosa and polymeric conjugation for improving stability and promoting receptor-mediator endocytosis [36, 37].

iii. Use of lipids with higher phase transition temperature like dipalmitoylphosphatidylcholine, distear-oylphosphatidylcholine and sphingomyelin along with cholesterol. They are resistant to hydrolysis and oxidation and provide stability owing to their higher rigidity and packing [38].

Thuan ThiDuong et al., developed Berberine-loaded liposomes using air-suspension coating (layering) method for reduction in exogenous cholesterol and production of anti-hyperlipidaemia therapeutic effects. The prepared formulation was in narrow size distribution with nano-size range, possess good drug entrapment and spherical morphology. The lipid-lowering activity was evaluated using rats and mice. 628% increment in oral bioavailability was obtained in comparison to plain drug. Moreover, reduction in low-density lipoprotein, total cholesterol, triglycerides and low-density lipoprotein cholesterol were in hyperlipidemic mice [39].

Shabari Girinath Kala and Santhivardhan Chinni prepared D-alpha-tocopheryl polyethylene glycol 1000 succinate (TPGS) liposomes of nintedanib esylate. It is a kinase inhibitor used to treat lung cancer. It suffered from first-pass metabolism and hence has low oral bioavailability (~4.7%). The liposomes were prepared using the thin-film hydration method. They have applied the design of experiments to check the influence of process and formulation parameters like phospholipids: cholesterol ratio, drug loading and sonication time. Prepared TPGS liposomes had a particle size of 125 ± 6.7 nm, entrapment efficiency of 88.6 ± 4.1% and zeta potential of + 46 ± 2.8 mV. Morphologically they were spherical in a state with partial amorphization. In vitro drug release follows Higuchi kinetics with sustained drug release of 92% in 36 h in vitro cytotoxicity test was performed using A-549 cells and C-6-labeled liposomes revealed more effective than the marketed formulation. The preparation was found stable in stability chamber and simulated fluids. Based on the pharmacokinetic data prepared liposomal shows bout 6% times greater oral bioavailability compared to marketed formulation. Hence the prepared formulation shows prolonged drug release with improved bioavailability [40].

Shuang Liu et al. prepared chitosan-coated nanoliposomes (CC-NLs) of betanin using soya lecithin and cholesterol by a reverse-phase evaporation method. The physicochemical properties of chitosan-coated material were compared with uncoated nanoliposomes. They have found lower values of absolute zeta potentials and larger particle sizes than uncoated NLs. Moreover, stability and target release rate was improved in CC-NLs compared to uncoated NLs. Further, betanin delivered by

CC-NLs had higher in vitro and cellular antioxidant activities than free betanin and betanin delivered by uncoated NLs [41].

Chen Yanga et al. developed alpha-linolenic acid nanoliposomes (ALA-NLs) decorated with carboxymethyl chitosan for improving the oral bioavailability of linolenic acid. Upon comparison with CMC-coated liposomes with uncoated liposomes, they have observed layer formation with spherical morphology, improved physicochemical properties and encapsulation efficiency of about 79% of ALA. Further release of ALA in a simulated gastrointestinal environment would be regulated in CMC-coated nanoliposomes. Moreover, in vivo testing found that greater area under the curve ALA concentration and its absorption of CMCS-ALA-NLs compared to ALA-NLs and ALA-emulsion. The absorption of ALA was improved by CMCS-ALA-NLs [42].

3.4 Phytosomes

Phytosomes are also known as phytoconstituents–phospholipids complex in which bioactive phytoconstituents form a strong hydrogen bonding and Van der Waals forces with polar region of phospholipids. They are derived from a stoichiometric chemical reaction between APIs and phospholipids. Various methods such as solvent evaporation, salting out and lyophilization method are employed using non-polar solvents such as ethanol, dichloromethane and tetrahydrofuran [43]. Ravi Gundadka Shriram et al. developed Silymarin a hepatoprotective agent phytosomes for improving oral bioavailability by solvent evaporation method. The prepared phytosomes were of porous particles with smooth surface and particle size was in the range of 218.4 ± 2.54 nm. A significant enhancement in the aqueous solubility was obtained which correlates with its high drug release rate. Moreover, the in vivo studies exhibited heptatoprotective effect with good efficacy of formulation in it during the CCl_4-induced hepatotoxicity rat model [44].

3.5 Lipid nanocapsules (LNCs)

LNCs are structurally hybrid arrangements between liposomes and polymeric nanoparticles. External shell is composed of solid lipids emulsified with surfactant and semiliquid enriched central core. Three principal components of LNCs are oils and mixture of a non-ionic surfactant as well as hyrdophobic surfactant. The core is generally made of liquid lipids which act as a drug depot and about 10–25% w/w while solid lipids form the shell. NLCs are generally prepared using medium-chain triglycerides such as caprylic acid and capric acid. Lecithin, which is a complex mixture of various phosphatidyl esters such as phosphatidylinositol, phosphatidylcholine, phosphatidylserine and phosphatidylethanolamine is widely used as a lipophilic surfactant. The main sources of lecithin are eggs, sunflower, soybean, lysolecithin and rapeseed [45]. For enhancing the stability of NLCs, up to 1.5% w/w of lecithin is used. It forms a rigid shell when cooled. Hence, its concentration directly influences the rigidity and thickness of the outer shell [46]. Apart from this, non-ionic surfactants like solutol, Cremophor RH40 and RH60 are also used [47].

3.6 Nanoemulsion and microemulsion

Nanoemulsions or microemulsions are dispersion systems of two immiscible liquids possessing varying droplet sizes. They are isotropic mixture consisting of hydrophilic solvents and co-cosurfactant/surfactants that help to increase the solubility of hydrophobic APIs. Nanoemulsion is generally interchanged by microemulsion. Both have tremendous differences in structural aspects as well as thermodynamic stability. These differences are due to the presence of surfactant concentration and the method of preparations. Nanoemulsion requires exogenous energy during manufacturing like micofludization, high shear homogenization, etc., due to low concentration of surfactant while microemulsion can form spontaneously as surfactant concentration is high. Microemulsions are thermodynamically more stable than nanoemulsion [48, 49].

Onkar B. Patil et al., developed effective and stable nanoemulsion of tadalafil (TDF) and ketoconazole (KTZ) for targeting liver. They have utilized Leciva S-95 as lipid, tween 80 which is a hydrophilic surfactant, and span 80 which is a lipophilic surfactant were utilized as a surfactant while poloxamer 108 as a co-surfactant. The prepared formulation possesses a spherical shape nano-size droplet with narrow size distribution. In vitro drug released data exhibited controlled release behaviors of both drugs in the formulation. This may indicate improvement in half-life and reduced toxicity for normal tissue cells. NEs showed improvement in cytotoxicity towards HepG2 cells by increasing the drug uptake [50]. Gabriela Garrastazu Pereira et al. formulated nanoemulsion of anticancer ω-3 fatty acid derivatives for oral administration. They formulated a stable nanoemulsion comprised of Labrafac™ as a lipidic phase, span 80 and tween 80 as a surfactant having droplet size 150 nm. They prepared the formulation by employing phase-inversion emulsification process and reduction in particle size by high-pressure homogenization. Prepared nanoemulsions, during in vivo tumor study in mice, showed a significant reduction in relative tumor volume [51]. Manohar Mahadev et al. fabricated quercetin nanoemulsion for enhancing the therapeutic effectiveness and oral bioavailability in diabetes mellitus. They have used tween 80, ethyl oleate and labrasol as surfactant, oil and co-surfactant, respectively, for the formulation of nanoemulsion and optimized the formula using Box–Behnken design. The formulation had a 125.51 nm particle size with a 0.215 poly dispersibility index with a spherical shape. Formulation exhibited greater drug release in comparison to pure drug. Moreover, animal studies revealed remarkable protective and therapeutic properties in the management of diabetes [52].

3.7 Self-emulsifying drug delivery system (SEDDS)

These systems are made using oil, surfactant/co-surfactant mixture (ratio of oil:surfactant is generally varying from 20:30 to 20:60). Upon oral administration, spontaneous nanoemulsion form in the GIT. These systems have the capacity to penetrate the mucus layer and reach the epithelial tissue thus helping the penetration of drug molecules having less permeability in general. SEDDS have the potential to facilitate the delivery of poorly permeable drugs. Nowadays, research is going on for the combination of SEDDS with polymers in the oral absorption of peptides. Polymer can improve the mucoadhesion in the mucus membrane which may, in turn, lead to prolonged therapeutic effectiveness. Net negative charges are present in the mucus carrier due to the presence of sialic and sulphonic acid and upon ionic interaction, oily droplets exhibit positive charges and improve adhesion and absorption of drug molecules [53]. Diego A. Bravo-Alfaro et al. formulated self-nanoemulsifying drug delivery systems of betulinic acid (BA), a bioactive molecule having antineoplastic, antiviral and anti-inflammatory activity. Betulinic acid has low water solubility. They used lauroglycol FCC and caprylic acid as a lipid phase and found greater solubility of BA. By applying pseudoternary phase diagrams Cremophor EL® and Labrafil M1944CS were selected as surfactant and co-surfactant. Prepared nanoemulsion possess approximately 22–56 nm particle size with 0.058–0.135 PDI. Moreover, they have found no changes in the particle size in the presence of simulated small intestinal phase conditions for 105 min. In vivo studies demonstrated about a 15-fold increment in the bioavailability of BA compared to free BA solution [54].

4. Mechanism of lipid nanoparticles

Regarding the typical triglyceride-based lipid nano-particles will undergo the same digestive processes as lipids consumed through food after being administered orally. Still, mechanism of oral bioavailability has now no longer been defined but some of the additives are standard for know-how the enhancement of absorption. Surface area, smaller particle size and morphology are extra suitable traits for oral absorption. Since lipids are regarded to improve oral absorption of drug and they can be prepared with less particle size, it has been concluded that this carrier system must use lipids as the excipient for greater and steady absorption through gastrointestinal pathway [55]. Additionally, solid-lipid nanoparticles (SLNs) surface area, interaction with epithelial membranes and bio adhesion to the GI wall appear to extend their absorption in the GIT, which probably improves oral absorption. There are three basic mechanisms for oral administration of lipids, lipophilic excipients and lipid-based formulation for increased absorption [56],

1. Pre-enterocyte level (solubilization of drug)

2. Intra-enterocyte level (chylomicron formulation)

3. Post-enterocyte level (lymphatic drug transport)

According to a claim that lipid nanoparticles have adhesive characteristics that allow them to adhere to the surface of enterocytes in the stomach and immediately release drugs for absorption into the cells. Parallel to this, SLN contributes significantly to the formation of micelles in the oral uptake by causing the release of bile salts and lipase/co-lipase, Additionally, the bile salts and micelles interact to form mixed micelles that facilitate the absorption of these colloidal species by enterocytes, which transport drugs inside cells, these mechanisms have been called the "Trojan horse" effect [57]. Micelles are created after absorption and present in the enterocyte, where they are re-esterified via the monoacyl glycerol or phosphatidic acid route to become chylomicrons and maintained by phospholipids. The penetration of mucus and unstirred water layer, however, is what restricts the rate of digestion. Following formation, the chylomicrons are subjected to the lymphatic transport system via mesenteric lymph before being drained by the thoracic duct [58, 59].

Following oral administration, several techniques for drug transport into the lymphatic system have been reported. These Peyer's patches contained M cells that are used for vaccine distribution through the transcellular and paracellular mechanisms [55], as well as therapeutic drugs and nanocarriers. The transcellular approach is the most fundamental technique for lipid-based carriers to be absorbed. Enterocytes are promoted to generate chylomicron when drug is delivered using lipid-based transporters, which further emulsify and incorporate the lipophilic drug molecules into the nonpolar core. This stimulates the intestinal lymphatics to absorb drugs that are just slightly water soluble.

Additionally, lipid-based carriers can enhance intestinal lymphatic lipid flux and lipoprotein production, both of which are regulated by the physiochemical characteristics of lipids and the presence of stabilizer. Lipid-based transcellular routes are additional. There are various transcellular mechanisms through which lipid-based drug delivery systems are transported into enterocytes, including macro-pinocytosis, caveolae-mediated, clathrin-mediated and clathrin and caveolae-independent endocytosis [60].

Griffin and O'Driscoll gave explanations for how the lipid-based formulations improved the oral absorption of lipophilic drugs specifically for peptide and protein-like drugs, in addition, to improving intestinal lymphatic transport and drug solubilization. These enclosed increased intestinal membrane permeability, fluidization of the intestinal membranes, reduce the enzymatic degradation, alteration of TJs, generation of lipid-protein interactions and alteration of enterocyte-based efflux and metabolic activities are some of these [61].

In addition to the above-mentioned factors, lipid-based formulations stimulate prolonged gastric emptying, which prolongs the stomach's time in the stomach and increases the rates at which drug molecules dissolve at the absorptive site, hence improving drug absorption [62]. As a result, lipid-based nanoparticles increase the oral bioavailability of lipophilic drugs through bio-adhesion mechanisms in addition to endogenous lipid absorption pathways, which include absorption through M cells of Peyer's patches, solubilization, permeability across the enterocyte, increased paracellular and transcellular transport, controlled drug release, delayed gastric emptying time, stimulation of lymphatic transport, avoidance of intestinal first-pass metabolism, etc.

The review demonstrated that due to the unique characteristics of lipid nanoparticles and its components (wide variety of lipid constituents such as P-gp inhibitor, permeability enhancer, endogenous solubilizing components, etc.) multiple mechanisms for absorption and permeation, no toxicity and its formulation opportunities including avoidance of organic solvents during production of complex and challenging formulation strategy for drugs that, when taken orally have poor water solubility [63], Drug (lipid-nano formulation) may be eliminated from the body after oral administration as a result of its lipophilicity, which is directly affected to the bioavailability of drug molecules and lipid nanoparticles. Changes in the components of lipids may affect the bioavailability of bioactive characteristics, including, such of those vaccines. However, adding the surface of lipid nanoparticles with a surface-active substance like PEG prolongs their stay in the bloodstream while preventing phagocytosis uptake.

5. Critical influencing factors

It is claimed that the type of lipid (chain lengths and saturation degree) is one of the most essential factors that affect CM transport. Lipophilicity of short, medium and long-chain fatty acids and CM binding capacity both are significantly correlated with chain length. Reports say that transport via the portal vein there is preferred short-chain fatty acid, whereas medium-chain or long-chain fatty acids are prone to be transported via the lymph. Self-nanoemulsifying drug delivery systems (SNEDSS) composed of long-chain fatty acids than medium chain-fatty acids in lymph add proof to support the dependency of chain length [64]. Halofantrine, a particularly lipophilic drug, was used in a research of lipid-based vehicles to demonstrate that the lymphatic affinity of the vehicles followed the order of C18 (15.8%) > C8–10 (5.5%) > C4 (2.22%) > C0 (0.34%) [65]. An increase in FA chain length is highly correlated with enhanced drug transport efficiency. This may be explained by higher affinity to intracellular CMs and lipoproteins by higher lipophilicity of long-chain fatty acid. Administered in oil solution of 1,3-dioctanoyl-2-linoleyl-*sn*-glycerol, abbreviation MLM to denote the position of "medium long medium" chains, enhances absorption of halofantrine while maintaining levels of lymphatic transport that are comparable to the level of sunflower oil solution. However, halofantrine formulation was made into SNEDSS which based on MLM and 1,3-dilinoyl-2-octanoyl-*sn*-glycerol, enclosed as LML to indicate "long-chain-long" chain lengths, lymphatic transport was found to be 17.9% and 27.4%, although the availability of plasma was 56.9% (MLM) and 37.2% (LML), respectively [66]. It is indicated that consideration of ratio and length of chain may be a way to change how drugs are distributed throughout various pathways.

Another factor is food effect that may enhance lymphatic transport and with bioavailability of plasma. Radio-labeled cannabinoid receptor agonist CRA13 have 72–75% oral bioavailability in fed dogs vs. 8–20% in fasted ones, with 43.7% through lymphatic transport [67]. After the meal has been taken total amount of halofantrine increases from 1.3% to 54% in lymphatic transport of the administered dose. Sometimes, consumption of food may slow down the process of absorption, but not necessarily affect systemic bioavailability and AUC. Regarding the food effect, there are some exceptions which should be noted. For example, after administration of high-fat food, the AUC of DDT with high CM binding efficiency enhances by 1.5-fold, however, under identical circumstances, diazepam with low CM binding efficiency shows no significant difference, lymphatic transport is higher for DDT but not for diazepam. Stimulation of CMs may have partly affected by the food effect. Intake of not only fat but high contents of carbohydrates also affects the higher production of CM [68]. Additionally, the bile salts produced during lipid digestion help to stabilize the mixed micelles that entrap the drug molecule. This is turn help to increase the drug absorption and CM formation inside the cell enterocytes. The importance of many endogenous bile salts is demonstrated by the drastically reduced halofantrine synthesis in lymph in bile duct salt-cannulated rats.

6. Lymphatic transport of lipid carriers

There are two pathways for entry to the lymphatic system: M-cell uptake of particles and absorption of lipidic molecules through lymph vessels. The vascular region throughout the body is surrounded by specialized lymphatic vessels that absorb the molecules giving entry to a complex network of lymphatic systems [69, 70]. The pore size of blood vessels is not enough for the uptake of large molecules of triglycerides and phospholipids. However, the lymphatic capillaries are single-layer, thin-walled and non-fenestrated due to which it is easily able to permit these large molecules [71]. Upon absorption through lymph vessels, the lymph fluid containing absorbed molecules enters the thoracic duct followed by subclavian vein and finally is drained into the circulatory system. This pathway bypasses the liver before entering the blood circulatory system thus avoiding first-pass hepatic metabolism [72]. When drug reaches the circulatory system, it is in form of micelles or mixed micelles which dissociate into monomers because of dilution with the large volume of lymph/blood (the surfactant concentration decreases due to dilution and results in a concentration below its CMC value) [73]. In other cases where the drug is carried in lipid vesicle form, the release of drug becomes prolonged. It has been reported in literature that the presence of triglyceride-rich lipoproteins diverts the absorption of drug exclusively through lymphatic route. Moreover, it has been also reported that greater lipoprotein synthesis particularly after postprandial administration diverts absorption of drugs dominantly through lymphatic system [67, 74]. This indicates that lipid derived either from diet or formulation determines the transport of drug either through lymphatic system or portal blood circulation [75]. This further relates to the new era for formulation development ruling out the necessity of traditional pathways like increasing solubilization capacity. It also brings new opportunities for various excipients that are emerging as bioactive recently in the last decade [76]. Further, excipients such as Cremophor EL and pluronic polymers have been shown to decrease chylomicron production and reduce the P-gp efflux transport of drug molecules [77, 78]. One of the versatile excipients in this category is tween 80 which has been found as excellent solubilizer, inhibitor of P-gp efflux and increase chylomicron production [76, 79]. Another pathway for lymphatic absorption through M cells has also been explored in the last two decades. These cells are able to recognize pathogens due to the presence of specific ligands on their surface. The particles of formulation have thus been engineered to mimic these ligands that are recognized by M-cells. Such ligands include peptides like Arg-Gly-Asp, glucans, proteins like lectins etc. [80–82]. Another peptide ligand investigated for M-cell uptake is RGD which recognizes a5b1 integrin on M-cells. However, due to its instability in gastrointestinal tract media, its analogue RGD peptidomimetic has been developed. This new moiety has been grafted on the surface of poly(lactic-*co*-glycolic acid) nanoparticles and tested for M-cell uptake. It was found that the efficacy of this new molecule remained the same as compared to its parent moiety (RGD) but the stability in GI media was improved [83, 84].

7. Conclusion

In recent decades, number of innovations have been developed in lipid-based drug delivery for oral route. Moreover, the advancements in technology transfer have also been seen favoring the production of these novel systems. The in vivo performance evaluation, in vitro drug release studies have also been improved allowing us to track the amount of drug that is able to cross the gastrointestinal tract and/or lymphatic absorption. This delivery system has proved as more useful for poorly water-soluble drugs especially for potent lipophilic drugs because of their biocompatibility and non-toxicity, solubility enhancing properties. Overall, lipid-based drug delivery is one of the safest options for the oral delivery of lipophilic drugs.

Conflict of interest

The authors declare no conflict of interest.

Author details

Jagruti Desai[1*], Tapan Desai[1] and Ashwini Patel[2]

1 Department of Pharmaceutics and Pharmaceutical Technology, Ramanbhai Patel College of Pharmacy, Charotar University of Science and Technology (CHARUSAT), Changa, India

2 Krishna School of Pharmacy and Research (Formerly Known as Babaria Institute of Pharmacy), Drs. Kiran and Pallavi Patel Global University, Vadodara, India

*Address all correspondence to: jagrutidesai.ph@charusat.ac.in

References

[1] Ansel HC, Popovich NG, Allen LV. Pharmaceutical Dosage Forms and Drug Delivery Systems. Philadelphia, PA: Lippincott Williams & Wilkins; 1995

[2] Paul K, Singh N, Jain S. Drug–lipid conjugates for enhanced oral drug delivery. AAPS PharmSciTech. 2019;**20**(2):1-11

[3] Roger E, Lagarce F, Benoit J-P. Development and characterization of a novel lipid nanocapsule formulation of Sn38 for oral administration. European Journal of Pharmaceutics and Biopharmaceutics. 2011;**79**(1):181-188

[4] Ensign LM, Cone R, Hanes J. Oral drug delivery with polymeric nanoparticles: The gastrointestinal mucus barriers. Advanced Drug Delivery Reviews. 2012;**64**(6):557-570

[5] He H, Lu Y, Qi J, Zhu Q, Chen Z, Wu W. Adapting liposomes for oral drug delivery. Acta Pharmaceutica Sinica B. 2019;**9**(1):36-48

[6] Pridgen EM, Alexis F, Farokhzad OC. Polymeric nanoparticle drug delivery technologies for oral delivery applications. Expert Opinion on Drug Delivery. 2015;**12**(9):1459-1473

[7] Shugarts S, Benet LZ. The role of transporters in the pharmacokinetics of orally administered drugs. Pharmaceutical Research. 2009;**26**(9): 2039-2054

[8] Amidon GL, Lennernäs H, Shah VP, Crison JR. A theoretical basis for a biopharmaceutic drug classification: The correlation of in vitro drug product dissolution and in vivo bioavailability. Pharmaceutical Research. 1995;**12**(3):413-420

[9] Desai J, Khatri N, Chauhan S, Seth A. Design, development and optimization of self-microemulsifying drug delivery system of an anti-obesity drug. Journal of Pharmacy & Bioallied Sciences. 2012;**4**(Suppl. 1):S21

[10] Mu H, Holm R. Solid lipid nanocarriers in drug delivery: Characterization and design. Expert Opinion on Drug Delivery. 2018;**15**(8):771-785

[11] Lane ME, O'Driscoll CM, Corrigan OI. Quantitative estimation of the effects of bile salt surfactant systems on insulin stability and permeability in the rat intestine using a mass balance model. Journal of Pharmacy and Pharmacology. 2005;**57**(2):169-175

[12] Desai J, Thakkar H. Mechanistic evaluation of lymphatic targeting efficiency of Atazanavir sulfate loaded lipid nanocarriers: In-vitro and in-vivo studies. Journal of Drug Delivery Science and Technology. 2022;**68**:103090

[13] Desai JL, Thakkar HP. Role of Lipid Nanocarriers in Lymphatic Targeting: Promises and Safety Considerations. Singapore: Springer; 2021. pp. 43-59

[14] Maher S, Brayden DJ, Casettari L, Illum L. Application of permeation enhancers in oral delivery of macromolecules: An update. Pharmaceutics. 2019;**11**(1):41

[15] Dahan A, Hoffman A. Rationalizing the selection of oral lipid based drug delivery systems by an in vitro dynamic lipolysis model for improved oral bioavailability of poorly water soluble drugs. Journal of Controlled Release. 2008;**129**(1):1-10

[16] Ahn H, Park J-H. Liposomal delivery systems for intestinal lymphatic drug

transport. Biomaterials Research. 2016;**20**(1):1-6

[17] Markovic M, Ben-Shabat S, Aponick A, Zimmermann EM, Dahan A. Lipids and lipid-processing pathways in drug delivery and therapeutics. International Journal of Molecular Sciences. 2020;**21**(9):3248

[18] Pouton CW, Porter CJ. Formulation of lipid-based delivery systems for oral administration: Materials, methods and strategies. Advanced Drug Delivery Reviews. 2008;**60**(6):625-637

[19] Vishwakarma N, Jain A, Sharma R, Mody N, Vyas S, Vyas SP. Lipid-based nanocarriers for lymphatic transportation. AAPS PharmSciTech. 2019;**20**(2):1-13

[20] Markovic M, Ben-Shabat S, Keinan S, Aponick A, Zimmermann EM, Dahan A. Lipidic prodrug approach for improved oral drug delivery and therapy. Medicinal Research Reviews. 2019;**39**(2):579-607

[21] Iqbal J, Hussain MM. Intestinal lipid absorption. American Journal of Physiology-Endocrinology and Metabolism. 2009;**296**(6):E1183-E1E94. DOI: 10.1152/ajpendo.90899.2008

[22] Carey MC, Small DM, Bliss CM. Lipid digestion and absorption. Annual Review of Physiology. 1983;**45**(1):651-677

[23] Chakraborty S, Shukla D, Mishra B, Singh S. Lipid–an emerging platform for oral delivery of drugs with poor bioavailability. European Journal of Pharmaceutics and Biopharmaceutics. 2009;**73**(1):1-15. DOI: 10.1016/j.ejpb.2009.06.001

[24] Yanez JA, Wang SW, Knemeyer IW, Wirth MA, Alton KB. Intestinal lymphatic transport for drug delivery. Advanced Drug Delivery Reviews. 2011;**63**(10-11):923-942. DOI: 10.1016/j.addr.2011.05.019

[25] Bazinet RP, Layé S. Polyunsaturated fatty acids and their metabolites in brain function and disease. Nature Reviews Neuroscience. 2014;**15**(12):771-785. DOI: 10.1038/nrn3820

[26] Cunha S, Amaral MH, Lobo JMS, Silva AC. Lipid nanoparticles for nasal/intranasal drug delivery. Critical Reviews in Therapeutic Drug Carrier Systems. 2017;**34**(3):257-282. DOI: 10.1615/CritRevTherDrug CarrierSyst.2017018693

[27] Anderluzzi G, Lou G, Su Y, Perrie Y. Scalable manufacturing processes for solid lipid nanoparticles. Pharmaceutical Nanotechnology. 2019;**7**(6):444-459. DOI: 10.2174/2211738507666190925112942

[28] Gordillo-Galeano A, Mora-Huertas CE. Solid lipid nanoparticles and nanostructured lipid carriers: A review emphasizing on particle structure and drug release. European Journal of Pharmaceutics and Biopharmaceutics. 2018;**133**:285-308. DOI: 10.1016/j.ejpb.2018.10.017

[29] Unnisa A, Chettupalli AK, Al Hagbani T, Khalid M, Jandrajupalli SB, Chandolu S, et al. Development of Dapagliflozin solid lipid nanoparticles as a novel carrier for oral delivery: Statistical design, optimization, in-vitro and in-vivo characterization, and evaluation. Pharmaceuticals. 2022;**15**(5):568. DOI: 10.3390/ph15050568

[30] Rao H, Ahmad S, Madni A, Rao I, Ghazwani M, Hani U, et al. Compritol-based alprazolam solid lipid nanoparticles for sustained release of alprazolam: Preparation by hot

melt encapsulation. Molecules. 2022;**27**(24):8894

[31] Weber S, Zimmer A, Pardeike J. Solid lipid nanoparticles (SLN) and nanostructured lipid carriers (NLC) for pulmonary application: A review of the state of the art. European Journal of Pharmaceutics and Biopharmaceutics. 2014;**86**(1):7-22. DOI: 10.1016/j.ejpb.2013.08.013

[32] Lertpairod J, Tiyaboonchai W. pH-sensitive beads containing curcumin loaded nanostructured lipid carriers for a colon targeted oral delivery system. Journal of Pharmaceutical Investigation. 2022;**52**(3):387-396. DOI: 10.1007/s40005-022-00572-0

[33] Irby D, Du C, Li F. Lipid–drug conjugate for enhancing drug delivery. Molecular Pharmaceutics. 2017;**14**(5):1325-1338. DOI: 10.1021/acs.molpharmaceut.6b01027

[34] Selmani A, Seibert E, Tetyczka C, Kuehnelt D, Vidakovic I, Kornmueller K, et al. Thiolated chitosan conjugated liposomes for oral delivery of selenium nanoparticles. Pharmaceutics. 2022;**14**(4):803. DOI: 10.3390/pharmaceutics14040803

[35] Arafat M, Kirchhoefer C, Mikov MM, Sarfraz MK, Löbenberg R. Nanosized liposomes containing bile salt: A vesicular nanocarrier for enhancing oral bioavailability of BCS class III drug. Journal of Pharmacy & Pharmaceutical Sciences. 2017;**20**:305-318. DOI: 10.18433/J3CK88

[36] Hosny KM, Ahmed OA, Al-Abdali RT. Enteric-coated alendronate sodium nanoliposomes: A novel formula to overcome barriers for the treatment of osteoporosis. Expert Opinion on Drug Delivery. 2013;**10**(6):741-746. DOI: 10.1517/17425247.2013.799136

[37] Gradauer K, Barthelmes J, Vonach C, Almer G, Mangge H, Teubl B, et al. Liposomes coated with thiolated chitosan enhance oral peptide delivery to rats. Journal of Controlled Release. 2013;**172**(3):872-878. DOI: 10.1016/j.jconrel.2013.10.011

[38] Uhl P, Pantze S, Storck P, Parmentier J, Witzigmann D, Hofhaus G, et al. Oral delivery of vancomycin by tetraether lipid liposomes. European Journal of Pharmaceutics and Biopharmaceutics. 2017;**108**:111-118. DOI: 10.1016/j.ejps.2017.07.013

[39] Duong TT, Yen TTH, Nguyen LT, Nguyen TD, Nguyen TQ, Nghiem TH, et al. Berberine-loaded liposomes for oral delivery: Preparation, physicochemical characterization and in-vivo evaluation in an endogenous hyperlipidemic animal model. International Journal of Pharmaceutics. 2022;**616**:121525. DOI: 10.1016/j.ijpharm.2022.121525

[40] Kala SG, Chinni S. Bioavailability enhancement of vitamin E TPGS liposomes of nintedanib esylate: Formulation optimization, cytotoxicity and pharmacokinetic studies. Drug Delivery and Translational Research. 2022;**12**(11):2856-2864. DOI: 10.1007/s13346-022-01148-z

[41] Liu S, Lian J, Xu Z, Ning Y, Shi M, Zhao Z, et al. Chitosan-coated nanoliposomes for efficient delivery of betanin with enhanced stability and bioavailability. Food Hydrocolloids. 2022;**132**:107871

[42] Yang C, Gong L, Li X, Li W, Meng X, Liu B. Carboxymethyl chitosan coated alpha-linolenic acid nanoliposomes: Preparation, stability and release in vitro and in vivo. Food Chemistry. 2023;**404**(Pt A):134526. DOI: 10.1016/j.foodchem.2022.134526

[43] Telange DR, Patil AT, Pethe AM, Fegade H, Anand S, Dave VS. Formulation and characterization of an apigenin-phospholipid phytosome (APLC) for improved solubility, in vivo bioavailability, and antioxidant potential. European Journal of Pharmaceutics and Biopharmaceutics. 2017;**108**:36-49. DOI: 10.1016/j.ejps.2016.12.009

[44] Shriram RG, Moin A, Alotaibi HF, Khafagy E-S, Al Saqr A, Abu Lila AS, et al. Phytosomes as a plausible nano-delivery system for enhanced oral bioavailability and improved hepatoprotective activity of Silymarin. Pharmaceuticals. 2022;**15**(7):790. DOI: 10.3390/ph15070790

[45] Huynh NT, Passirani C, Saulnier P, Benoît J-P. Lipid nanocapsules: A new platform for nanomedicine. International Journal of Pharmaceutics. 2009;**379**(2):201-209. DOI: 10.1016/j.ijpharm.2009.04.026

[46] Dabholkar N, Waghule T, Rapalli VK, Gorantla S, Alexander A, Saha RN, et al. Lipid shell lipid nanocapsules as smart generation lipid nanocarriers. Journal of Molecular Liquids. 2021;**339**:117145. DOI: 10.1016/j.molliq.2021.117145

[47] Dulieu C, Bazile D. Influence of lipid nanocapsules composition on their aptness to freeze-drying. Pharmaceutical Research. 2005;**22**(2):285-292. DOI: 10.1007/s11095-004-1196-0

[48] Singh Y, Meher JG, Raval K, Khan FA, Chaurasia M, Jain NK, et al. Nanoemulsion: Concepts, development and applications in drug delivery. Journal of Controlled Release. 2017;**252**:28-49. DOI: 10.1016/j.jconrel.2017.03.008

[49] Callender SP, Mathews JA, Kobernyk K, Wettig SD. Microemulsion utility in pharmaceuticals: Implications for multi-drug delivery. International Journal of Pharmaceutics. 2017;**526**(1-2):425-442. DOI: 10.1016/j.ijpharm.2017.05.005

[50] Patil OB, Manjappa AS, Kumbhar PS, Bhosale SP, Disouza JI, Salawi A, et al. Development of stable self-nanoemulsifying composition and its nanoemulsions for improved oral delivery of non-oncology drugs against hepatic cancer. OpenNano. 2022;**7**:100044. DOI: 10.1016/j.onano.2022.100044

[51] Garrastazu Pereira G, Rawling T, Pozzoli M, Pazderka C, Chen Y, Dunstan CR, et al. Nanoemulsion-enabled oral delivery of novel anticancer omega-3 fatty acid derivatives. Nanomaterials. 2018;**8**(10):825. DOI: 10.3390/nano8100825

[52] Mahadev M, Nandini HS, Ramu R, Gowda DV, Almarhoon ZM, Al-Ghorbani M, et al. Fabrication and evaluation of quercetin nanoemulsion: A delivery system with improved bioavailability and therapeutic efficacy in diabetes mellitus. Pharmaceuticals. 2022;**15**(1):70

[53] Bennett KM, Walker SL, Lo DD. Epithelial microvilli establish an electrostatic barrier to microbial adhesion. Infection and Immunity. 2014;**82**(7):2860-2871. DOI: 10.1128/IAI.01681-14

[54] Bravo-Alfaro DA, Ochoa-Rodríguez LR, Villaseñor-Ortega F, Luna-Barcenas G, García HS. Self-nanoemulsifying drug delivery system (SNEDDS) improves the oral bioavailability of betulinic acid. Journal of Molecular Liquids. 2022;**364**:119946

[55] Li H, Zhao X, Ma Y, Zhai G, Li L, Lou H. Enhancement of gastrointestinal absorption of quercetin by solid lipid nanoparticles. Journal of Controlled

Release. 2009;**133**(3):238-244. DOI: 10.1016/j.jconrel.2008.10.002

[56] Zhuang C-Y, Li N, Wang M, Zhang X-N, Pan W-S, Peng J-J, et al. Preparation and characterization of vinpocetine loaded nanostructured lipid carriers (NLC) for improved oral bioavailability. International Journal of Pharmaceutics. 2010;**394**(1-2):179-185. DOI: 10.1016/j.ijpharm.2010.05.005

[57] Dumont C, Bourgeois S, Fessi H, Jannin V. Lipid-based nanosuspensions for oral delivery of peptides, a critical review. International Journal of Pharmaceutics. 2018;**541**(1-2):117-135. DOI: 10.1016/j.ijpharm.2018.02.038

[58] Wang TY, Liu M, Portincasa P, Wang DQH. New insights into the molecular mechanism of intestinal fatty acid absorption. European Journal of Clinical Investigation. 2013;**43**(11):1203-1223

[59] Muchow M, Maincent P, Müller RH. Lipid nanoparticles with a solid matrix (SLN®, NLC®, LDC®) for oral drug delivery. Drug Development and Industrial Pharmacy. 2008;**34**(12):1394-1405. DOI: 10.1080/03639040802130061

[60] Thanki K, Gangwal RP, Sangamwar AT, Jain S. Oral delivery of anticancer drugs: Challenges and opportunities. Journal of Controlled Release. 2013;**170**(1):15-40. DOI: 10.1016/j.jconrel.2013.04.020

[61] Griffin B, O'Driscoll C. Opportunities and challenges for oral delivery of hydrophobic versus hydrophilic peptide and protein-like drugs using lipid-based technologies. Therapeutic Delivery. 2011;**2**(12):1633-1653. DOI: 10.4155/tde.11.128

[62] Elgart A, Cherniakov I, Aldouby Y, Domb AJ, Hoffman A. Lipospheres and pro-nano lipospheres for delivery of poorly water soluble compounds. Chemistry and Physics of Lipids. 2012;**165**(4):438-453. DOI: 10.1016/j.chemphyslip.2012.01.007

[63] Humberstone AJ, Charman WN. Lipid-based vehicles for the oral delivery of poorly water soluble drugs. Advanced Drug Delivery Reviews. 1997;**25**(1):103-128. DOI: 10.1016/S0169-409X(96)00494-2

[64] Imada C, Takahashi T, Kuramoto M, Masuda K, Ogawara K-i, Sato A, et al. Improvement of oral bioavailability of N-251, a novel antimalarial drug, by increasing lymphatic transport with long-chain fatty acid-based self-nanoemulsifying drug delivery system. Pharmaceutical Research. 2015;**32**(8):2595-2608. DOI: 10.1007/s11095-015-1646-x

[65] Poovi G, Damodharan N. Lipid nanoparticles: A challenging approach for oral delivery of BCS class-II drugs. Future Journal of Pharmaceutical Sciences. 2018;**4**(2):191-205. DOI: 10.1016/j.fjps.2018.04.001

[66] Caliph SM, Charman WN, Porter CJ. Effect of short-, medium-, and long-chain fatty acid-based vehicles on the absolute oral bioavailability and intestinal lymphatic transport of halofantrine and assessment of mass balance in lymph-cannulated and non-cannulated ratsE. Journal of Pharmaceutical Sciences. 2000;**89**(8):1073-1084. DOI: 10.1002/1520-6017(200008)89:8<1073::aid-jps12>3.0.co;2-v

[67] Trevaskis NL, Shackleford DM, Charman WN, Edwards GA, Gardin A, Appel-Dingemanse S, et al. Intestinal lymphatic transport enhances the post-prandial oral bioavailability of a novel cannabinoid receptor

agonist via avoidance of first-pass metabolism. Pharmaceutical Research. 2009;**26**(6):1486-1495. DOI: 10.1007/s11095-009-9860-z

[68] Desmarchelier C, Borel P, Lairon D, Maraninchi M, Valéro R. Effect of nutrient and micronutrient intake on chylomicron production and postprandial lipemia. Nutrients. 2019;**11**(6):1299. DOI: 10.3390/nu11061299

[69] Zhang XY, Lu WY. Recent advances in lymphatic targeted drug delivery system for tumor metastasis. Cancer Biology & Medicine. 2014;**11**(4):247-254. DOI: 10.7497/j.issn.2095-3941.2014.04.003

[70] Reddy L, Murthy R. Lymphatic transport of orally administered drugs. Indian Journal of Experimental Biology. 2002;**40**:1097-1109

[71] Leak L. The structure of lymphatic capillaries in lymph formation. In: Federation Proceedings. Virginia. 1976

[72] Zuther JE, Norton S. Lymphedema Management: The Comprehensive Guide for Practitioners. New York. 2017

[73] Yokoyama M. Block copolymers as drug carriers. Critical Reviews in Therapeutic Drug Carrier Systems. 1992;**9**(3-4):213-248

[74] Khoo SM, Edwards GA, Porter CJ, Charman WN. A conscious dog model for assessing the absorption, enterocyte-based metabolism, and intestinal lymphatic transport of halofantrine. Journal of Pharmaceutical Sciences. 2001;**90**(10):1599-1607. DOI: 10.1002/jps.1110

[75] Williams HD, Trevaskis NL, Charman SA, Shanker RM, Charman WN, Pouton CW, et al. Strategies to address low drug solubility in discovery and development. Pharmacological Reviews. 2013;**65**(1):315-499. DOI: 10.1124/pr.112.005660

[76] Seeballuck F, Lawless E, Ashford MB, O'Driscoll CM. Stimulation of triglyceride-rich lipoprotein secretion by polysorbate 80: In vitro and in vivo correlation using Caco-2 cells and a cannulated rat intestinal lymphatic model. Pharmaceutical Research. 2004;**21**(12):2320-2326. DOI: 10.1007/s11095-004-7684-4

[77] Seeballuck F, Ashford MB, O'Driscoll CM. The effects of Pluronic® block copolymers and Cremophor® EL on intestinal lipoprotein processing and the potential link with P-glycoprotein in Caco-2 cells. Pharmaceutical Research. 2003;**20**(7):1085-1092. DOI: 10.1023/a:1024422625596

[78] Manjunath K, Venkateswarlu V. Pharmacokinetics, tissue distribution and bioavailability of nitrendipine solid lipid nanoparticles after intravenous and intraduodenal administration. Journal of Drug Targeting. 2006;**14**(9):632-645. DOI: 10.1080/10611860600888850

[79] O'Driscoll C, Griffin B. Biopharmaceutical challenges associated with drugs with low aqueous solubility—The potential impact of lipid-based formulations. Advanced Drug Delivery Reviews. 2008;**60**(6):617-624. DOI: 10.1016/j.addr.2007.10.012

[80] Li X, Yu M, Fan W, Gan Y, Hovgaard L, Yang M. Orally active-targeted drug delivery systems for proteins and peptides. Expert Opinion on Drug Delivery. 2014;**11**(9):1435-1447. DOI: 10.1517/17425247.2014.924500

[81] Man AL, Prieto-Garcia ME, Nicoletti C. Improving M cell mediated transport across mucosal barriers: Do certain bacteria hold the keys?

Immunology. 2004;**113**(1):15-22. DOI: 10.1111/j.1365-2567.2004.01964.x

[82] Devi RV, Basil-Rose MR. Lectins as ligands for directing nanostructured systems. Current Drug Delivery. 2018;**15**(4):448-452. DOI: 10.2174/1567201815666180108101246

[83] Wang W, Camenisch G, Sane DC, Zhang H, Hugger E, Wheeler GL, et al. A coumarin-based prodrug strategy to improve the oral absorption of RGD peptidomimetics. Journal of Controlled Release. 2000;**65**(1-2):245-251. DOI: 10.1016/s0168-3659(99)00241-2

[84] Fievez V, Plapied L, Rieux A, Pourcelle V, Freichels H, Wascotte V, et al. Targeting nanoparticles to M cells with non-peptidic ligands for oral vaccination. European Journal of Pharmaceutics and Biopharmaceutics. 2009;**73**(1):16-24. DOI: 10.1016/j.ejpb.2009.04.009

Chapter 6

Xylan-Based Hydrogels: A Polymeric Carrier for Sustained and Targeted Delivery of Drugs

Samit Kumar, Amit Kumar and Dinesh K. Mishra

Abstract

In spite of good advancement for diagnosis and treatment, cancer is the second most common disease after cardiovascular disorders, may be responsible for maximum deaths in the world. Cancer is a leading cause of death worldwide, accounting for nearly 10 million deaths in 2020. Among cancers, colon or colorectal cancer is the second most common form of cancer globally with 916,000 deaths reported annually. Colon is the largest part of large intestine extending from ileocecal junction to anus. The delivery of drugs to the targeted site such as colon requires protection to the drug. As the most of the drugs are unstable in the gastric environment of the stomach and are susceptible to absorb in the upper gastrointestinal tract (GIT). This causes poor drug bioavailability and diminishes their efficacy against inflammatory bowel diseases (IBD). Thus, to deliver a drug to the targeted site such as colon via GIT requires protection from an undesirable release in the upper GIT to achieve maximal pharmacological effect, while administered orally. As a consequence, protection of drugs can be achieved by xylan-based hydrogel polymeric carriers, which are of non-toxic and biocompatible nature, and which can also undergo in-vivo biodegradation easily.

Keywords: xylan, hydrogels, polymer, colon cancer, targeted drugs delivery

1. Introduction

Cancer is a leading cause of death worldwide, accounting for about 10 million in 2020. After lung cancer, colorectal cancer is the second most common form of cancer globally with 916,000 deaths reported annually [1]. Colorectal is a part of large intestine, extending from ileocecal junction to anus. The delivering of a drug to the targeted site for instance colon is a shattering problem as the most of the drugs have been reported to be unstable in the gastric environment of stomach and is more susceptible to absorb in the upper GIT. This causes diminished drug bioavailability and reduced their efficacy against inflammatory bowel disease (IBD). Thus drug delivery to the targeted site through GIT requires protection from an undesirable release in the upper GIT to achieve maximal pharmacological effect, while administered orally [2]. The protection of drugs can be achieved by using natural polymeric carrier-based hydrogels, such as xylan-based hydrogels, which are of non-cytotoxic [3], biocompatible nature, and which can also undergo in-vivo biodegradation easily. Hydrogels can provide spatial and sequential control over the release of various therapeutic agents, including small-molecule drugs, macromolecular drugs, and cells [4]. On account of their tunable physical properties, controllable biodegradability and capability to protect labile drugs from degradation, hydrogels serve as a molecule in which various physiochemical interactions with the encapsulated drugs control their release. Therefore, by imparting designed functionality and providing appropriate treatments of xylan-rich hemicellulose by-products can effectively be used for targeted drug delivery via hydrogel preparation. Thus, the *aim of the present research is to focus on the isolation of xylans, their derivatizations, synthesis of hydrogels, and their applications*.

2. Methods of isolation of xylan-rich hemicelluloses

Hemicelluloses are the second most abundant non-crystalline linear or branched polysaccharides after cellulosic one, which can be isolated from plant resources (**Figure 1**) or some bio-based industrial processes. It is a predominant byproduct of chemical and mechanical pulps [5, 6] in pulp industries and is severely wasted without an appropriate treatment. However, they could be used as a renewable matrix material with tunable functionality and biocompatibility in the field of pharmacy, cosmetic, food, etc. Hemicelluloses have lower molar masses than cellulose. Xylan is the principal structural hemicellulosic polysaccharides, present as 15–30% and 7–10% in hardwood and softwood, respectively. The major chain of xylan is composed of D-xylopyranosyl residues as backbone, which is linked by β-(1 → 4) glycosidic linkages, is similar to that of cellulose with a missing C-6 group. However, in marine

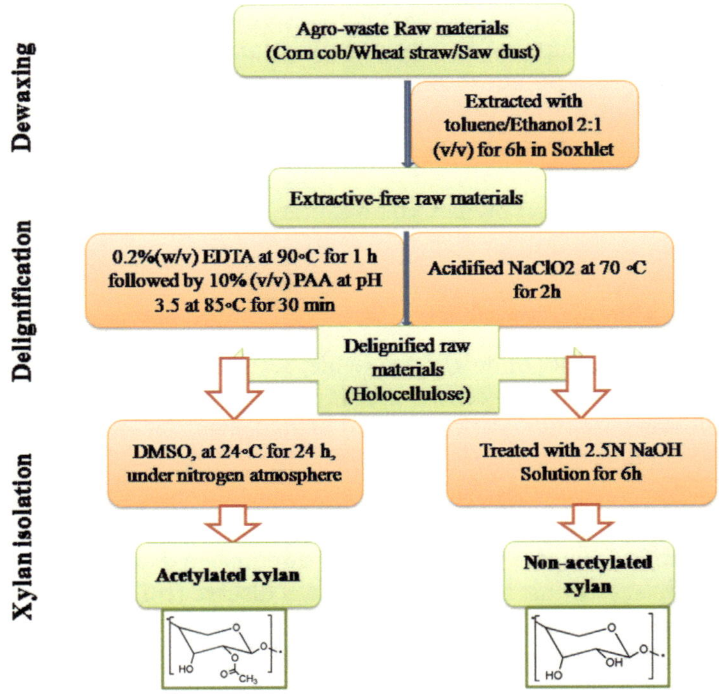

Figure 1.
Working plan for delignification and xylan isolation.

algae, xylan additionally contains β-(1 → 3) linkages. The β-(1 → 4)-D-xylopyranose unit of xylan is randomly substituted by glycosyl and acetyl groups depending on the source of the feedstock and extraction method [7, 8]. Depending upon the extraction method such as non-alkaline and alkaline treatment, xylan can be classified as acetylated (xylopyranose unit is substituted with acetyl groups) and non-acetylated (without substitution). Thus isolation of xylan can either be done by alkaline treatment or non-alkaline treatment.

The isolation of xylan from agro-waste raw materials is depicted in **Figures 1** and **2**. To isolate the xylan, the raw materials were milled into powder with uniform size of narrow distribution by mechanical agitation. The powdered raw materials were dewaxed with a mixture of toluene and ethanol in a ratio of 2:1 (v/v) in Soxhlet extractors for 12 hours. The solvent-soluble non-volatile materials were removed during the extraction known as dewaxing or extractive free process. The dewaxed/extractive free raw materials were delignified either with acidified $NaClO_2$ or with per acetic acid (PAA).

2.1 Delignification of biomass with per acetic acid

Seeing as, PAA is decomposed with metal ions thereby, the extractive free raw materials was initially treated with 0.2% (w/v) EDTA at 90°C for 1 hour to remove

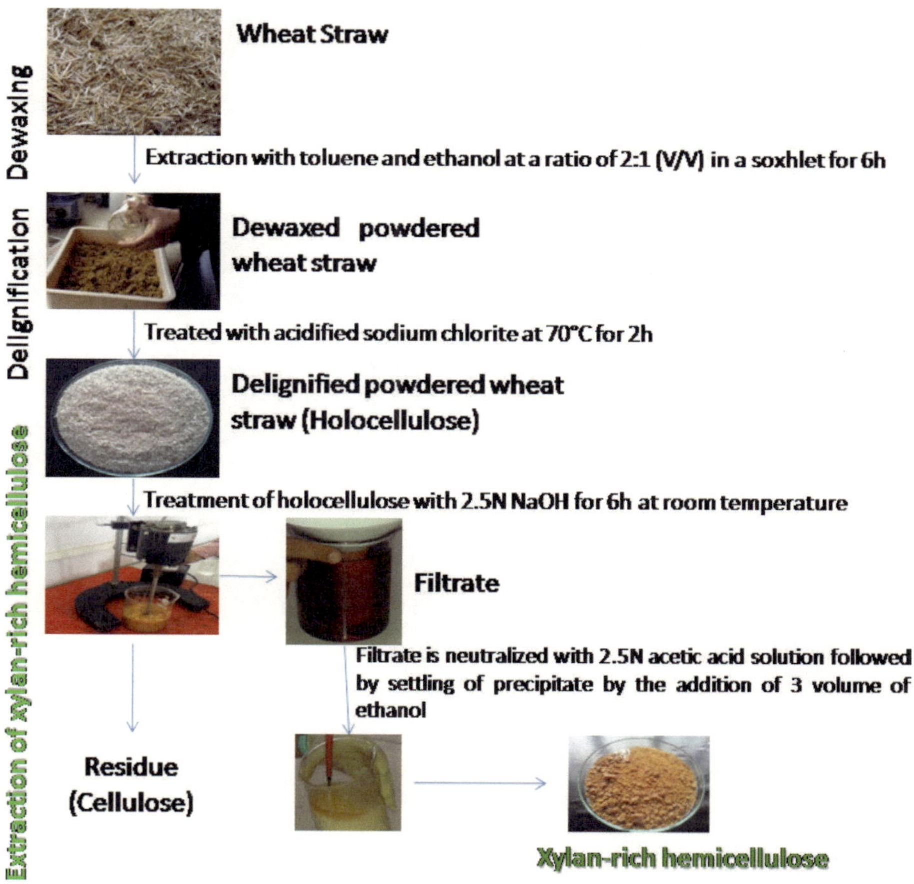

Figure 2.
Represents the steps involved in extraction of xylan-rich hemicellulose.

the metal ions prior to delignification [9]. The delignification of the extractive free materials was performed with 500 mL of 10% (v/v) PAA at pH 3.5 (adjusted with NaOH solution), at 85°C for 30 minutes with constant stirring. The system was cooled in an ice bath followed by dilution twice with distilled water. The delignified biomass (holocellulose) was collected by filtration and washing with warm distilled water and finally with acetone. The holocellulose was dried at 60°C in vacuum oven.

2.2 Delignification of biomass with acidified sodium chlorite

The delignification of biomass can also be done by acidified $NaClO_2$ at 70°C for 2 hours. The biomass obtained after delignification contains cellulose as well as hemicellulose and thus, it is collectively known as holocellulose [10].

2.3 Isolation of acetylated xylan

A sample of 6 g of delignified biomass (holocellulose) which was done either by PAA or by $NaClO_2$ was treated with 130 mL of DMSO, at room temperature for 24 hours, under inert atmosphere with constant stirring. Subsequent to the treatment, the suspension was filtered through a polystyrene membrane (porosity 60 μm) followed by washing with ~20 mL of distilled water. The filtrate was added to 600 mL of ethanol at pH 3.5 (adjusted with formic acid) and left for 12 hours at 4°C. The precipitated xylan-rich hemicelluloses were isolated by centrifugation and washing properly with methanol. The xylan-rich hemicelluloses were dried in a vacuum oven at 50°C for 24 hours. The total yield was calculated gravimetrically on oven dried basis of extractive-free biomass.

2.4 Isolation of non-acetylated xylan

The non-cellulosic product such as xylan-rich hemicelluloses was extracted from delignified biomass (holocellulose) which was obtained from agro-waste raw materials [11, 12].

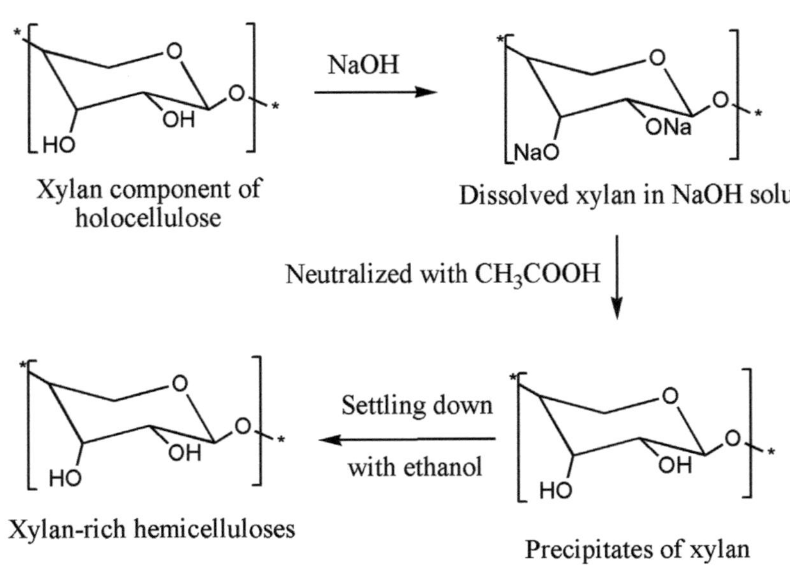

Figure 3.
Represents the chemical reactions involved.

The holocellulose was treated with 10% (2.5 N) NaOH solution with a solid to liquid ratio of 1:20 for 6 hours at room temperature. The NaOH treatment to holocellulose dissolves the xylan-rich hemicelluloses properly. The dissolved hemicellulose was filtered through Whatman No. 44 filter paper to separate it in the form of extract. The extract was further neutralized with acetic acid to get a precipitate of xylan-rich hemicellulose. The precipitate was separated by settling down after ethanol addition. Subsequently, several washing steps were performed using ethanol and filtered and dried at 60°C in vacuum oven to get xylan-rich hemicellulose. The percentage yield was calculated on oven dried basis of extractive-free raw materials. The schematic diagram of steps involved in preparation of xylan-rich hemicelluloses is represented (**Figures 2** and **3**).

3. Modification of xylan-rich hemicellulose

The extracted xylan-rich hemicellulose can easily be functionalized because of the presence of abundance of the hydroxyl moiety in its structure. The chemical modification of xylan provides more possibilities to tailor its properties, which aims to improve its applicability. Various xylan derivatives with better properties are successfully obtained after chemical modifications recently. Various methods to prepare xylan derivatives are discussed below.

3.1 Derivatization of xylan as carboxymethyl xylan (CMX)

The carboxymethyl xylan (CMX) synthesis is carried out by using sodium chloroacetate as a carboxylate group donor to xylan. On dissolution of xylan-rich hemicelluloses in NaOH solution (i.e., under alkali treatment), NaOH reacts with the hydroxyl group of xylan and generates a strong nucleophile as alkoxide ion. The alkoxide ion from the alkali xylan attacks the chloroacetate via SN2 reaction resulting in the carboxymethylation of xylan as a product. The product obtained is neutralized with acetic acid and washed with ethanol. The resulting product is filtered, centrifuged, and dried in vacuum oven [13, 14]. The degree of carboxymethylation depends on the number of hydroxyl group substituted with carboxymethyl groups. Furthermore, the product of glycolic acid and NaCl could be generated as by-products at high concentrations of sodium chloroacetate and NaOH [15] removed in the form of extract. The involved chemical reactions are represented as **Figure 4**.

3.2 Derivatization of xylan as dialdehyde xylan (DAX)

Oxidation is one of the prominently used pathways for derivatization. Oxidation of xylan is an easy and practically available method on the lab-scale now. The final

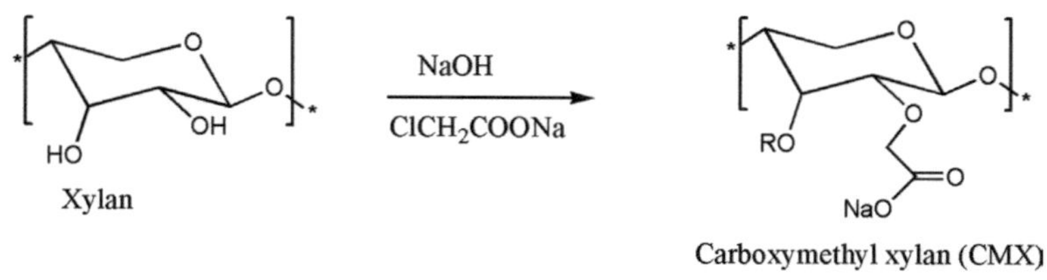

Figure 4.
Modification of xylan as carboxymethyl xylan (CMX).

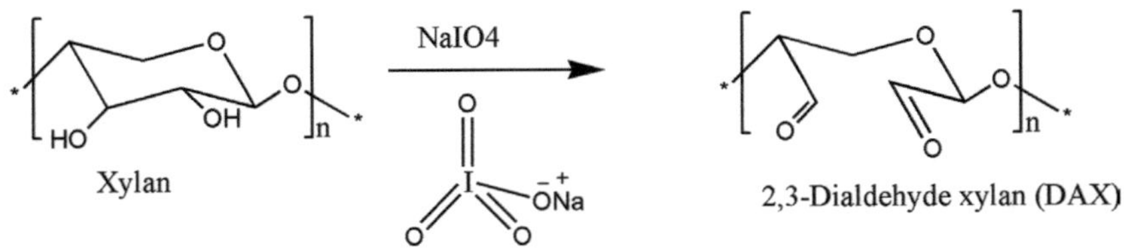

Figure 5.
Chemical reactions for the formation of DAX.

products from the oxidation of xylan called modified xylan have been proved an important role in material enhancement and functionalization.

A very well-known oxidation such as 2,2,6,6-tetramethylpiperidine 1-oxyl radical (TEMPO) oxidation used in cellulosics' material chemistry but is not pertinent to xylan, as xylan have D-xylopyranosyl residue as their building blocks, are lacking of primary hydroxyl group, which are the primary target of the TEMPO oxidation. Therefore, in oxidative xylan modification primarily sodium periodate is used, as it is easily and practically applied on the lab scale. Periodate oxidative cleavage of vicinal diol (i.e., cleavage of C2–C3 bond) is resulting in "dialdehyde polymers", which have a number of interesting applications in tissue engineering, drug delivery and as flocculating agents, and for ion-exchange separation. The resulting dialdehyde polymers exist as 2,3-hemialdal forms, which can be used for further functionalization [6, 16] particularly to prepare hydrogels. The preparation of DAX has been shown in **Figure 5**.

3.3 Derivatization of xylan as xylan methacrylate (XMA)

Another method for xylan modification is developed by Lin et al. [17] where xylan was dissolved in dimethyl sulfoxide (DMSO) at 95°C followed by addition of the catalyst 4-dimethylaminopyridine (DMAP) and cooling the mixture at room temperature. The reaction mixture was stirred for 30 minutes at room temperature. Later

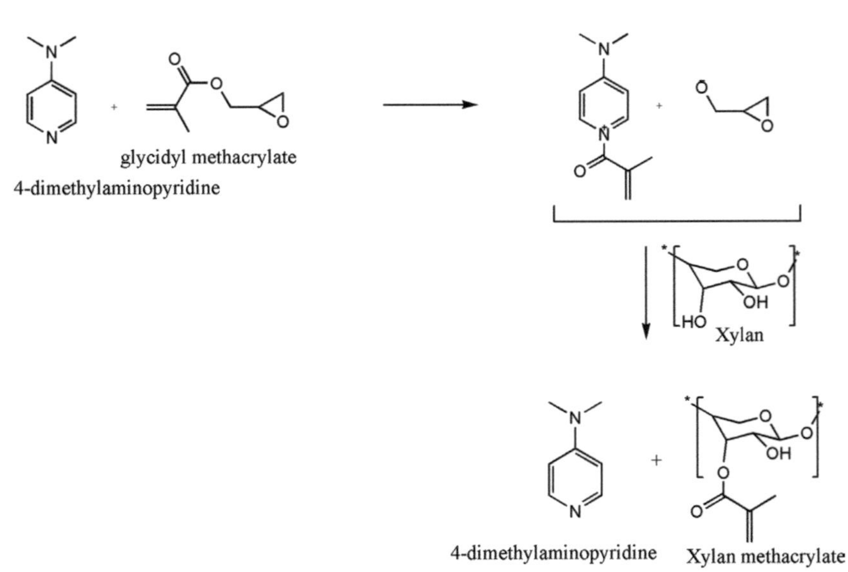

Figure 6.
Chemical reactions for the formation of xylan methacrylate.

on, glycidyl methacrylate was added and the final reaction mixture was stirred for 24 hours. The reaction mixture was precipitated with anhydrous ethanol and filtered. The obtained precipitate was washed with anhydrous ethanol three times. In this way modified xylan (MX) was obtained as xylan methacrylate as light brown in color. The schematic diagram is represented as **Figure 6**.

4. Preparation of hydrogel using modified xylan

Hydrogels are physical or chemical cross-linked three-dimensional polymer networks which swell upon by absorbing water without dissolving in it. The shape and the volume of hydrogels can be reversibly changed by various external stimuli such as pH, temperature, light, and electric and magnetic fields. Xylan is a renewable natural polymer bearing the advantages over other polymers in terms of non-toxicity, biocompatibility, biodegradability, and natural abundance. The ease of functionalization or chemical cross-linking of the hydroxyl moieties present in the backbone of xylan make it an attractive precursor for hydrogel preparation. Recently, xylan-based hydrogels have gained attention because of the multi-responsive behavior toward pH, organic solvents, and ions.

4.1 Preparation of hydrogel using carboxymethyl xylan as a precursor

Hydrogel using CMX, a modified xylan is prepared by dissolving it in distilled water and stirring it at 60°C in a water bath followed by addition of ammonium persulfate (APS) solution, acrylic acid, and methylene-bis-acrylamide (MBA). A series of chemical reaction takes place in the mixture which is continued for about 4 hours and results as hydrogels which is taken out and washed with water properly and cut into small pieces [17]. The chemical reactions for the preparation of hydrogel are presented in **Figure 7**.

4.2 Preparation of hydrogel using dialdehyde xylan as a precursor

In this method, prepared dialdehyde xylan (DAX) as shown in **Figure 5**, a biocompatible gel material employed as a biopolymer-based crosslinker to enable the formation of 3D gel network. The transparent, clean, and non-toxic DAX-crosslinked hydrogel could be obtained from the Schiff base reaction between aldehyde groups of DAX and amino groups of gelatin (G) [16, 18]. The demonstrated xylan-based hydrogel through a simple approach opened a new door for skin care products from natural and renewable biomass (**Figure 8**).

4.3 Preparation of hydrogel using carboxymethyl cellulose (CMC) as a precursor

Carboxymethyl cellulose (CMC) is used as a precursor for preparation of stimuli-responsive hydrogels. The carboxymethyl group adds a negative charge to the pyranose backbone of xylan, and it significantly increases the cross-linking points and reactive sites. Thus, thermal radical reactions are often employed with the cross-linker to prepare CMC-based homopolymer and copolymer hydrogels. Overall, the CMC-based hydrogels are used as carriers for drugs and biological macromolecules.

CMC-based hydrogel is prepared by dissolving the carboxymethyl cellulose to distilled water followed by the addition of potassium persulfate (KPS) at 70°C for

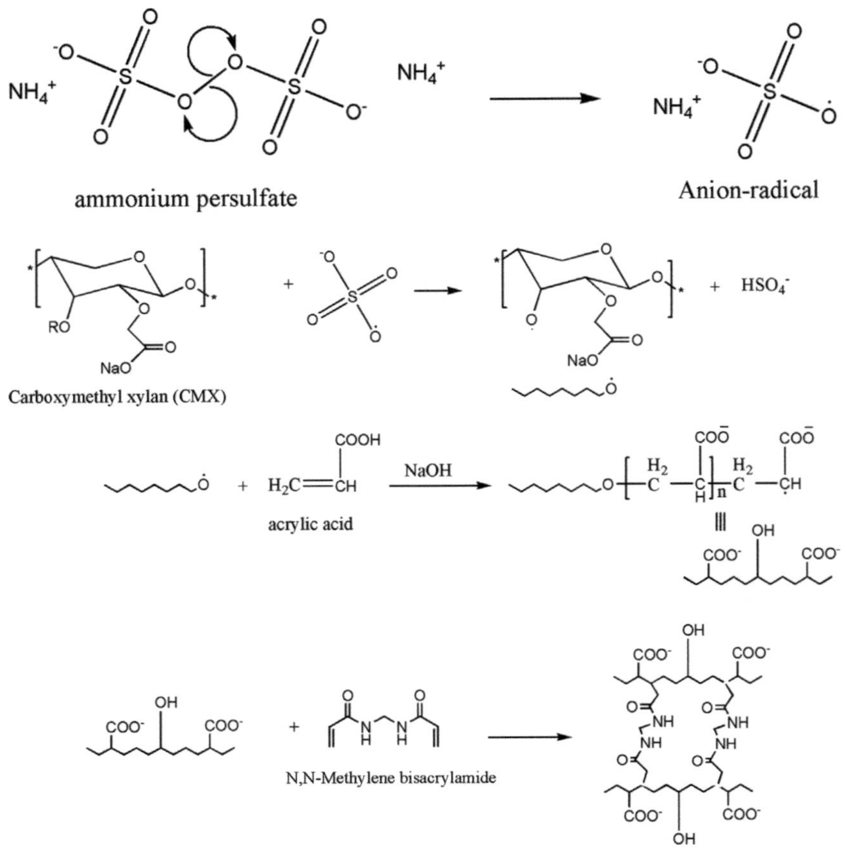

Figure 7.
Reactions involved in the preparation of hydrogel from CMX.

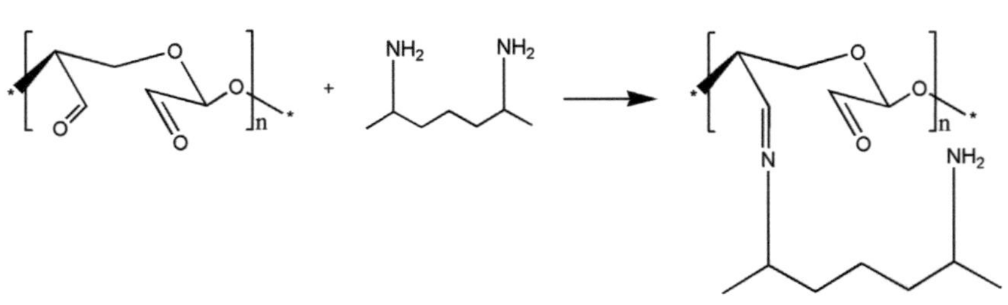

Figure 8.
Reaction involved in the preparation of hydrogel from DAX.

half an hour. The neutralized acrylic acid (AA) is added into the reaction mixture and subsequently the continuing stirred for about 2 hours. Thereafter, the pH of the reaction mixture is raised upto 8 by the addition of NaOH solution. The resulting outcome is precipitated by the addition of acetone. The precipitates of CMC-g-PNaA are dried in a vacuum oven for 24 hours at 60°C.

The CMC-g-PNaA (2% w/v) is further dissolved in distilled water by using a mechanical stirrer at 300 rpm for 6 hours. Then, 50 mL of CMC-g-PNaA solution is added dropwise in the 100 mL aqueous solution of $FeCl_3$ (0.02 mol). The mixture converts into spherical hydrogel beads which are filtered, washed with distilled water,

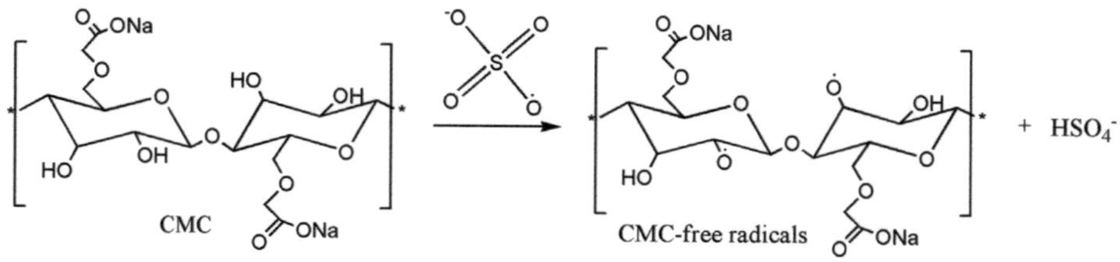

Figure 9.
Chemical reactions of CMC react with radical-anion to form CMC-free radicals.

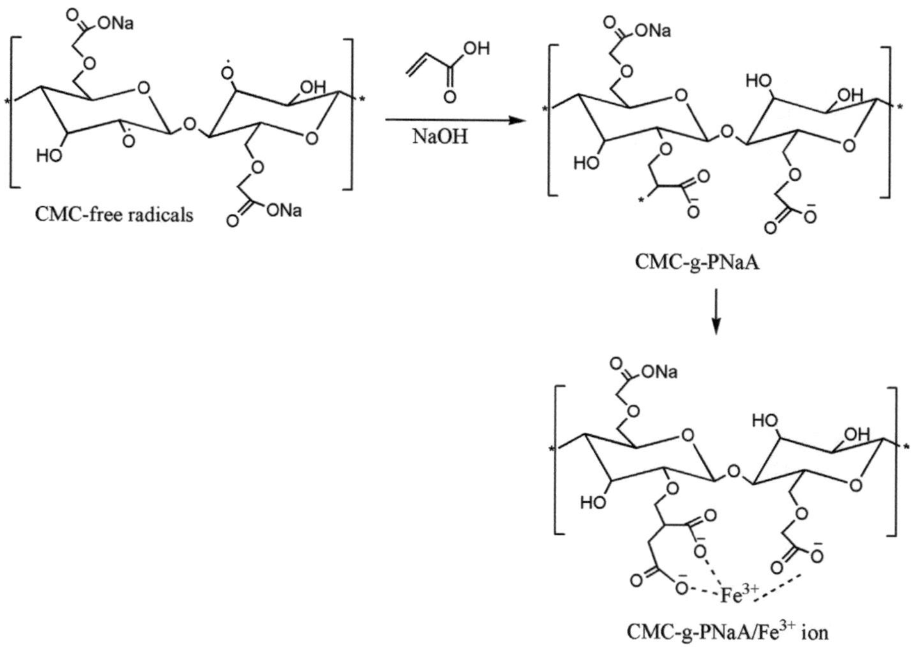

Figure 10.
Chemical reactions of CMC-free radicals with AA and finally with ferric ions.

and dried in a vacuum oven for 24 hours [19]. The chemical reactions involved in preparation of hydrogel from CMC are shown in **Figures 9** and **10**.

5. Optimization of physico-chemical properties of hydrogels

The hydrogels had been prepared using different ratios of precursors and cross-linkers. The prepared hydrogels had been optimized on the basis of biocompatibility, biodegradability, swelling ratio, mechanical strength, and pore size. The pore-size of hydrogels could be improved by using different inorganic or organic pore-forming agents. The chain length and the molecular weight of organic pore-forming agents such as polyethylene glycol 2000, carbamide, and polyvinyl pyrrolidone had an important influence on the pore size, the compressive strength, and the swelling ratio. However, among inorganic pore-forming agents such as NaCl, $CaCO_3$, and $NaHCO_3$, hydrogels with $NaHCO_3$ displayed a great performance in terms of the pore size of the hydrogels, mechanical properties, and drug release. Moreover, the pore-forming agents had little influence on the thermal stability of the hydrogels. The strength of hydrogels could also be enhanced by the formation of coordination bonds between Zn^{2+} and anionic groups such as $-COO^-$ when hydrogel is immersed in the solution of $ZnCl_2$ [20].

6. Applications of xylan-based hydrogels

Xylan-rich-hemicellulose-based hydrogels have many promising applications for the researchers and scientists as:

6.1 Super adsorbent

Colored effluents of industries can be highly toxic and carcinogenic, causing a great danger to living organisms. As organic dye effluents have complex chemical structure, high hydrophilicity and stability, resistant to their removal poses difficulties for wastewater treatment [21]. Technologies such as coagulation and flocculation, oxidation, adsorption, membrane separation, and electro-coagulation methods [22, 23] have been used to treat colored wastewater. Among these, the adsorption method is regarded as one of the most attractive processes because of its easy operation and high removal efficiency. The xylan-based hydrogels showed outstanding adsorption capacity for organic dyes removal instead of its excellent properties of biodegradability and renewability [24–26]. Sun and co-workers were prepared a novel adsorbent composite hydrogel of acylated xylan and silanized graphene oxide via free radical polymerization reactions. The composite hydrogel based-adsorbent showed excellent removal capacity of Cu^{2+} ions from an aqueous solution. Study of adsorption thermodynamics showed the adsorption of Cu^{2+} ions was endothermal and spontaneous, and the adsorption amount rose with an increase in temperature. In addition, higher desorption percentages of Cu^{2+} ions from the used hydrogel were also achieved up to 77.3% after recycling for six times. Thus, all obtained results were indicated that the prepared hydrogel is promising for water treatment and collection of metal ions [27].

6.2 Sensitive response to H_2O_2 detection

Acetylated xylan-based magnetic Fe_3O_4 nano-composite hydrogels were prepared by fabricating Fe_3O_4 particles within a hydrogel matrix. The hydrogel matrix was synthesized by graft copolymerization reaction of acetylated xylan (porous nature of hydrogels were increased by introducing the acetyl functional group) with acrylamide and N-isopropylacrylamide under ultraviolet irradiation. The magnetic hydrogels were accessible to excellent catalytic activity and provided a sensitive response to H_2O_2 detection even at low concentration. The approach to prepare magnetic hydrogels endows with promising applications in the field of environmental chemistry [28].

6.3 Photodynamic antimicrobial chemotherapy (PACT)

The use of most of the existing photosensitizers has been harshly hampered because of their significant self-quenching effect, poor water solubility, lack of selectivity against bacterial cells, and possible damage to the surrounding tissues. Therefore, to overcome the limitations, the PS encapsulated hydrogels were prepared recently. Recently, hydrophilic photosensitizer (PS) for instance 5, 10, 15, 20-tetrakis (1-methylpyridinium-4-yl)porphyrin tetraiodide (TMPyP) incorporated xylan-based hydrogels were synthesized which showed prolonged release of PS up to 24 hours with a cumulative release of 100%. TMPyP-loaded hydrogel were effective against *Pseudomonas aeruginosa*, *Escherichia coli*, *Staphylococcus aureus* strains, and *Bacillus cereus*, while ineffective in the dark. This PACT showed to be promising antimicrobial treatment to overcome the challenges of multidrug resistant bacteria [29].

6.4 Skin care

The bio-compatibility [11] and cyto-compatibility [6] of xylan based hydrogels were confirmed through experiments and thereby the fabricated hydrogels may be used as a potential material in skin. Fu and co-workers were prepared attractive hydrogels by using dialdehyde xylan (DAX) as a crosslinker for substrate gelatine (G). The properties of hydrogels were further improved in terms of texture, antibacterial, and cyto-compatibility by the introduction of glycerol (Gly) and nicotinamide (NCA) and the prepared DAX-G-Gly-NCA hydrogel showed highly fascinating materials in the application of skin care [6].

6.5 Targeted drug carriers

The delivery of drugs to the colorectal is the major problem in the treatment of colorectal cancer because of the instability of drugs in the gastric environment of upper GIT. This problem can be solved if the release time of drugs extended or drugs are binded strongly with the matrix material. Hore and Kohne [30] showed delayed drug release by enhancing the binding of a loaded drug to the hydrogel matrix. The multi-responsive (temperature, pH, and magnetic) xylan-based hydrogels encapsulate the magnetic nanoparticles which would facilitate drug release in specific region and realize drug controlled delivery remotely [11]. In a study, the drug loading to the hydrogel is done by immersing the dried hydrogel to the phosphate buffer saline (PBS) solution having pH 7.4. The drug loading and cumulative drug release properties of a hydrogel could be improved significantly using pore-forming agents. Suitable pore-forming agents gave rise to the enhancement of the drug release properties of the hydrogels due to the introduction of desirable pores within the network of the hydrogels. Study showed that the cumulative drug release has been substantially improved up to 71.05%, when hydrogel prepared with $NaHCO_3$ pore-forming agent [31]. Gao and co-workers [11] prepared a pH susceptible xylan-based hydrogels with *N*-isopropylacrylamide (NIPAm) and acrylic acid (AA) using *N,N′*-methylene-bis-acrylamide (MBA) as a cross-linker and 2,2-dimethoxy-2-phenylacetophenone as a photoinitiator by using ultraviolet irradiation. The prepared hydrogels showed efficient encapsulation efficiency of acetylsalicylic acid (upto 97.6%) and cumulative release of 26.35 and 90.12% in the gastric and intestinal fluid, respectively. The porous xylan-β-cyclodextrin based hydrogels were synthesized by using glycol diglycidyl ether as a crosslinker in alkaline medium. The model drugs of curcumin and 5-fluorouracil (5-FU) were loaded 26 and 56%, respectively. Furthermore, the hydrogels were showed the highest cumulative release of 37% curcumin and 56% 5-FU and after 24 hours [32].

7. Conclusions

The most of the drugs have been reported to be unstable in the gastric environment and are susceptible to absorption in the upper gastrointestinal tract (GIT) therefore; delivery of a drug to the targeted site via GIT requires protection. The protection of drugs can be achieved by encapsulation within polymeric network of xylan based-hydrogels. The drug-loading and drug-release profile can further be enhanced by pore-forming agent. The non-cytotoxic and biocompatible nature of hydrogels endow to skin care application. The photosensitizers encapsulated hydrogels showed promising antimicrobial treatment to overcome the challenges of multidrug resistant bacteria. The acetylated xylan-based polymeric network of hydrogels encapsulates the magnetic nanoparticles which endow the excellent catalytic activity and provide a sensitive response to H_2O_2 detection even at low concentration.

Acknowledgements

Authors would like to acknowledge the AKS University for the financial support and facilities in carrying out this research work.

Conflicts of interest

The authors declare no conflict of interest.

Author details

Samit Kumar[1*], Amit Kumar[2] and Dinesh K. Mishra[1]

1 Department of Chemistry, Faculty of basic Sciences, AKS University, Satna, Madhya Pradesh, India

2 Department of Dairy Chemistry, G.N. Patel College of Dairy Technology, Kamdhenu University, Banaskantha, Gujarat, India

*Address all correspondence to: samitiitr07@gmail.com

References

[1] https://www.who.int/news-room/fact-sheets/detail/cancer

[2] Sinha VR, Kumria R. Microbially triggered drug delivery to the colon. European Journal of Pharmaceutical Sciences. 2003;**18**(1):3-18

[3] Tanodekaew S, Channasanon S, Uppanan P. Xylan/polyvinyl alcohol blend and its performance as hydrogel. Journal of Applied Polymer Science. 2006;**100**(3):1914-1918

[4] Li J, Mooney DJ. Designing hydrogels for controlled drug delivery. Nature Reviews Materials. 2016;**1**(12):1-17

[5] Fischer K, Schmidt I. Hemicellulose in dissolving pulp and its behavior during its processing to viscose. Macromolecular Symposia. 2008;**262**:85-88

[6] Fu GQ, Zhang SC, Chen GG, Hao X, Bian J, Peng F. Xylan-based hydrogels for potential skin care application. International Journal of Biological Macromolecules. 2020;**158**:244-250

[7] Ebringerová A, Heinze T. Xylan and xylan derivatives–biopolymers with valuable properties, 1. Naturally occurring xylans structures, isolation procedures and properties. Macromolecular Rapid Communications. 2000;**21**(9):542-556

[8] Kumar S, Negi YS. Corn cob xylan-based nanoparticles: Ester prodrug of 5-aminosalicylic acid for possible targeted delivery of drug. Journal of Pharmaceutical Sciences and Research. 2012;**4**(12):1995

[9] Brienzo M, Siqueira AF, Milagres AM. Search for optimum conditions of sugarcane bagasse hemicellulose extraction. Biochemical Engineering Journal. 2009;**46**(2):199-204

[10] Kumar S, Upadhyaya JS, Negi YS. Preparation of nanoparticles from corn cobs by chemical treatment methods. BioResources. 2010;**5**(2):1292-1300

[11] Gao C, Ren J, Zhao C, Kong W, Dai Q, Chen Q, et al. Xylan-based temperature/pH sensitive hydrogels for drug controlled release. Carbohydrate Polymers. 2016;**151**:189-197

[12] Kumar S, Negi YS. Nanoparticles synthesis from corn cob (xylan) and their potential application as colon-specific drug carrier. In: Macromolecular Symposia. Vol. 320. Weinheim: WILEY-VCH Verlag; 2012. pp. 75-80

[13] Queirós LC, Sousa SC, Duarte AF, Domingues FC, Ramos AM. Development of carboxymethyl xylan films with functional properties. Journal of Food Science and Technology. 2017;**54**(1):9-17

[14] Li N, Sun D, Su Z, Hao X, Li M, Ren J, et al. Rapid fabrication of xylan-based hydrogel by graft polymerization via a dynamic lignin-Fe^{3+} plant catechol system. Carbohydrate Polymers. 2021;**269**:118306

[15] Sun XF, Zeng Q, Wang H, Hao Y. Preparation and swelling behavior of pH/temperature responsive semi-IPN hydrogel based on carboxymethyl xylan and poly (N-isopropyl acrylamide). Cellulose. 2019;**26**(3):1909-1922

[16] Amer H, Nypelö T, Sulaeva I, Bacher M, Henniges U, Potthast A, et al. Synthesis and characterization of periodate-oxidized polysaccharides: Dialdehyde xylan (DAX). Biomacromolecules. 2016;**17**(9):2972-2980

[17] Lin Y, Fang G, Deng Y, Shen K, Huang C, Wu T. A pH-sensitive xylan-based superabsorbent hydrogel for the removal of methylene blue from water. BioResources. 2019;**14**(3):5573-5585

[18] Chemin M, Rakotovelo A, Ham-Pichavant F, Chollet G, da Silva Perez D, Petit-Conil M, et al. Synthesis and characterization of functionalized 4-O-methylglucuronoxylan derivatives. Holzforschung. 2015;**69**(6):713-720

[19] Kumar B, Priyadarshi R, Deeba F, Kulshreshtha A, Gaikwad KK, Kim J, et al. Nanoporous sodium carboxymethyl cellulose-G-poly (sodium acrylate)/ $FeCl_3$ hydrogel beads: Synthesis and characterization. Gels. 2020;**6**(4):49

[20] Kong W, Huang D, Xu G, Ren JL, Liu CF, Zhao LH, et al. A new design strategy for graphene oxide/ polyacrylamide/aluminium ion-crosslinked carboxymethyl hemicelluloses nanocomposite hydrogels with highly tough and elastic properties. Chemistry: An Asian Journal. 2016;**11**:1697-1704

[21] Mohammed N, Grishkewich N, Berry RM, Tam KC. Cellulose nanocrystal–alginate hydrogel beads as novel adsorbents for organic dyes in aqueous solutions. Cellulose. 2015;**22**(6):3725-3738

[22] Wang Q, Tian S, Cun J, Ning P. Degradation of methylene blue using a heterogeneous Fenton process catalyzed by ferrocene. Desalination and Water Treatment. 2013;**51**(28-30):5821-5830

[23] Katheresan V, Kansedo J, Lau SY. Efficiency of various recent wastewater dye removal methods: A review. Journal of Environmental Chemical Engineering. 2018;**6**(4):4676-4697

[24] Zhou Y, Fu S, Liu H, Yang S, Zhan H. Removal of methylene blue dyes from wastewater using cellulose-based superadsorbent hydrogels. Polymer Engineering & Science. 2011;**51**(12):2417-2424

[25] Yu SJ, Wang XX, Pang HW, Zhang R, Song WC. Boron nitride-based materials for the removal of pollutants from aqueous solutions: A review. Chemical Engineering Journal. 2018;**333**:343-360

[26] Xiang Z, Tang N, Jin X, Gao W. Fabrications and applications of hemicellulose-based bio-adsorbents. Carbohydrate Polymers. 2022;**278**:118945

[27] Sun XF, Xie Y, Shan S, Li W, Sun L. Chemically-crosslinked xylan/graphene oxide composite hydrogel for copper ions removal. Journal of Polymers and the Environment. 2022;**30**:3999-4013

[28] Dai QQ, Ren JL, Peng F, Chen XF, Gao CD, Sun RC. Synthesis of acylated xylan-based magnetic Fe_3O_4 hydrogels and their application for H_2O_2 detection. Materials. 2016;**9**(8):690

[29] Elkihel A, Christie C, Vernisse C, Ouk TS, Lucas R, Chaleix V, et al. Xylan-based cross-linked hydrogel for photodynamic antimicrobial chemotherapy. ACS Applied Bio Materials. 2021;**4**(9):7204-7212

[30] Hoare TR, Kohane DS. Hydrogels in drug delivery: Progress and challenges. Polymer. 2008;**49**(8):1993-2007

[31] Chang M, Liu X, Meng L, Wang X, Ren J. Xylan-based hydrogels as a potential carrier for drug delivery: Effect of pore-forming agents. Pharmaceutics. 2018;**10**(4):261

[32] Gami P, Kundu D, Seera SDK, Banerjee T. Chemically crosslinked xylan–β-cyclodextrin hydrogel for the in vitro delivery of curcumin and 5-fluorouracil. International Journal of Biological Macromolecules. 2020;**158**:18-31

Chapter 7

Porphyrinoid Photosensitizers for Targeted and Precise Photodynamic Therapy: Progress in Fabrication

Devika Sivakumar, Rakhi Raju, Y.T. Kamal, Shahana Salam, Sabna Kotta and Rahul Soman

Abstract

This chapter focuses on basic facts and details of photodynamic therapy (PDT). PDT's ability to cause cytotoxicity has led to its applications for a variety of medical conditions other than cancer treatment. This adaptable technology has some advantages in treating severe illness situations such as cancer, alopecia, angina pectoris, and periodontitis. It stands out even more because of the interaction of three elements: light, a photosensitizer (PS), and cellular oxygen. By preventing PS accumulation in normal vegetative cells, targeted photodynamic therapy plays an important role in achieving better accumulation of PS in a specific area. This section discusses various types of targeting methods, such as active targeting, passive targeting, and peptide-mediated targeting. Aid in both diagnosing and curing diseases, gaining widespread acceptance. It is a promising therapeutic approach with a lot of potential.

Keywords: photodynamic therapy, porphyrin photosensitizers, targeted drug delivery, theranostics, photodynamic antimicrobial chemotherapy

1. Introduction

Photodynamic therapy, also known as PDT, is a versatile treatment strategy, commonly used for cancer mitigation that combines three non-toxic components to cause the death of the target cell: light, a photosensitizer (PS), and tissue oxygen [1]. As we know conventional cancer therapy has various drawbacks due to serious adverse effects [2]. However, in the case of PDT such side effects are comparatively minimal and relatively less documented. PDT always ensures that cells are effectively targeted and damaged through necrosis or apoptosis [3].

Photosensitizers (PS) are organic or inorganic molecules that can be triggered by visible light and can produce reactive oxygen species (ROS) [4]. The PS can absorb the light energy and excite from the ground to its higher energy excited state. As shown in **Figure 1**, during the relaxation process, ROS production occurs by utilizing tissue/cellular oxygen to

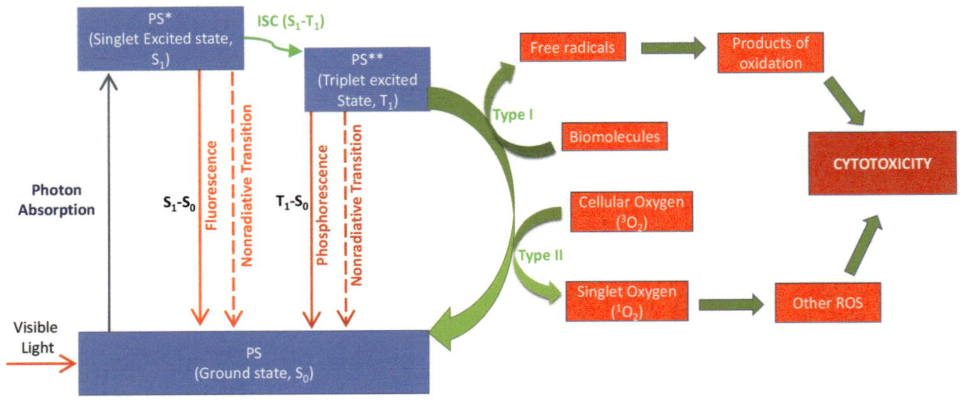

Figure 1.
Modified Jablonski diagram showing the mechanism of PDT.

cause cellular damage using apoptosis or necrosis [5]. The key benefits of this mechanism are that only localized cells are destroyed and limiting the toxicity in the tumor environment. The selectivity of PS to the target tissue is a key factor while designing a PDT system, otherwise irrespective of tissues, PS can damage the normal vegetative tissues also [6].

There are a few porphyrinoid-based PS with interesting ROS-producing abilities and better selectivity to the target tissue. A few US and Indian-approved porphyrinoid PS includes Photofrin II, ALA (prodrug), and Foscan. PDT now has a wide range of applications, ranging from illness prevention to diagnosis [3]. Every day, a new class of porphyrinoid photosensitizers is being discovered, allowing for the treatment of an expanding range of illnesses. PDT offers the advantage of treating solid tumors at all phases of the disease, from early to advanced, and that too non-invasively. Rather it has been shown to treat a variety of diseases ranging from skin disorders to cardiovascular and ocular diseases. Targeting takes place in both passive and active methods, with nanoparticles, peptides, proteins, and polyclonal as well as monoclonal antibodies (mAb), or any other systems that direct PS toward targeted cancer cells or tissue and avoid the localization of PS inside healthy normal cells. Passive targeting uses the EPR effect to deliver the medicine to the target location, whereas active targeting uses proteins, ligands, and pores to cross the cells and deliver the drug to the target site [7].

The ability of photosensitizers to act as diagnostic and theranostic agents is one of their growing applications. The concept has only lately gained popularity, although PDT has already established it through fluorescence imaging. Diagnostics refers to the use of fluorescence, MRI, NIR, photoacoustic PET, and SPECT imaging to aid in the diagnosis of a certain disease or metabolic pathway. Theranostic in the sense of possessing both diagnostic and disease-mitigating capabilities. Real-time imaging can assess dosimetry, medication efficacy, kinetics, singlet oxygen production, light delivery, oxygen pitch, blood gush, neighboring cells, and the status of the targeted cells or tissues [8].

For example, nano texaphyrin, a novel theranostic compound linked with a prostate-specific membrane antigen (PSMA) used in targeted radionucleotide imaging and focal photodynamic therapy. The creation of an activatable theranostic is currently the primary emphasis. As an inert chemical, some stimuli, such as pH and temperature, will activate inside the target. Another classic example is Photofrin having both photosensitizing and fluorescence capabilities.

Furthermore, the cost of this therapeutic procedure is not too expensive. With personalized PDT, PS dose, frequency, and side effects can be minimized. It will aid in the provision of individualized treatments, which is now more vital than ever. PDT is becoming more popular in the field of biotechnology, which will result in less pollution and greater human health compliance [9].

2. Photodynamic therapy

Tetrapyrrolic pigments with porphyrinoid origin are frequently used as photosensitizing agents in PDT [3]. The reactive oxygen species (ROS) required for the photodynamic effect can be produced efficiently by these porphyrinoid systems. Apart from that, these porphyrin-based systems exhibit fluorescence. The fluorescent photosensitizers with cancer-targeting properties can be used to perform cancer diagnosis and fluorescence-guided surgery with fluorescence imaging techniques. Porphyrinoids can form strong coordination complexes with a variety of metals including gadolinium. This approach can be effectively utilized for developing porphyrin-based magnetic resonance imaging (MRI) contrasting agents for MRI imaging as a diagnostic tool. The current treatment modalities change more toward theranostic approaches. These multifunctional substances have both medicinal and diagnostic capabilities in a single molecule and are the major focus of the current research [10, 11]. Theranostic will be heavily used in future tailored therapies and medication delivery. It could be called "P4 medications," or in other words, preventive, personalized, participatory, and predictive medicine [12, 13]. In addition to fluorescence-guided imaging, other diagnostic techniques, such as magnetic resonance imaging and photoacoustic imaging, can be tried depending on the PS when constructing PDT [14, 15]. One of the most difficult challenges in the molecular design of PS for PDT is the ability to selectively target a specific sick tissue or organ. Different carrier techniques or formulation approaches can be tested to improve cancer targeting to provide a selectively focused effect [16, 17]. Various methods, such as carbon nanodots, pH- and temperature-sensitive nanoparticles, and liposomes, have been developed to deliver medications deeply into tumors [18, 19]. Apart from cancer, PDT has greater acceptance in the treatment of conditions, such as acne vulgaris alopecia, and vitiligo [20, 21]. As a result, PDT is a viable therapeutic approach with all of its benefits.

2.1 Components of PDT

Here we will be discussing three essential components of PDT as shown in **Figure 2** (1) photosensitizer; (2) light; (3) tissue oxygen.

2.1.1 Photosensitizer

Photosensitizers (PS) are either endogenous or exogenous substances; they should not possess any toxicity at specified doses in absence of light [22]. A classic example of endogenous PS is Protoporphyrin IX, which is obtained by metabolizing 5-ALA [23, 24]. The tissue penetration capability of light is shown in **Figure 3**, so the absorption and emission characteristics of PS have a significant role in their photodynamic action. The molecular structural factors of PS are important in their transport and localization.

2.1.2 Light source

The light of a particular wavelength, where the PS has a very good ε value plays an important role in PDT. The selection of light source was done by considering other

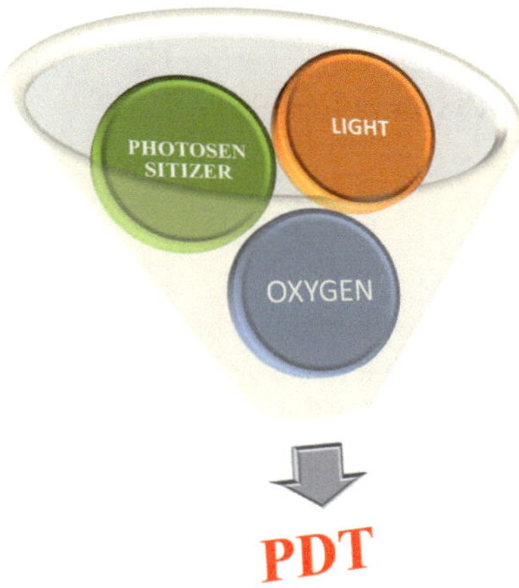

Figure 2.
Components of PDT.

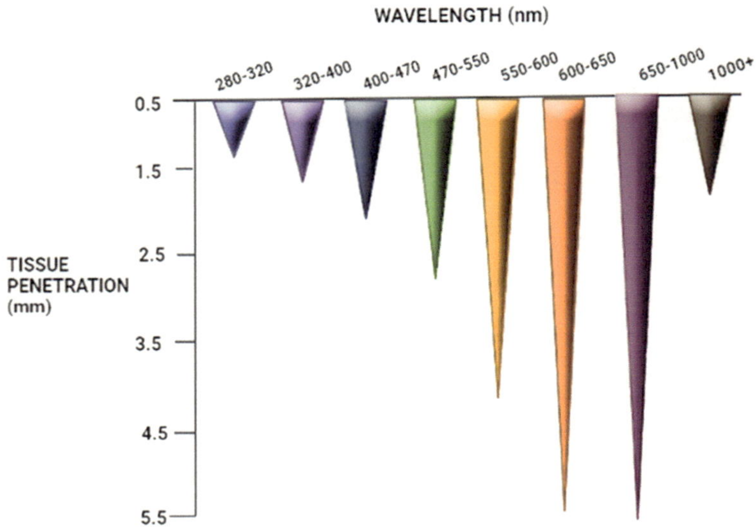

Figure 3.
Comparative tissue penetration ability of different wavelengths of light [25].

factors also, such as the target location, photosensitizer used, and fluence rate of light (*i.e.,* number of photons per unit area) (**Figure 3**). A stable light source with excellent conformity helps in targeted PDT by enhancing tumor control impact and reducing collateral damage to nearby tissues. Uniform lighting can be obtained by mounting micro-lens or diffusing cover on the tip of optical fibers [26, 27]. **Figure 3** demonstrates different wavelength lights and their tissue penetration ability [25].

2.1.3 Tissue oxygen

The third major component in PDT is molecular oxygen. In many cases, reduced blood flow to grown tumors leads to hypoxia [28]. Molecular oxygen is one of the important components in therapy to produce ROS. There are two methods to increase the availability of oxygen in an affected specific area, *that is*, indirect and direct introduction of oxygen. Conversion of intracellular hydrogen peroxide to oxygen by enzyme catalysis and to combat tumor hypoxia, oxygen carriers such as perfluorocarbons and hemoglobin are frequently introduced into photodynamic therapy [29].

2.2 History of PDT

The process of PDT entails selectively making tissues light-sensitive. From antiquity to the current era, light has been used as a therapeutic aid in medicine and surgery. Ancient Greece, Egypt, and India, all had phototherapy, but it was lost for many centuries before being rediscovered by western civilization around the turn of the twentieth century [8, 30, 31].

The Danish doctor Niels Finsen was the first to describe the use of modern phototherapy. To cure Lupus vulgaris, a skin disorder caused by tuberculosis, he used Finsen Lamp, a heat-filtered carbon-arc lamp, to effectively demonstrate photodynamic therapy. In 1903, he won the Nobel prize in medicine [30].

Oscar Raab, a student of Professor Hermann Von Tappeiner from Munich in 1901, was the first who described the idea of phototoxicity caused by the interaction of light and acridine orange. He observed the fatal effects of light and acridine orange combination on paramecium species (malaria-causing protozoa). Following the initial reports, PDT research found additional possible photosensitizers, primarily those connected to porphyrins. The timeline to PDT is explained very well in **Figure 4** [32, 33].

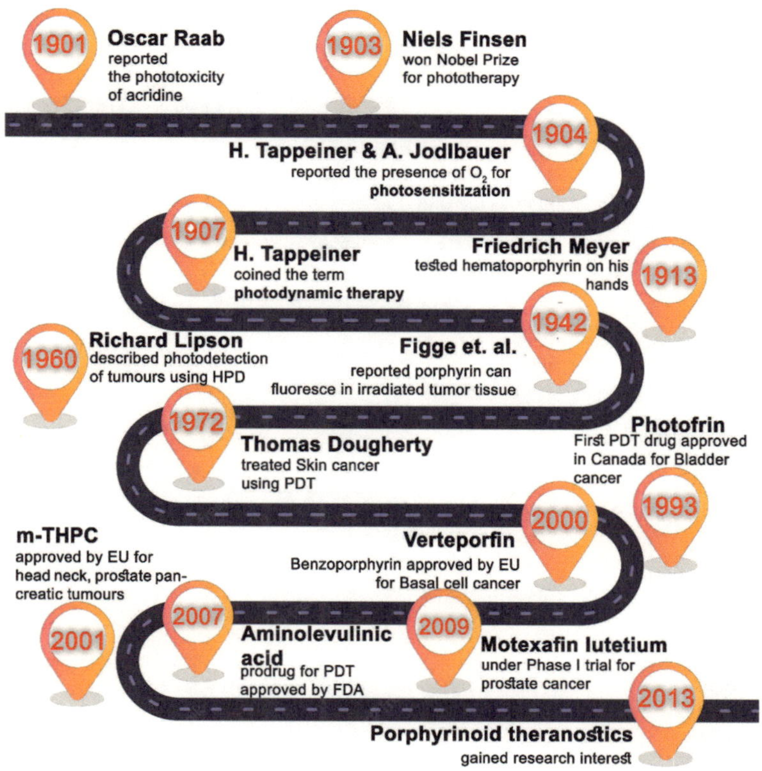

Figure 4.
Roadmap to photodynamic therapy.

Later research in Von Tappeiner's lab popularized the term "Photodynamic action" and demonstrated the significance of oxygen in PDT. In 1907, Tappeiner first proposed the name "*Photodynamic therapy*" in one of his books to describe the process of oxygen-dependent photosensitization. Before 1907 itself, the group recorded the fluorescence of porphyrins from tumors, and tumor targeting through PDT was achieved [34, 35]. During the 1970s, T. Dougherty studied the photosensitizing ability of Fluorescein diacetate [8, 16]. Then K. Weishaupt and T. Dougherty discovered the requirement of singlet oxygen during the process of PDT [36]. Thus, in the initial days, more efficiently singlet oxygen-producing molecules with better deep skin penetration capacity were used as photosensitizers.

The scientist Hans Fischer got a Nobel prize in 1930 for his research on the synthesis of hemin and chlorophyll [37, 38]. Later, T. Dougherty rediscovered the potentials

Generic Name	BRAND NAME / Manufacturer	W.L.* (nm)	Approved by (Country)	Potential applications	Ref.
Porfimer sodium	PHOTOFRIN / Axcan Pharma Inc	632	US-FDA, HPFB (CANADA), EMEA	Cervical, esophageal, lung, and cervical cancer	[40]
5-Aminolevulinic acid	LEVULAN / Dusa Fudan-zhangjiang	632	EMEA, US-FDA, CFDA (CHINA)	Human papilloma virus, actinic keratosis	[40, 41]
Methyl amino levulinate	METVIX / Photocure Asa	632	EMEA, HPFB (CANADA), US-FDA	Basal cell carcinoma (BCC), actinic keratosis	[42]
Hexaminolevulinate hydrochloride	CYSVIEW / Photocure USA	632	EMEA, US-FDA	Bladder cancer	[43]
Verteporfin	VISUDYNE / Novartis	690	NoMA (NORWAY), CFDA (CHINA)	Age-related macular degeneration, BCC	[44]
Temoporfin	FOSCAN / Biolitec Pharma Ltd.	652	EMEA, NoMA (NORWAY), IMA (ICELAND)	Neck and head cancer	[45, 46]
Hematoporphyrinmonomethyl ether	HEMOPORFIN / Shanghai Fudan -Zhangjiang Bio-Pharmaceutical Co., Ltd.	630	CFDA (CHINA)	Prader-Willi syndrome	[47]
2-(1-Hexyloxyethyl)-2-devinyl pyropheophorbide-a	PHOTOCHLOR / Roswell Park Cancer Institute	665	US-FDA (under clinical trial)	Lung cancer, neck, and head cancer	[48]

**W.L. = Excitation wavelength in nm.*

Table 1.
List of PSs approved clinically and reached until the clinical trial for PDT.

of hematoporphyrin derivatives (HpD), which is also having singlet oxygen-producing capacity and tissue penetrating ability, purified it, and named it Photofrin [8, 10]. A significant development in the realm of photodynamic treatment was the Canadian health protection branch's 1993 approval of Photofrin (porfimer sodium) as PS in PDT. Later, Photofrin was approved by the FDA and other organizations, mostly for the treatment of lung and esophageal cancer. Recently, numerous trials involving this specific chemical have also been ongoing. Several nations, including the US, Japan, the Netherlands, China, and India, have approved additional substances, such as 5-aminolaevulinic acid (ALA), its esters, and benzoporphyrin derivatives.

Modern classifications of photosensitizers include first-, second-, and third-generation photosensitizers. Hematoporphyrin derivatives (HpD), including its purified form Photofrin II, are considered first-generation. The HpD showed higher absorption (ε) in the lower wavelength region, and they showed relatively less tumor localization after purification. The second-generation PS has a well-defined chemical structure and improved absorption in the red region spectrum. They are Levulan, Foscan, Visudyne, texaphyrin, and protoporphyrin IX (PpIX), etc. Most of them have porphyrinoid structures. Another most commonly used prodrug in this class is the precursor of PpIX, named δ-aminolaevulinic acid (ALA) and its ester derivatives. Third-generation PS is in pipeline and going through the development stage and clinical trials. Few of them are PS with targeting ability formulated in nanoparticles and have NIR absorption and emission ability, for example, various chlorin e6 (Ce6) based nanoparticles [39]. Chlorin-based photosensitizers are gaining a lot of importance due to their ability to show better absorption in the red region, for example, photochlor, a chlorin-based PS under clinical trial (**Table 1**). Recently, PK Panda et al. reported a class of contracted chlorins with very good singlet oxygen quantum yield and better *in-vitro* PDT ability [49, 50].

The PDT was the new moniker given to it by Jhon Toth. For the treatment of pre-cancerous skin lesions on the scalp and face, PDT become an efficient non-invasive, inexpensive targeted therapy approach in recent years. Used to treat different diseases

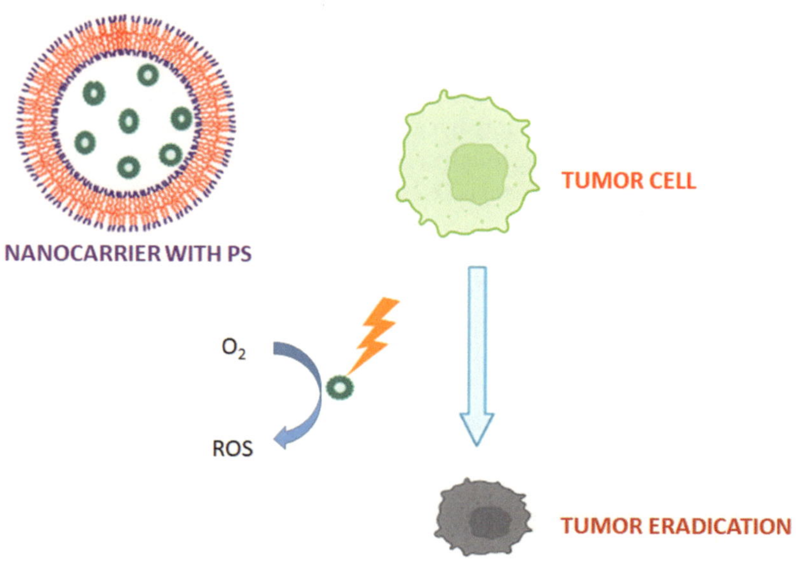

Figure 5.
Advances in PDT based on nano-platforms, by functionalized nanomaterials integrated with photosensitizers toward enhanced efficacy by tumor-selectivity of photodynamic therapy [9].

like cancer, acne vulgaris, periodontitis, age-related muscular degeneration, high-grade dysplasia, etc. [51] PDT has reached a higher level now, extending up to the introduction of phototheranostics, and nano photodynamic immunotherapy for disease mitigation. The role of targeting tumors to induce the PDT effect is shown in **Figure 5** [9].

Photofrin, an oligomer of hematoporphyrin derivative (HpD), was approved as the first porphyrinic photosensitizer for treatment (**Table 1**) [52]. These are the least polar compounds that are comparable with hematoporphyrin and showed a high tumor localizing capacity. Soon, later sodium porfimer (Photofrin II), was approved worldwide and replaced the above HpD because of its stability and purity. The efficiency of PDT relays on complex dosimetry. PDT can treat various types of cancers, such as skin, breast, bladder, glioblastoma, and lung cervical. PDT is used widely in cancer therapy as it is a non-invasive, targetable, cost-effective treatment methodology with less dosing frequency [53].

.In 2011, ALA, a precursor of PpIX, and its esters, specifically methyl 5-aminolevulinate, were approved for the treatment of actinic keratosis (AK). In 2016, the FDA approved ALA 10% gel for AK in the face and scalp. The FDA approved 5- ALA for PDT applications in the treatment of high-grade gliomas (HGG) in 2017. The 5- ALA-assisted fluorescence surgery destroyed more tumors than standard surgery. As a result, ALA was approved as a diagnostic tool. As shown in **Table 1**, two ALA ester derivatives were also approved clinically. In 2020, ALA was approved for the treatment of AK in the neck and trunk, as well as for the treatment of acne vulgaris [54]. In the sphere of research and clinical activities, NIR fluorescence imaging is a bioimaging technology that is rapidly increasing [55]. FDA-approved fluorophores include indocyanine green (800 nm fluorophore) and methylene blue (700 nm NIR fluorophore) [56].

2.3 Mechanism of PDT

As discussed, photodynamic therapy (PDT) opens a promising treatment approach for the management of a variety of solid tumors. Here, cell death is caused by oxidative damage to the cellular organelles through the reactive oxygen species (ROS). It has been demonstrated that cell death in PDT works by apoptosis [programmed cell death] and necrosis [Unprogrammed cell death] [57]. For example, necrotic cell death was observed in the PDT of human lung adenocarcinoma cells using Palladium 2 – tetraphenyl porphycene [58]. Lutetium texaphyrins showed induction of cellular apoptosis through selective modulation of Bcl-2 family proteins. The choice of cell death mechanisms (i.e., whether apoptosis or necrosis) in PDT varies based on:

- Nature of the cell
- Intracellular PS localization
- Amount/dose of light introduced to activate the PS locally [59].

PDT works by the accumulation of photosensitizer (PS) in the tumor or targeted diseased tissue before being exposed to the laser or visible light of a specific wavelength. The applied light should be of a higher wavelength and have to match the absorption band of PS. As shown in **Figure 3**, the higher wavelength light possesses better penetration and less absorption will get lost inside the tissues [60]. By absorbing the light, PS dye gets electronically excited and comes to its singlet excited state.

The specially designed PS dyes show better intersystem crossing ability and move to a triplet excited state. Before intersystem crossing, the singlet state PS drops its energy either as light emission (fluorescence) or through heat production (nonradiative relaxation) [61]. From the triplet excited state, PS relaxes in different ways, among them two mechanisms are beneficial for the generation of ROS. They are generally classified as Type I and II.

In type I, the excited state PS can generate radicals which will then retaliate with cellular oxygen to form ROS, such as superoxide radical anions ($O_2^{\cdot -}$), hydrogen peroxide (H_2O_2), and hydroxyl radicals (OH).

The type II mechanism happens by directly transferring the energy to cellular oxygen (molecular oxygen in triplet state $^3O_2$) and converts to singlet oxygen ($^1O_2$) [33]. Singlet oxygen, the putative cytotoxic agent is one of the major outcomes of such photochemical reactions (**Figure 1**).

Even though the singlet oxygen has only around a 10–55 nm radius of destruction inside cells and a very short lifetime of 10–320 ns [62], it can enable a considerable and complicated chain of events that modify the immune response. These events progress to local, regional, and systemic levels, making it feasible to reliably regulate tumor growth. Same time PDT can also trigger cell signaling and leads to killing cells directly. These all totally depend on the physiochemical properties, concentration, and intracellular location of the PS. Besides that, the availability and concentration of cellular oxygen also play a key role in PDT [30]. Various steps involved during photodynamic therapy include:

2.3.1 Subcellular localization of the photosensitizer

The photosensitizer is brought into the target cellularly or subcellular level or intracellularly using mechanisms like low-density lipoprotein binding, receptor-mediated phagocytosis or pinocytosis, uptake via epidermal growth factor/tyrosine kinase receptors, etc. PS molecules can also accumulate inside various cell organelles like mitochondria, golgi apparatus, ribosomes, cytoplasm, etc. [59]. For example, in the case of Photofrin, rather than accumulating inside the cell membrane, it can bind with the mitochondria [61]. It is observed that, usually, PS localize selectively into the tumors, because of i) its leaky microvasculature, ii) its low extracellular pH, iii) it contains a large number of macrophages, iv) its large interstitial volume, v) it contains more lipoproteins and receptors, and vi) its poor lymphatic drainage [63].

2.3.2 Activation of the photosensitizer by light

Once the PS is localized in the tumor cells, the appropriate light with the desired wavelength can electronically excite the dye. This can give rise to type I or type II reactions as **Figure 1**. The formed singlet oxygen and other ROS will carry out cellular destruction through the chromosomal and cytoplasmic breaking of the localized cell [61]. The outcome of PDT will limit to the localized cells only, it will not be progressing to the neighboring cells, due to the short lifetime of the produced singlet oxygen and as it is active around 10–55 nm in cells [64].

2.3.3 Necrosis and apoptosis: modes of cell death

As discussed, Necrosis and apoptosis were found to be the major mode of cytotoxicity after PDT [65]. Necrosis is the sudden cell death occurring through the influence of external factors, while apoptosis is natural cell death. It is believed that a

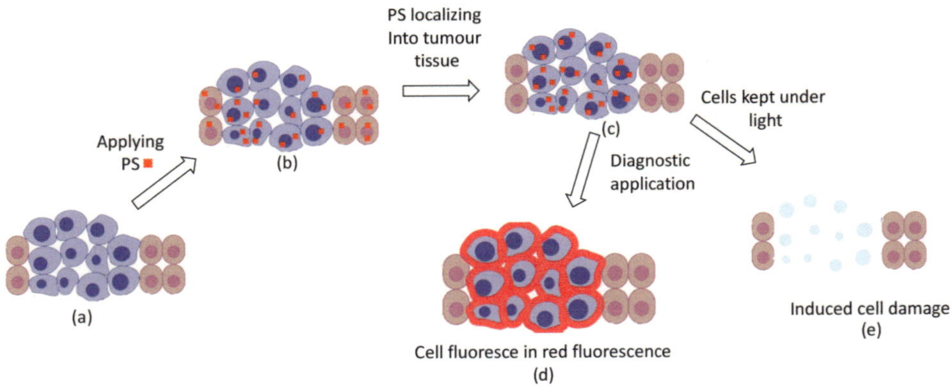

Figure 6.
A series of events during PDT (a) a cluster of cancer cells (blue) and normal cells (light rose); (b) PS accumulates in both the cells; (c) after a period PS localize into tumor tissue; (d) porphyrinoid PS fluoresce inside cancer tissue; (e) laser/visible light can induce PDT action.

low dose of light will cause apoptosis and meanwhile higher dose will cause necrosis. Found that around 70% of cytotoxicity was due to apoptosis and 99% was because of necrosis (**Figure 6**) [66].

In the case of tumor-specific PS with good fluorescence, the ability can be effectively employed for tumor detection and fluorescence-guided surgery. On the other hand, fluorescence-guided surgery can be achieved by effective utilization of different fluorophores and PS in a nanocarrier (e.g., liposomes, niosmes, cubosomes, and other nanoparticles), which readily accumulate in tumor tissue [17]. Lee et al. utilized such combined fluorescence-assisted surgery and PDT toward glioblastoma using indocyanine-green and chlorin-e6 in a nanocluster [67].

3. Design of targeted PDT

The specificity of photosensitizer toward the tumor or diseased tissue is always questionable. As discussed, once the photosensitizers get activated by the light they will produce ROS. The formed ROS can easily destroy the cell structures of pathogenic mammalian cells or microbes. But ROS-mediated toxicity is not limited to pathogens if the PS located in normal vegetative tissue can lead to lethal action [9]. A targeted drug delivery approach is only a solution to minimize vegetative tissue destruction. In the process of designing the targeted PDT, the selection of photosensitizer also plays a key role. Both the free radical (type I) and singlet oxygen (type II) mediated mechanisms are equally harmful and end up with a series of reactive oxygen species (ROS). Currently, there are different approaches adopted to direct these highly active photosensitizers to our site of action. Among them, molecular design-based targeting and nanocarrier approaches are two leading methodologies [26]. In the targeted approach, we have to impart a targeting aid to lead the molecule toward the diseased tissue. The most studied drug delivery approach is the vesicle or nanocarrier-mediated technique [68].

3.1 The concept of targeting

Paul Ehrlich first pioneered the theory of targeting [69]. Targeted delivery is a process of binding a drug into a specific site of the body, to minimize the toxicity

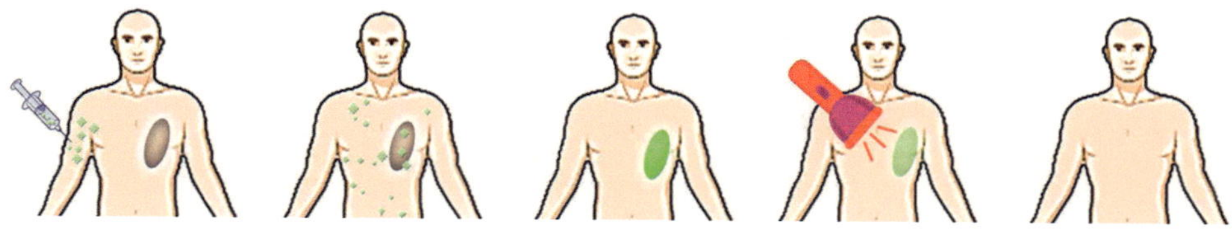

Figure 7.
The concept of treatment of PDT with targeted PS into tumor tissue [70].

by avoiding the localization of the drug into other body parts (**Figure 7**) [71]. By efficient targeting, the concentration of active ingredients should be more at the site of diseased tissue, this helps in reducing the dose and side effects due to decreased body distribution and accumulation of the drug. Drug targeting has many advantages over conventional delivery of drugs; such as better therapeutic effect, reduced expense by decreasing the dose, increase concentration of drug at the specific target site, minimizing the adverse effect, and preventing the accumulation of drugs in the non-targeting site.

.In the case of PDT, the PS has disadvantages such as it can accumulate in the normal vegetative tissues and can cause unfavorable conditions, for example, phototoxicity, photophobia, etc. The only solution to avoid such dangerous situations associated with PDT is targeted photodynamic therapy. Targeted PDT helps in preventing such types of adverse reactions [72, 73]. As per reports PS, they self-have an inherent tumor-targeting ability, but in many cases, it fails to achieve efficient targeting. Better targeting is achieved by the encapsulation of the PS into a proper nanocarrier to improve its accumulation in a specific target site. S. Nair et al. developed a unique nanomedicine to inhibit the migration of metastatic breast cancer cells. The team fabricated a core shell with PLGA nanocore encapsulated with temoporphin (mTHPC) as PS [74]. Manzoor et al. developed a photosensitizer (Ce6 or m-THPC) conjugated nanoparticle with an optical and magnetic contrast agent. Interestingly the system showed better targeting ability with higher singlet oxygen-producing efficiency and fluorescence quantum yield [75]. The process of targeting can be divided into active targeting and passive targeting based on their mechanisms as shown in **Figure 8**.

In passive targeting, the nanocarriers (in the case of tumor targeting) move across and target the cell based on the properties of the tumor microenvironment (TME), which is distinct from the normal tissue. So, passive targeting happens based on the biodistribution (i.e., physicochemical factors and pathophysiological factors) of the target tissue [76]. The limitations of passive targeting are ineffective transfection at the target site and quick clearance of some smaller drug particles due to variable blood flow in the target site.

Active targeting can be used to overcome such limitations to improve the binding of PS to the specific targeted site [77]. It is the process of drug delivery to a specific targeting site, based on the interaction between the ligands, receptors, etc. [78]. **Figure 8** depicts passive and active PDT schematically.

3.2 .Passive targeting

In passive accumulation, the drugs or drugs in nanocarriers will naturally penetrate the targeted tissue due to the change in the milieu of the target site concerning its healthy surroundings. Here the driving force to reach the target site include various physicochemical factors of drug or nanocarrier, material composition, size, and

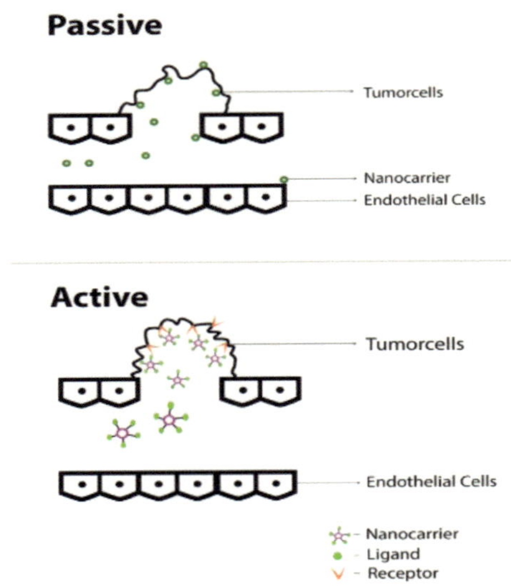

Figure 8.
Presentation of the passive and active PDT schematically [75].

surface characters (e.g., cationic or anionic nature) and pathophysiological factors of the target site, such as TME as well as EPR effect. For example, the lower diameter of nanovesicles promotes passive targeting of rapidly growing carcinoma due to the enhanced permeability and retention effect (EPR) [79]. Maeda and Matsumura first narrated the EPR effect, the macromolecules or smaller nanoparticles can progressively accumulate into the tumor, due to the leaky vasculature and poor lymphatic drainage in the tumor tissue [80, 81].

To maximize the effectiveness of PDT, the nanocarrier has the potential to enhance the selectivity and sensitivity of PS by altering the distribution pattern. In the tumor area, the permeability is high to promote the rapid multiplication of the tumor, and at the same time, the lymphatic drainage is poor in the area. As a result of that, the macromolecules and nanoparticles are not cleared and get accumulated in the tumor site. The biophysical and morphological characteristics of the nanocarriers play a significant role in the targeted distribution of PS-loaded nanocarriers. Due to its large size, it will not quickly revert to the bloodstream and thus results in its accumulation in the specific tumor site.

To facilitate longer circulation periods and enhance accumulations at the desired region, hydrophilic polymers, surfactants, or biodegradable copolymers are typically used to coat nanoparticles. Because of poor biodistribution of hydrophobic PS, low cellular uptake, and low efficiency in treating bulky tumors, nanoparticles are developed [82]. Liposomes, polymer micelles, polymeric nanoparticles, gold nanoparticles, and carbon-based nanoparticles are used as drug carriers to enhance the drug loading capacity, improve drug delivery, increase bioavailability, etc. [83].

Liposomes are spherical structured vesicles with hydrophobic cavities and hydrophilic cavities. Such vesicular structures will help to increase drug loading efficiency and therapeutic efficiency. It will enter the cancer cell by endocytosis and maintain the constant release of PS at a specific site and it is achieved by passive targeting. The liposome can be activated by modifying its surface with ligands.

Passive PSs are more readily available, less expensive, and simpler to administer. For example, amphiphilic cationic porphyrin-based photosensitizers. The efficacy of a PS in PDT depends on its amphiphilicity; hydrophilicity will promote the distribution and improved clearance rate, while lipophilicity will aid in cellular uptake. PS can accumulate in the targeted area by the passive target [78].

3.3 Active targeting

In active targeting, the pharmacophore directs to the specific receptor site by peripherally decorated targeting moieties in the delivery vesicle [84]. The process of active targeting is a promising methodology. It helps to overcome the limitations of the passive targeting method by improving the binding of PS to a specific tumor site. So, this method reduces the major adverse effects of PDT by avoiding the accumulation of PS in the non-targeting area. Various research in nanotechnology significantly contributed to the area of active targeting. Well-developed selective tumor-targeting ligands, such as monoclonal antibodies (mAb), antibody fragments, peptides, aptamers (single-stranded oligonucleotides), and nucleic acid are coupled with nanoparticles [72]. Such targeting ligand-incorporated nanoparticles or vesicles shows active binding of PS into tumor receptors. Usually in PDT to enhance the tumor cell uptake of PS, these modified nanoparticles will target overexpressed tumor receptors like folate receptor, transferrin receptor, CD44, and growth factor receptor (EGFR) [85]. For example, targeted photodynamic therapy (TPDT) was attained by encapsulating PS into polymeric micelles for breast cancer treatment and diagnosis [86]. Breast cancer is the most common cancer in women around the world, and it is currently treated with traditional methods such as chemotherapy, radiotherapy, and surgery. The challenges in using PDT in breast cancer were poor water solubility and the non-specificity of PSs. These problems frequently reduced the overall efficacy of this novel cancer treatment. But PDT driven with monoclonal antibody targeted drug delivery systems based on gold NP showed improved specificity of PSs in breast cancer tumors. In approximately 25% of breast cancer cases, HER2 monoclonal antibodies are conjugated with gold nanoparticles, and this antibody binds to the HER2 receptors that are overexpressed on the cellular surface [87]. In recent years, monoclonal antibody-based targeted drug delivery gains much attention because of its high accuracy in targeting and better therapeutic activity. For example, porphyrin-trastuzumab complexes are effectively used to deliver the PS to a specific target site. Trastuzumab is an FDA-approved Mab against HER2 (Epidermal growth factor 2 receptor)-positive breast cancer [88, 89].

Another major overexpressed receptor in tumors is the transferrin receptor (TfR), it can be targeted using antibodies against TfR and transferrin itself. HpD with albumin and transferrin conjugates showed better-prolonged phototoxicity. Nowadays transferrin-conjugated liposome is one of the important targeting aids, but M. O Senge reported that temoporfin-loaded transferrin-conjugated liposomes do not improve the efficiency of invitro PDT [90]. On the other hand, L. E. Xodo and coworkers developed a successful RAS-driven active targeting system with cationic porphyrins and studied it in pancreatic adenocarcinoma cells. The confocal microscopic results showed the photoactivated PS binds and induces apoptosis even in nanomolar concentration by RAS gene suppression system [91].

3.4 Peptide-mediated targeting

Peptide-mediated targeting in PDT is also known as peptide-based supramolecular photodynamic therapy. As the name represents here the PS and the peptide molecules are allowed to self-assemble either covalently or non-covalently, thus directing the PS into the cancer lesion site effectively [92]. As discussed above to achieve the targeted photodynamic therapy, one should localize the PS into the intracellular space where ever required. But such targeting is hard to achieve in many cases due to various structural and morphological characteristics of the PS, such as molecular size, shape, penetrability, and solubility. Here comes the importance of peptide targeting. It's reported that the number of receptors in the tumor periphery is more, so the small peptides can bind with it. Thus, a PS-bound peptide can effectively deliver them to the target site.

Small peptides are having various advantages, such as ease in synthesis, good penetrability even into the BBB, small size, rapid tumor access, ease in linking to a spacer through amide bonds, and high clearance rate [93]. Some of the major examples of peptides used widely for PDT-mediated anti-cancer therapy include:

- *Disruptin*: a decoy peptide to destabilize activated EGFR used in colon cancer [94].

- *Transportan 10 (TP10)*: an amphiphilic peptide mainly improves the pharmacokinetics and pharmacodynamics of drugs mainly used for cervical cancer and osteosarcoma [95].

- *Ras-related protein (RALA)*: a type of small G protein and inactive GDP-bound states, plays a key role in cell proliferation and motility used for prostatic and breast cancer targeting [91].

- *The peptide P28 protein is derived from bacteria azurin:* It is a post-translational, multi-target anticancer agent used for fibrosarcoma and various other solid tumors [96].

- *P12 peptide*: A 14 amino acid peptide from fibronectin, used for solid tumor targeting [97, 98].

H. Lin *et al* formulated a pH-responsive peptide targeted PDT. Here protoporphyrin IX (PpIX) coupled with the N terminal of the P12 peptide to form a PpIX-P12 conjugate. This peptide conjugate targets the acidic microenvironment of the tumor-as

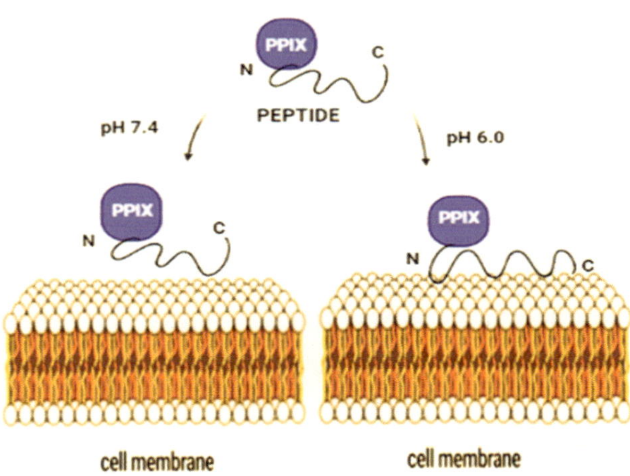

Figure 9.
pH-responsive targeted PDT; protoporphyrin IX (PpIX) coupled with P12 peptide (PpIX-P12 conjugate) binds the cancer cells in the acidic microenvironment [99].

shown in **Figure 9**. It could localize specifically into the tumor cell and a greater phototoxic effect was shown within the acidic medium. The team first explained the activity through in vitro studies and found that PpIX-P12 is having the drift to get attached to cancerous cells. Thus, they proved that this will be an asset in treating solid tumors [99].

.Another example is the use of epidermal growth factor (EGF) peptide-labeled formulations showed better killing efficiency than unlabeled formulations. The peptide is combined with gold nanoparticles (EGF pep-Au NP) encapsulated with silicone phthalocyanine (PS-4). The nanoformulation efficiently targeted the early endosomes, and *in vitro* studies showed that this combination was twofold effective in destroying tumor cells as compared to conventional systems. As the silicone phthalocyanines have the potential to generate fluorescence, they also conducted *in vivo* investigations to support their claim and were able to perform fluorescence imaging to ensure targeting [100].

Formation of a dual targeting PS-peptide amphiphile conjugate containing encapsulated doxorubicin for increased chemo-photodynamic cancer therapy. When the Doxorubicin-PS-Peptide nano micelle enters the tumor via R8 peptide. The doxorubicin and PpIX were released as a result of cathepsin B-triggered hydrolysis [77]. X. Z. Zhang et al. created a cell membrane targeting PpIX-PS by loading a charge-reversible self-delivery chimeric peptide. This self-assembled peptide can achieve a long-term photodynamic effect for about 14 hours, by delivering the PS through enhanced permeability and retention effect. Under an acidic environment, the peptide-PS complex changes the charge and in the presence of light, ROS is generated which leads to direct necrosis [101].

A chip made of a chimeric peptide and PpIX was developed by C. Hong et al. This chip has a hydrophilic PEG chain, and a bioactive peptide series with a double targeting ability. This double-targeted chip can bind with the mitochondria and plasma membrane, hence creating a synergistic effect. During the introduction of light, generated ROS can cause tumor necrosis [102]. Another example of a synergistic effect is the development of a nanorod with dual targeting capacity (plasma membrane and Nucleus). The PS loaded inside the self-assembling chimeric peptide upon light irradiation, generated ROS can induce necrosis and thereby cell death [103].

The disadvantages of ALA targeting can be mitigated by incorporating an ALA prodrug and a zwitterionic stealth peptide into a nanoparticle. The ALA-conjugated prodrug nanoparticles were created through conjugation with a thiolated stealth peptide sequence called CPPPPEKEKEKEKEKEKEDGR. The release of ALA prodrugs is dependent on lysosomal/endosomal pH 5.5 [104].

The development of a protease activatable-cell-penetrating peptide-PS conjugate can induce proteolysis using peptide activity at the tumor site which will result in the release of the PS into the tumor site. The fluorescence produced by the conjugate after getting accumulated into the tumor will aid in tumor diagnosis and image-driven PDT [105].

Tumor hypoxia during PDT is a significant issue that affects efficacy; to address this, an arginine-peptide complex that is compatible with a *m*THPP to generate a stable nanoparticle has been designed. This combination will both release nitric oxide and can deliver PS directly into the tumor microenvironment. Nitric oxide will be released, which will help to enhance cellular oxygen levels and prevent cells from respiring through their mitochondria. Thereby resolving the difficulty [106].

4. Diagnostics and theranostics

The detection of illness is broadly known as diagnosis, and biomedical imaging is one of the commonly used diagnostic tools. Biomedical imaging is a fast-growing area of research and various advanced imaging techniques include Near-Infrared (NIR) fluorescence Imaging, shortwave infrared (SWIR) fluorescence imaging, positron emission tomography (PET), magnetic resonance imaging (MRI), single-photon emission computed tomography (SPECT), *invivo* nuclear magnetic resonance (NMR) imaging and photoacoustic imaging [107]. Many of the imaging techniques are still at the research level, in 2020 first PET Imaging drug Gallium (68Ga) gozetotide accepted for prostate cancer in men [108]. In 1960 itself Lipson proved that the hematoporphyrin derivative discovered by T. Doughtery has the fluorescence property to diagnose tumors (**Figure 4**) [8]. He observed hematoporphyrin derivatives produce fluorescence selectively from cancer cells. Currently, porphyrinoids and their derivatives are utilized in a variety of diagnostic imaging areas, including MRI, PET/SPECT, and NIR imaging [109].

During the course of treatment for several disorders, including cancer, rheumatoid arthritis, and neurodegenerative diseases, there may be some variation (tissue alteration, physiological change, and change in medication disposition). Therefore, during therapy, frequent monitoring is necessary which theranostics can fulfill [110]. Thus, theranostics is a fast-growing research area, that combines diagnosis with narrowly focused therapy to provide patients with individualized care [111]. The use of theranostic agents can improve disease destruction with high localized cytotoxicity and minimal collateral damage. The fluorescence that is released can be used to diagnose diseases as photo diagnosis and molecular imaging, known as photosensitizer fluorescence detection (PFD). The combination of PFD and PDT will diagnose and treat the diseases. But PFD has some limitations such as autofluorescence and tissue absorption leading to decreased tissue penetration (**Figure 3**). So, such limitations can be reduced by using NIR (from 700 nm to 1000 nm) and SWIR (from 1000 nm to 2500 nm) radiations, because of their high image resolution they can deeply penetrate the tissues [112]. For example, Lanthanide (Ln) porphyrinoids show near-infrared emission and can be used for fluorescence imaging [113].

Gadolinium-porphyrin-based polymer nanotheranostics showed excellent fluorescence imaging properties, good singlet oxygen-producing efficiency, and excellent long-term colloidal stability. As shown in **Figure 10**, the nanotheranostics acted like a therapeutic tool, fluorophore, and MRI contrasting agent [114]. The coupling of porphyrinoids with nanoparticles has greater importance in cancer targeting and theranostics. Different theranostic formulations of porphyrin nanomaterials based on silica nanoparticles, fullerene, virus capsids, protein, steroids, carbohydrates, iron oxide nanoparticles, polymers, graphene oxide, and liposomes have a greater future in cancer treatment [115].

.Instead of this nano theranostics, various single molecular theranostics also gained research interest. In 2014 Zijian Guo reported a single molecule cancer theranostics *i.e.,* platinum (II)–gadolinium (III) complexes with better biocompatibility [116]. Texaphyrin, an expanded porphyrinoid, which is developed' by Sessler *et al.* showed applications in PDT. Now finding its uses as MRI contrast agents and anticancer agents [117]. Recently the same group reported Indium-111radiolabelleddmetallatedd luteum texaphyrin for prostate-specific membrane antigen (PSMA) targeting. This novel texaphyrin system showed high-resolution SPECT imaging and better PDT action toward prostate carcinoma [118]. The challenges in porphyrin-based compounds toward their theranostic or biological applications are their poor water solubility, this can be addressed by the use of cationic and anionic porphyrinoids. In the case of the lipophilic porphyrinic systems, the problem can be addressed by designing the proper nanocarrier drug delivery system such as liposomes, micelles, and silica nanoparticles [119].

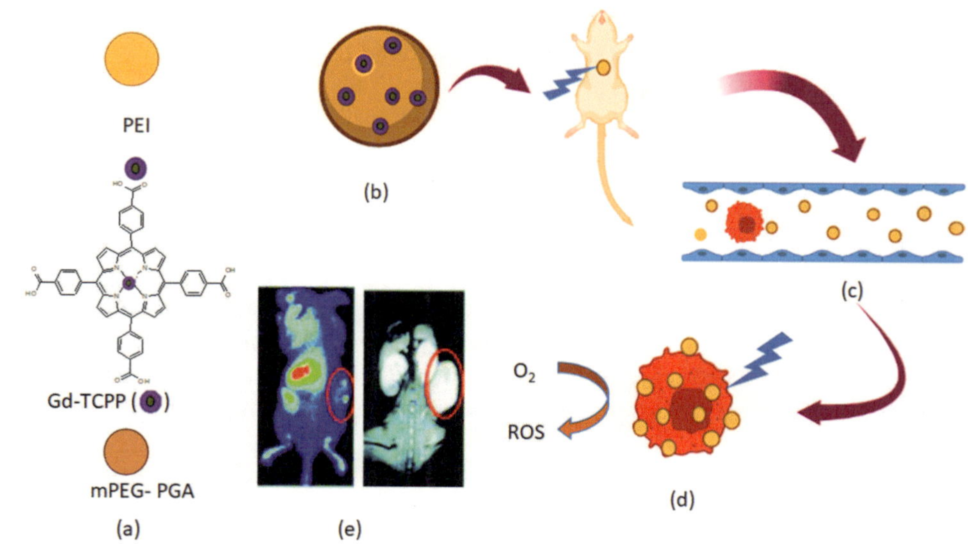

Figure 10.
Schematic representation of (a) components and (b) formulation of gadolinium-porphyrin-based polymer nanotheranostics; (c) its invivo administration, (d) PDT action, and (e) fluorescence (FL) and MRI imaging [114].

Recent years of research in the metal-organic framework (MOF) gained considerable attention in catalysis and hydrogen storage cells [120]. Various nano-MOF (NMOFs) showed interesting biomedical applications in drug delivery, imaging, chemotherapy, photodynamic and photothermal therapy [120–122]. For example NMOF (Zr-NMOFs) is used for bioimaging and targeted photodynamic therapy [123]. Nowadays, covalent organic frameworks (COFs) have a promising future in the field of PDT. Integrating a dye-labeled oligonucleotide onto porphyrin-based COF nanoparticles are incredibly effective in cancer treatment and diagnosis. This COF-based nanoplatform operates well in vitro, and in vivo and is superior to theranostic probes based on other nanomaterials, such as metal-organic frameworks, in terms of stability, biocompatibility, and high integration [124].

The principles of PDT are not limited to cancer therapy, it can be used in many diseases like rheumatoid arthritis (RA), skin diseases and microbial infections, etc. Tetra sulphonatophenyl porphyrin has many applications in the field of cancer and other inflammatory diseases. The combination of tetra sulphonatophenyl porphyrin and nanoparticle is used as a diagnostic and theranostic agent for many cancer and other diseases [125].

5. Photodynamic antimicrobial chemotherapy (PACT/aPDT)

PDT is not only used in cancer therapy; as previously stated, it can also be used to treat a variety of other diseases. Nowadays, the most common and commercially available photodynamic agent is 5-amino laevulinic acid for acne treatment, which is gaining popularity among millennials [30, 54]. Acne vulgaris is caused due to the clogging of hair follicles by bacteria, dirt, dust, and sebum. The main bacteria causing acne is *Propionibacterium acne*. PDT is a very effective tool in destroying this kind of antimicrobial-resistant microbes and thus can reduce the severity of acne vulgaris.

In the past itself, it is proved that porphyrins can improve perifollicular inflammatory reaction and trigger the aspect of keratinocyte-derived IL-8 by producing cytotoxic singlet oxygen [20].

Photodynamic antimicrobial chemotherapy (PACT) is more adventitious than regular microbial treatment as it can effectively destroy every infection causing micro-organisms. Even antimicrobial-resistive microbes can be destroyed using PACT [77]. The mechanism of action of PACT is mainly similar to that of the PDT mechanism. PACT also acts in the presence of photosensitizers such as hemato-porphyrin derivative monomers, dimers, and oligomers, as well as cationic PS acting in the wavelength range of 610–630 nm, the light of appropriate dose and wavelength, and molecular oxygen. These three react to produce singlet oxygen, which is capable of causing cytotoxicity in microbial cells. The mode of cell death may vary from necrosis to apoptosis depending upon the intensity of applied photons.

PACT has various applications including treating oral bacterial infections and to that treating COVID-19. The use of PACT in various diseases includes:

- In the field of dentistry, PACT has been used widely to eradicate the microbes existing as biofilms, creating oral diseases such as periodontitis, gingivitis, and mucosal infections [126, 127].

- To prevent the spread of COVID-19 infection and in the making of photoactive fabrics like masks, suits, and gloves aPDT has been established using protopor-phyrin-IX [128].

- Treatment of fungal infection- skin mycoses caused by the fungus *Trichophyton rubrum* with high antimicrobial resistance [129].

- PDT effect in *Candida albicans* species affecting immunocompromised people has been demonstrated using newly synthesized PSs, tin (IV) porphyrins with axial ligand modifications as well as hydroxyl and 4-nitrophenolate moieties. These compounds demonstrated high cellular penetration and destruction of *C. Albicans* species [130].

5.1 Other disease cured by PDT includes

Chronic central serous chorioretinopathy is a retinal disorder that begins often at a very young age. The disease represents damage to the retinal pigment epithelium and photoreceptors. Synergistic application of PDT using verteporfin as the PS with other corresponding treatment modalities has been proven for curing the disease [131]. Loss of melanocytes gives rise to depigmentation leading to a skin disease called vitiligo. The remedy was not at all satisfying till now. In PDT using ALA with 0.5% of the drug has been proven to cure vitiligo [132, 133].

There have been reports of atherosclerosis treatment. It has been demonstrated that modest phototherapy along with PDT using a black TiO_2 nanoprobe decreases intracellular lipid levels in atherosclerotic foam cells without inducing apoptosis. The nanoprobe was filled with PS porphine and hyaluronic acid to achieve the desired effect. PPT and PDT worked together to significantly reduce the thickness of the lipid cell layer [134].

6. Future prospective

A promising area for cancer research is porphyrinoid photodynamic treatment, which has several potential theranostic uses. Porphyrinoids have potential in PDT, as we covered in the chapter, and theranostic is currently a study field that is expanding. These macrocyclic compounds have fluorescent characteristics that are useful for fluorescence imaging in diagnostic procedures. These substances are a prospective tool for MRI and PET imaging because of their ability to chelate with Mn, Fe, Gd, and Tc [135]. The treatment of multidrug-resistant tumors and antibiotic-resistant bacteria is always challenging, and PDT is an ideal alternative in such cases [49]. Researchers are now working on the condition called hypoxia occurring in the tumor—lack or decrease in oxygen content (hypoxia) in the TME, nanomedicines are currently employed to handle the strategy [136].

PDT plays an important role in the field of veterinary medicine because it shows encouraging results for the treatment of different animal pathologies such as bovine mastitis, malassezia, and cutaneous hemangiosarcoma [137]. Photodynamic therapy has many promising advantages to improve the quality of current treatment modalities along with easy diagnosis. Aptamer-targeted photodynamic therapy is a futuristic tool for tumor targeting, current studies showed 500-fold increased light-activated cytotoxicity and improved tissue-specific killing of cancer [138]. With light irradiation, the aptamer-modified PSs or PSs-containing nanocarriers produce significant levels of reactive oxygen species and provide improved photodynamic therapeutic efficacy in malignancies [138, 139].

7. Conclusion

Light has been used in medicine since ancient times, extending up in the form of PDT these days. Malignant cells can be killed quickly and efficiently by combining the three nontoxic aforementioned components. In the presence of molecular oxygen, porphyrinoids with the ability to localize inside the target tissue, NIR region light with deeper tissue penetration will effectively produce necrosis and apoptosis. The main advantage of this modality is that it seems to be highly adaptable to individualized treatment. The disadvantage of the therapy is that it destroys normal vegetative cells, causing the patient to become light-sensitive. This issue can be mitigated by using a more site-specific and targeted drug delivery method. Targeting can be accomplished using both passive and active mechanisms via appropriate nanoformulations. The PDT is becoming more popular among millennials due to its ease of use and faster healing time. Acne treatment with PDT is gaining more demand because it does not leave scars and aids in the fading of acne scars. The discovery of novel and effective photosensitizers with theranostic applications will improve PDT's efficacy in disease prevention, diagnosis, and monitoring. Targeted delivery with PDT is an uncharted territory that can only be carved out by a formulation scientist.

Conflict of interest

The authors declare no conflict of interest.

Abbreviations

ALA	δ-Amino laevulinic acid
APDT	antimicrobial photodynamic therapy
BCC	basal cell carcinoma
Ce6	chlorin e6
COFs	covalent organic frameworks
EGFR	epidermal growth factor receptor
EMEA	European medicine evaluation agency
EU	European Union
EPR effect	enhanced permeability and amp; retention effect
FDA	United States Food and Drug Administration
Ga	gallium
GD 2	glycoprotein D2
HER-2	human epidermal growth 2
HP	hematoporphyrin
HpD	hematoporphyrin derivatives
HPFB	The Health Products and Food Branch of Health Canada
Mab	monoclonal antibody
MOF	metal-organic framework
MRI	magnetic resonance imaging
NIR	near-infrared
Nm	nanometers
NMPA	National Medical Products Administration
NMOF	Nano metal-organic framework
NoMA	The Norwegian Medicines Agency
Ns	nanoseconds
PACT	photodynamic antimicrobial therapy
PDT	photodynamic therapy
PEG	polyethylene glycol
PET	positron emission tomography
PFD	photosensitizer fluorescence detection
PpIX	protoporphyrin IX
PS	photosensitizer
RA	rheumatoid arthritis
ROS	reactive oxygen species
SPECT	single photon emission computerized tomography
SWIR	shortwave infrared fluorescence imaging
TFR	transferrin receptor
TME	tumor microenvironment
WL	wavelength

Author details

Devika Sivakumar[1†], Rakhi Raju[1†], Y.T. Kamal[2*], Shahana Salam[3], Sabna Kotta[4,5*] and Rahul Soman[1*]

1 Department of Pharmaceutics, Bioorganic Materials Research Laboratory, Amrita School of Pharmacy, Amrita Institute of Medical Sciences and Research Centre, AIMS Health Sciences Campus, Amrita Vishwa Vidyapeetham, Kochi, Kerala, India

2 Department of Pharmacognosy, College of Pharmacy, King Khalid University, Abha, Saudi Arabia

3 Department of Chemistry, College of Pharmacy, Prince Sattam Bin Abdulaziz University, Al-Kharj, Saudi Arabia

4 Faculty of Pharmacy, Department of Pharmaceutics, King Abdulaziz University, Jeddah, Saudi Arabia

5 Center of Excellence for Drug Research and Pharmaceutical Industries, King Abdulaziz University, Jeddah, Saudi Arabia

*Address all correspondence to: kthajudeen@kku.edu.sa; skotta@kau.edu.sa and somansmail@gmail.com

† These authors contributed equally.

References

[1] Stanely B, Brown EA, Walker I. The present and future role of photodynamic therapy in cancer treatment. The Lancet Oncology. 2004;**5**(8):497-508

[2] National Cancer Institute. Side Effects of Cancer Treatment – NCI. 2020. Available from: https://www.cancer.gov/about-cancer/treatment/types/radiation-therapy/side-effects

[3] Pandey RK, Dougherty TJ, Kessel D. Handbook of Photodynamic Therapy: Updates on Recent Applications of Porphyrin-Based Compounds. Singapore: World Scientific; 2016

[4] Oinuma T, Nakamura T, Nishiwaki Y. Report on the National Survey of Photodynamic Therapy (PDT) for Gastric Cancer in Japan (a secondary publication). Laser Therapy. 2016;**25**(2):87-98

[5] Lee D, Kwon S, Jang S, Park E, Lee Y, Koo H. Overcoming the obstacles of current photodynamic therapy in tumors using nanoparticles. Bioactive Materials. 2022;**8**:20-34

[6] Tierney EP, Melody JE, Gordon J, David O. Photodynamic therapy for actinic keratoses: survey of patient perceptions of treatment satisfaction and outcomes. Journal of Cosmetic & Laser Therapy. 2008;**10**(2):81-86

[7] Kessel D. Photodynamic therapy: a brief history. Journal of Clinical Medicine. 2019;**8**(10):1581

[8] Sarbadhikary P, George BP, Abrahamse H. Recent advances in photosensitizers as multifunctional theranostic agents for imaging-guided photodynamic therapy of cancer. Theranostics. 2021;**11**(18):9054

[9] Hong JE, Dae GC, Min S. Targeted and effective photodynamic therapy for cancer using functionalized nanomaterials. Acta Pharmaceutica Sinica B. 2016;**6**(4):297-307

[10] Won M, Seyoung K, Hao L, Sessler JL, Jin YL, Amit S, et al. An ethacrynic acid-brominated BODIPY photosensitizer (EA-BPS) construct enhances the lethality of reactive oxygen species in hypoxic tumor-targeted photodynamic therapy. Angewandte Chemie International Edition. 2021;**60**(6):3196-3204

[11] Zhou Y, Xiaolong L, Zhifei D. Porphyrin-loaded nanoparticles for cancer theranostics. Nanoscale. 2016;**8**(25):12394-12405

[12] Jeelani S, Jagat RC, Thangadurai RM, Asokan GS, Dany A, Anand B. Theranostics an emerging paradigm-a review. Journal of Pharmacy & Bioallied Sciences. 2014;**6**(Suppl. 1):S6

[13] Jakka S, Michael R. An economic perspective on personalized medicine. The HUGO Journal. 2013;**7**(1):1-6

[14] Gross S, Assaf G, Avigdor S, Michal N, Yoram S. Monitoring photodynamic therapy of solid tumors online by BOLD-contrast MRI. Nature Medicine. 2003;**9**(10):1327-1331

[15] Hester SC, Ke M, Christopher DN, Srivalleesha M. Role of ultrasound and photoacoustic imaging in photodynamic therapy for cancer. Photochemistry and Photobiology. 2020;**96**(2):260-279

[16] Dougherty TJ. An update on photodynamic therapy applications. Journal of Clinical Laser Medicine & Surgery. 2002;**20**(1):3-7

[17] Qidwai A, Nabi B, Kotta S, Narang JK, Baboota S, Ali J. Role of nanocarriers in photodynamic therapy.

J. Photodiagnosis and Photodynamic Therapy. 2020;**30**:101782

[18] Sekar R, Nagaraj B, Saktishree J, Santhoshkumar J, Pandian E, Amballa C, et al. Recent Developments in Heteroatom/Metal-Doped Carbon Dot-Based Image-Guided Photodynamic Therapy for Cancer. Pharmaceutics. 2022;**14**(9):1869

[19] Dayyih AA, Alawak M, Ayoub AM, Amin MU, Dayyih WA, Engelhardt K, et al. Thermosensitive liposomes encapsulating hypericin: Characterization and photodynamic efficiency. International Journal of Pharmaceutics. 2021;**609**:121195

[20] Barbaric J, Abbott R, Posadzki P, Car M, Gunn LH, Layton AM, et al. Light therapies for acne: abridged Cochrane systematic review including GRADE assessments. British Journal of Dermatology. 2018;**178**(1):61-75

[21] Cao Z, Xiaojing L, Linglin Z, Yunfeng Z, Zhongxia Z, Guolong Z, et al. Treatment of androgenetic alopecia with 5-aminolevulinic acid photodynamic therapy: A randomized, placebo-controlled, split-scalp study of efficacy and safety. Photodiagnosis and Photodynamic Therapy. 2021;**36**:102491

[22] Plotino G, Grande NM, Montserrat M. Photodynamic therapy in endodontics. International Endodontic Journal. 2019;**52**(6):760-774

[23] Kennedy JC, Pottier RH, Pross DC. Photodynamic therapy with endogenous protoporphyrin: IX: basic principles and present clinical experience. Journal of Photochemistry and Photobiology B: Biology. 1990;**6**(1-2):143-148

[24] Maiya BJ. Photodynamic therapy (PDT). Resonance. 2000;**5**(6):15-29

[25] Ruggiero E, Silvia A, Abraha H, Luca SD. Transactions. 2016;**45**(33): 13012-13020

[26] Garland MJ, Cassidy CM, David W, Donnelly RF. Future Medicinal Chemistry. 2009;**1**(4):667-691

[27] Kim MM, Arash D. Photochemistry and Photobiology. 2020;**96**(2):280-294

[28] Brancaleon L, Moseley H. Lasers in Medical Science. 2002;**17**(3):173-186

[29] Liu J, Wenbo B, Shi J. Chemical Reviews. 2017;**117**(9):6160-6224

[30] Gold MH. History of photodynamic therapy. In: Photodynamic Therapy in Dermatology. New York, NY: Springer; 2011. pp. 1-4

[31] Yawalkar MM, Menon S, Swart HC, Dhoble SJ. Fundamentals of photodynamic therapy. In: Photophysics and Nanophysics in Therapeutics. England: Elsevier; 2022. pp. 51-88

[32] Dolmans DE, Dai F, Rakesh KJ. Photodynamic therapy for cancer. Nature Reviews Cancer. 2003;**3**(5):380-387

[33] Moan J, Peng Q. An outline of the history of PDT. Photodynamic Therapy. 2003;**2**:1-18

[34] Gunaydin G, Gedik ME, Ayan S. Photodynamic therapy—current limitations and novel approaches. Frontiers in Chemistry. 2021;**9**:691697

[35] Jesionek A, Von Tappeiner H. Historische entwicklung der photodynamischen therapie. Archiv für Klinische Medizin. 1905;**82**:223-227

[36] Weishaupt KR, Charles JG, Dougherty TJ. Identification of singlet oxygen as the cytotoxic agent in photo-inactivation of a murine tumor. Cancer Research. 1976;**36**(7_Part_1):2326-2329

[37] Fischer H. Chlorophyll. Chemical Reviews. 1937;**20**(1):41-68

[38] Stern AJ. N-H TAUTOMERISM IN PORPHYRINS AND CHLORINS. Annals

of the New York Academy of Sciences. 1973;**206**(1):752-761

[39] Baskaran R, Junghan L, Yang S-G. Clinical development of photodynamic agents and therapeutic applications. Biomaterials Research. 2018;**22**(1):1-8

[40] Alexiades M. Photodynamic therapy. Procedures in Cosmetic Dermatology: Lasers, Lights, and Energy Devices. 2023;**1**:127

[41] Bai-Habelski JC, Medrano K, Palacio A, Reinhold U. No room for pain: a prospective study showing effective and nearly pain-free treatment of actinic keratosis with simulated daylight photodynamic therapy (SDL-PDT) using the IndoorLux® system in combination with BF-200 ALA (Ameluz®). Photodiagnosis and Photodynamic Therapy. 2022;**37**:102692

[42] Gardlo K, Thomas R. Metvix (PhotoCure). Current Opinion in Investigational Drugs (London, England: 2000). 2002;**3**(11):1672-1678

[43] Bazargani ST, Hooman D, Schuckman AK, Cory MH, Siamak D. MP23-20 blue light cystoscopy for diagnosis of urothelial bladder cancer: results from a prospective multicenter registry. The Journal of Endourology, Videourology. 2016;**195**(4S):e269-e270

[44] Keam SJ, Lesley JS, Monique PC. Verteporfin. Drugs. 2003;**63**(22): 2521-2554

[45] Senge MO, Brandt JC. Temoporfin (Foscan®, 5, 10, 15, 20-tetra (m-hydroxyphenyl) chlorin)—a second-generation photosensitizer. Photochemistry and Photobiology. 2011;**87**(6):1240-1296

[46] Li X, Zheng B-D, Peng X-H, Li S-Z, Ying J-W, Zhao Y, et al. Phthalocyanines as medicinal photosensitizers: Developments in the last five years. Coordination Chemistry Reviews. 2019;**379**:147-160

[47] Dong W, Zhang X, Lu Z. Effect of 532nm photodynamic therapy with hemoporfin on the expression of vascular endothelial growth factor in cultured human vascular endothelial cells. Photodiagnosis and Photodynamic Therapy. 2020;**30**:101793

[48] Cheruku RR, Turowski SG, Durrani FA, Tabaczynski WA, Cacaccio J, Missert JR, et al. Tumor-Avid 3-(1'-Hexyloxy) ethyl-3-devinylpyrpyropheophorbide-a (HPPH)-3Gd (III) tetraxetan (DOTA) Conjugate Defines Primary Tumors and Metastases. Journal of Medicinal Chemistry. 2022;**65**(13):9267-9280

[49] Soman R, Chandra B, Ishfaq AB, Raveendra BM, Panda PK. Process for the preparation of fluorescent B(III)sub chlorins dyes and utility as theranostics for biomedical applications. Indian Patent with Application 202041048863. 2020

[50] Soman R, Brijesh C, Ishfaq BA, Kumar BS, Hossain SS, Nandy S, et al. A2B-and A3-Type Boron (III) Subchlorins Derived from meso-Diethoxycarbonyltripyrrane: Synthesis and Photophysical Exploration. The Journal of Organic Chemistry. 2021;**86**:10280-10287

[51] Correia JH, Rodrigues JA, Sara P, Dong T, Yang Z. Photodynamic therapy review: Principles, photosensitizers, applications, and future directions. Pharmaceutics. 2021;**13**(9):1332

[52] Kou J, Dou, Yang L. Porphyrin photosensitizers in photodynamic therapy and its applications. Oncotarget. 2017;**8**(46):81591

[53] Chilakamarthi U, Lingamallu G. Photodynamic therapy: past, present, and future. The Chemical Record. The Chemical Record. 2017;**17**(8):775-802

[54] Zeitouni NC, Bhatia N, Ceilley RI, Cohen JL, Del Rosso JQ, Moore AY, et al. Photodynamic Therapy with 5-aminolevulinic Acid 10% Gel and Red Light for the Treatment of Actinic Keratosis, Nonmelanoma Skin Cancers, and Acne: Current Evidence and Best Practices. The Journal of Clinical Aesthetic Dermatology. 2021;**14**(10):E53-E65

[55] Hong G, Antaris AL, Dai H. Near-infrared fluorophores for biomedical imaging. Nature Biomedical Engineering. 2017;**1**(1):1-22

[56] Gibbs SL. Near infrared fluorescence for image-guided surgery. Quantitative Imaging in Medicine and Surgery. 2012;**2**(3):177

[57] Hosokawa S, Goro T, Ken-ichi S, Satoru T, Jun O, Yoshinori T, et al. Photodiagnosis and Photodynamic Therapy. 2020;**29**:101627

[58] Cañete M, Ortega C, Gavalda A, Cristobal J, Juarranz A, Nonell S, et al. A red-light-activated sulfonamide porphycene for highly efficient photodynamic therapy against the hypoxic tumor. International Journal of Oncology. 2004;**24**(5):1221-1228

[59] Dąbrowski JM, Arnaut LG. Photodynamic therapy (PDT) of cancer: from local to systemic treatment. Photochemical & Photobiological Sciences. 2015;**14**(10):1765-1780

[60] Ruggiero E, Castro S A-d, Abraha H, Luca S. Upconverting nanoparticles for the near-infrared photoactivation of transition metal complexes: new opportunities and challenges in medicinal inorganic photochemistry. Dalton Transactions. 2016;**45**(33):13012-13020

[61] Kwiatkowski S, Knap B, Przystupski D, Saczko J, Kędzierska E, Knap-Czop K, et al. Photodynamic therapy–mechanisms, photosensitizers, and combinations. Biomedicine & Pharmacotherapy. 2018;**106**:1098-1107

[62] Maggioni D, Marco G, Laura D, Donato I, Di MV, Laura S, et al. A luminescent poly (amidoamine)–iridium complex as a new singlet-oxygen sensitizer for photodynamic therapy. Inorganic Chemistry. 2015;**54**(2):544-553

[63] Patrice T, editor. Photodynamic Therapy. Vol. 2. Royal Society of Chemistry. London. 2003

[64] Ryter SW, Charles JG, Angela F, MRF A, Marian L, Natalie R, et al. Cellular stress responses following photodynamic therapy. In: Photodynamic Therapy. Florida: CRC Press; 2020. pp. 55-62

[65] Escudero A, Carolina CC, Carmen MC, Elena R-B, Christian RB, Noureddine K. Photodynamic therapy: Photosensitizers and nanostructures. Materials Chemistry Frontiers. 2021;**5**(10):3788-3812

[66] Teng CW, Amirshaghaghi A, Cho SS, Cai SS, De Ravin E, Singh Y, et al. Combined fluorescence-guided surgery and photodynamic therapy for glioblastoma multiforme using cyanine and chlorin nanocluster. Journal of Neuro-Oncology. 2020;**149**(2):243-252

[67] Clare WT, Amirshaghaghi A, Cho SS, Cai SS, Ravin ED, Singh Y, et al. Combined fluorescence-guided surgery and photodynamic therapy for glioblastoma multiforme using cyanine and chlorin nanocluster. Journal of Neurooncology. 2020;**149**(2):243-252

[68] Olivier FD, Véronique Pt F. Journal of Controlled Release. 2010;**148**(2):135-146

[69] Tewabe A, Abate A, Tamrie M, Seyfu A, Siraj EA. Targeted drug delivery—from the magic bullet to nanomedicine: principles, challenges, and future perspectives. Journal of Multidisciplinary Healthcare. 2021;**14**:1711

[70] Karges J. Clinical development of metal complexes as photosensitizers for photodynamic therapy of cancer. Angewandte Chemie International Edition. 2022;**61**(5):e202112236

[71] Koyakutty M, Dominic JR, Henricus J, Slavka K, Shantikumar N. Amrita Center for Nanosciences and Molecular Medicine Move, Nanosciences "Targeted nano-photo medicines for photodynamic therapy of cancer. U.S. Patent Application 13/377,764. 2012.

[72] Solban N, Imran R, Tayyaba H. Targeted photodynamic therapy. Lasers in Surgery and Medicine: The Official Journal of the American Society for Laser Medicine and Surgery. 2006;**38**(5):522-531

[73] Verma S, Gregory M, Wzhiming M, Tayyaba H. Photochemistry and Photobiology. Strategies for enhanced photodynamic therapy effects. 2007;**83**(5):996-1005

[74] Malarvizhi GL, Parwathy C, Archana PR, Ranjith R, Neha G, Shantikumar N, et al. A rationally designed photo-chemo core-shell nanomedicine for inhibiting the migration of metastatic breast cancer cells followed by photodynamic killing. Nanomedicine: Nanotechnology, Biology and Medicine. 2014;**10**(3):579-587

[75] Koyakutty M, Dominic R, Henricus JC, Kascakova S, Shantikumar N. Amrita Center for Nanosciences and Molecular Medicine Move, nanosciences Targeted nano photo medicines for photodynamic therapy of cancer U.S. Patent 20220296714. 2022

[76] Bugaj AM. Targeted photodynamic therapy–a promising strategy of tumor treatment. Photochemical & Photobiological Sciences. 2011;**10**(7): 1097-1109

[77] Byrne JD, Tania B, Lisa B-P. Advanced Drug Delivery Reviews. Active targeting schemes for nanoparticle systems in cancer therapeutics. 2008;**60**(15):1615-1626

[78] Bae YH, Kinam P. Targeted drug delivery to tumors: myths, reality and possibility. Journal of Controlled Release. 2011;**153**(3):198

[79] Park J, Lee Y-K, Park I-K, Seung RH. Current limitations and recent progress in nanomedicine for clinically available photodynamic therapy. Biomedicine. 2021;**9**(1):85

[80] Matsumura Y, Hiroshi M. A new concept for macromolecular therapeutics in cancer chemotherapy: mechanism of tumor tropic accumulation of proteins and the antitumor agent smancs. Cancer Research. 1986;**46**(12_Part_1):6387-6392

[81] Bazak R, Mohamad H, Samar EA, Wael H, Tamer R. Passive targeting of nanoparticles to cancer: A comprehensive review of the literature. Molecular and Clinical Oncology. 2014;**2**(6):904-908

[82] Torchilin VP. Passive and active drug targeting: drug delivery to tumors as an example. Drug Delivery. 2010;**197**:3-53

[83] Fahmy SA, Mohamed H, Jens S. Liposome photosensitizer formulations for effective cancer photodynamic therapy. Pharmaceutics. 2021;**13**:1345

[84] Naidoo C, Cherie A, Heidi A. Photodynamic therapy for metastatic melanoma treatment: A review. Technology in Cancer Research & Treatment. 2018;**17**:1533033818791795

[85] Piktel E, Niemirowicz K, Watek M, Wollny T, Debtula P, Bucki R. Recent insights in nanotechnology-based drugs and formulations designed for effective anti-cancer therapy. Journal of Nanobiotechnology. 2016;**14**(1):1-23

[86] Hanish M, Ann Kruger C, Abrahamse H. Review: Organic nanoparticle based active targeting for photodynamic therapy treatment of breast cancer cells. Oncotarget. 2020;**11**:2120

[87] Stuchinskaya TMM, Michael JC, Dylan RE, David AR. Targeted photodynamic therapy of breast cancer cells using antibody-phthalocyanine-gold nanoparticle conjugates. Photochemical & Photobiological Sciences. 2011;**10**(5): 822-831

[88] Phillips D. Toward targeted photodynamic therapy. Pure and Applied Chemistry. 2011;**83**(4):733-748

[89] Kang X, Guo X, Niu X, An W, Li S, Liu Z, et al. Photothermal therapeutic application of gold nanorods-porphyrin-trastuzumab complexes in HER2-positive breast cancer. Scientific Reports. 2017;**7**(1):1-14

[90] Paszko E, Vaz GMF, Ehrhardt C, Senge MO. Transferrin conjugation does not increase the efficiency of liposomal Foscan during in vitro photodynamic therapy of esophageal cancer. European Journal of Pharmaceutical Sciences. 2013;**48**(1-2):202-210

[91] Ferino A, Nicoletto G, D'Este F, Zorzet S, Lago S, Richter SN, et al. Photodynamic therapy for Ras-driven cancers: Targeting G-quadruplex RNA structures with bifunctional alkyl-modified porphyrins. Journal of Medicinal Chemistry. 2020;**63**(3):1245-1260

[92] Li Y, Mingyang Z, Haijie H, Baohong Z, John BM, Defu C, et al. Peptide-based supramolecular photodynamic therapy systems: From rational molecular design to effective cancer treatment. Chemical Engineering Journal. 2022;**436**:135240

[93] Parrasia S, Szabò I, Zoratti M, Biasutto L. Peptides as Pharmacological Carriers to the Brain: Promises, Shortcomings and Challenges. Molecular Pharmaceutics. 2022;**19**(11):3700-3729

[94] Mehta RK, Shukla S, Ramanand SG, Somnay V, Bridges AJ, Lawrence TS, et al. Disruptin, a cell-penetrating peptide degrader of EGFR: Cell-Penetrating Peptide in Cancer Therapy. Translational Oncology. 2021;**14**(8):101140

[95] Klimpel A, Lützenburg T, Neundorf I. Recent advances of anti-cancer therapies including the use of cell-penetrating peptides. Current Opinion in Pharmacology. 2019;**47**:8-13

[96] Garizo AR, Bernardes N, Chakrabarty AM, Fialho AM. Microbial Infections and Cancer Therapy. Dubai, U.A.E: Jenny Stanford Publishing; 2019. pp. 319-338

[97] Song P, Du W, Li W, Zhu L, Zhang W, Gao X, et al. Preparation, characterization, and in vitro evaluation of amphiphilic peptide P12 and P12-DOX nanomicelles as antitumor drug carriers. Nanomaterials and Nanotechnology. 2020;**10**:1847980420911519

[98] Li X, Xie C, Zha S, Tam WS, Mingjun J, Ka-Leung W. Biocompatible Porphyrin-Peptide Conjugates as Theranostic Agents Targeting the

Epstein-Barr Virus. ChemPlusChem. 2022;**87**:e202200184

[99] Lin H, Runhong Z, Yu T, He J. An acid-targeting peptide can be used as a carrier for photodynamic therapy (PDT). Materials Today Communications. 2022;**31**:103659

[100] Meyers JD, Cheng Y, Broome AM, Agnes RS, Schluchter MD, Margevicius S, et al. Peptide-targeted gold nanoparticles for photodynamic therapy of brain cancer. Particle & Particle Systems Characterization. 2015;**32**(4): 448-457

[101] Cheng YJ, Qin SY, Liu WL, Ma YH, Chen XS, Zhang AQ, et al. Dual-Targeting Photosensitizer-Peptide Amphiphile Conjugate for Enzyme-Triggered Drug Delivery and Synergistic Chemo-Photodynamic Tumor Therapy. Advanced Materials Interfaces. 2020;**7**(19):2000935

[102] Cheng H, Zheng R-R, Fan G-L, Fan J-H, Zhao L-P, Jiang X-Y, et al. Mitochondria and plasma membrane dual-targeted chimeric peptide for single-agent synergistic photodynamic therapy. Biomaterials. 2019;**188**:1-11

[103] Cheng H, Yuan P, Guiling F, Linping Z, Rongrong Z, Yang B, et al. Chimeric peptide nanorods for plasma membrane and nuclear targeted photosensitizer delivery and enhanced photodynamic therapy. Applied Materials Today. 2019;**16**:120-131

[104] Wu J, Lin Y, Li H, Jin Q, Ji J. Zwitterionic stealth peptide-capped 5-aminolevulinic acid prodrug nanoparticles for targeted photodynamic therapy. Journal of Colloid and Interface Science. 2017;**485**:251-259

[105] Li SY, Cheng H, Qiu W-X, Liu L-H, Chen S, Hu Y, et al. Protease Activable Cell-Penetrating Peptide-Protoporphyrin Conjugate for Targeted Photodynamic Therapy In Vivo. ACS Applied Materials & Interfaces. 2015;**7**(51):28319-28329

[106] Hou Y, Yafei K, Qikun J, Zhou S, Yu J, He Z , et al. Arginine-peptide complex-based assemblies to combat tumor hypoxia for enhanced photodynamic therapeutic effect. Nano Research. 2022;**15**(6):5183-5192

[107] Webb A. Introduction to Biomedical Imaging. John Wiley & Sons. New Jersey; 2022

[108] FDA Approves First PSMA-Targeted PET Imaging Drug for Men with Prostate Cancer | FDA. 2020.Available from: https://jnm.snmjournals.org/content/jnumed/62/2/11N.2.full.pdf

[109] Tsolekile N, Nelana S, Oluwafemi OS. Porphyrin as diagnostic and therapeutic agent. Molecules. 2019;**24**(14):2669

[110] Radhakrishnan R, Kamalasanan K. Pharmaceutical perspectives of selection criteria and toxicity profiling of nano theranostics agents. Drug Delivery Nanosystems for Biomedical Applications. London. 2018. p. 45-74

[111] Kelkar SS, Reineke MT. Theranostics: combining imaging and therapy. Bioconjugate Chemistry. 2011;**22**(10):1879-1903

[112] Kun L, Huang J, He R, Wang Q, Chai Y, Shen M. Comparison of Vis-NIR and SWIR hyperspectral imaging for the non-destructive detection of DON levels in Fusarium head blight wheat kernels and wheat flour. Infrared Physics & Technology. 2020;**106**:103281

[113] Jin GQ, Chau CV, Arambula JF, Gao S, Sessler JL, Zhang J-L. Lanthanide porphyrinoids as molecular theranostics. Chemical Society Reviews. 2022;**51**:6177-6209

[114] Chen W, Zhao J, Hou M, Yang M, Changqing Y. Gadolinium–porphyrin-based polymer nanotheranostics for fluorescence/magnetic resonance imaging guided photodynamic therapy. Nanoscale. 2021;**13**(38):16197-16206

[115] Qindeel M, Sargazi S, Hosseinikhah SM, Rahdar A, Barani M, Thakur VK, et al. Porphyrin-Based Nanostructures for Cancer Theranostics: Chemistry, Fundamentals and Recent Advances. ChemistrySelect. 2021;**6**(48):14082-14099

[116] Zhu Z, Wang X, Li T, Aime S, Sadler PJ, Guo Z. Platinum (II)–Gadolinium (III) Complexes as Potential Single-Molecular Theranostic Agents for Cancer Treatment. Angewandte Chemie. 2014;**126**(48):13441-13444

[117] Sessler JL, Miller RA. Texaphyrins: new drugs with diverse clinical applications in radiation and photodynamic therapy. Biochemical Pharmacology. 2000;**59**(7):733-739

[118] Cheng MHY, Overchuk M, Rajora MA, Lou JWH, Chen Y, Pomper MG, et al. Targeted Theranostic 111In/Lu-Nano texaphyrin for SPECT Imaging and Photodynamic Therapy. Molecular Pharmaceutics. 2021;**19**(6): 1803-1813

[119] Aggarwal A, Samaroo D, Jovanovic IR, Singh S, Tuz MP, Mackiewicz MR. Porphyrinoid-based photosensitizers for diagnostic and therapeutic applications: An update. Journal of Porphyrins and Phthalocyanines. 2019;**23**(07n08): 729-765

[120] Zhou HC, Long JR, Yaghi OM. Introduction to metal–organic frameworks. Chemical Reviews. 2012;**112**(2):673-674

[121] Furukawa H, Cordova KE, O'Keeffe M, Yaghi OM. The Chemistry and Applications of Metal-Organic Frameworks. Science. 2013;**341**(6149):1230444

[122] Kandambeth S, Dey K, Banerjee R. Covalent Organic Frameworks: Chemistry beyond the Structures. Journal of the American Chemical Society. 2018;**141**(5):1807-1822

[123] Meng HM, Hu X-X, Ge-Zhi Kong C, Yang TF, Li Z-H, Zhang X-B. Aptamer-functionalized nanoscale metal-organic frameworks for targeted photodynamic therapy. Theranostics. 2018;**8**(16):4332

[124] Gao P, Wang M, Chen Y, Pan W, Zhou P, Wan X, et al. A COF-based nanoplatform for highly efficient cancer diagnosis, photodynamic therapy and prognosis. Chemical Science. 2020;**11**(26):6882-6888

[125] Zhao C, Rehman FU, Yang Y, Li X, Zhang D, Jiang H, et al. Bio-imaging and Photodynamic Therapy with Tetra Sulphonatophenyl Porphyrin (TSPP)-TiO2 Nanowhiskers: New Approaches in Rheumatoid Arthritis Theranostics. Scientific Reports. 2015;**5**(1):1-11

[126] Cieplik F, Deng D, Crielaard W, Buchalla W, Hellwig E, Al-Ahmad A, et al. Antimicrobial photodynamic therapy – what we know and what we don't. Critical Reviews in Microbiology. 2018;**44**(5):571-589

[127] Comeau P, Burgess J, Qi NR, Lee A, Manso A. The antimicrobial, physical, and chemical properties of a riboflavin-loaded dental resin intended for antimicrobial photodynamic therapy. Photodiagnosis and Photodynamic Therapy. 2022;**40**:103124

[128] Almeida H, Amparo M, Maria FFF, Neves GPMS. Antimicrobial

Photodynamic Therapy in the Control of COVID-19. Antibiotics. 2020;**9**(6):320

[129] Shen JJ, Jemec GBE, Arendrup MC, Saunte DML. Photodynamic therapy treatment of superficial fungal infections: A systematic review. Photodiagnosis and Photodynamic Therapy. 2020;**31**:101774

[130] Soman R, Raghav D, Sujatha S, Rathinasamy K, Arunkumar C. Axial Ligand Modified High Valent Tin (IV) Porphyrins: Synthesis, Structure, Photophysical Studies and Photodynamic Antimicrobial Activities on Candida Albicans. RSC Advances. 2015;**5**(75):61103-61117

[131] Roca JA, Wu L, Fromow-Guerra J, Rodríguez FJ, Berrocal MH, Rojas S, et al. Yellow (577 nm) micropulse laser versus half-dose verteporfin photodynamic therapy in eyes with chronic central serous chorioretinopathy: results of the Pan-American Collaborative Retina Study (PACORES) Group. British Journal of Ophthalmology. 2018;**102**(12):1696-1700

[132] Simons RE, Danna LZ, Jafferany M. Psychodermatology of vitiligo: Psychological impact and consequences. Dermatologic Therapy. 2020;**33**(3):e13418

[133] Zhang Y, Lin H, Guo XJ, Zou XB. A case series pilot study on the combination of 5-aminolevulinic acid and photodynamic therapy (ALA-PDT) for treatment of vitiligo. Anais Brasileiros de Dermatologia. 2018;**93**:539-545

[134] Dai T, He W, Tu S, Han J, Yuan B, Yao C, et al. Black TiO2 nanoprobe-mediated mild phototherapy reduces intracellular lipid levels in atherosclerotic foam cells via cholesterol regulation pathways instead of apoptosis. Bioactive Materials. 2022;**17**:18-28

[135] Mallidi S, Anbil S, B A-L, Obaid G, Ichikawa M, Hasan T. Beyond the Barriers of Light Penetration: Strategies, Perspectives and Possibilities for Photodynamic Therapy. Theranostics. 2016;**6**(13):2458

[136] Sun Y, Dongyang Z, Wang G, Wang Y, Cao L, Sun J, et al. Recent progress of hypoxia-modulated multifunctional nanomedicines to enhance photodynamic therapy: opportunities, challenges, and future development. Acta Pharmaceutica Sinica B. 2020;**10**(8):1382-1396

[137] Sellera FP, Nascimento CL, Ribeiro MS. Clinical applications of antimicrobial PDT. In: Photodynamic Therapy in Veterinary Medicine: From Basics to Clinical Practice. Springer; 2016. pp. 169-196

[138] Yan J, Gao T, Lu Z, Yin J, Zhang Y, Pei R. Aptamer-targeted photodynamic platforms for tumor therapy. ACS Applied Materials & Interfaces. 2021;**13**(24):27749-27773

[139] Couto GK, Seixas FK, Iglesias BA, Collares T. Perspectives of photodynamic therapy in biotechnology. Journal of Photochemistry and Photobiology B: Biology. 2020;**213**:112051

Section 3

Characterization and Analysis

Chapter 8

Synthesis of Glycoconjugates in Potentiating Pharmacological and Pharmaceutical Activity

Smita Kumbhar and Manish Bhatia

Abstract

The full range of glycoconjugates made up of glycans, or carbohydrate chains, that are covalently joined to lipid or protein molecules is known as the glycome. Glycoconjugates are created, through the process of glycosylation (vary in length, glycan sequence, and the connections that connect them). The creation of therapies can now take advantage of new knowledge about the structure and operation of the glycome, which may enhance our capacity to control inflammation and immune responses, maximize the efficacy of therapeutic antibodies, and enhance immune responses to cancer. These instances highlight the promise of the young discipline of "glycomedicine." The prevalence of glycoconjugates in nature and their significance in various biological processes have prompted the development of numerous synthesizing techniques for these molecules. Today, synthetic glycoconjugates are utilized to address a wide range of biological concerns linked to glycoconjugates. This study seeks to update earlier reviews on the topic as well as gather and compile the most recent developments in the fields of glycopeptide, glycoprotein, and glycolipid synthesis. Finally, we hope that this study may stimulate fruitful research in this significant area of medicinal chemistry by highlighting the triumphs and shortcomings of prior research.

Keywords: Glycoconjugates, N-linked glycosylation, O-linked glycans, C-linked glycans, pharmacological activity, pharmaceutical activity

1. Introduction

Glycoconjugates are a class of sugars, or glycans, that are bonded covalently to various chemical species, such as proteins, peptides, lipids, and other compounds. The production of glycoconjugates occurs through the process of glycosylation [1]. Glycoconjugates, which include glycoproteins, glycopeptides, peptidoglycans, glycolipids, glycosides, and lipopolysaccharides, among other groups, are very important biological compounds. They take part in cell-cell interactions, matrix interactions, cell-cell interactions, and detoxification activities [2].

In general, the carbohydrate part(s) of a glycoconjugate play a vital role in its function; noteworthy examples of this are blood proteins and neural cell adhesion molecule, where minute differences in the carbohydrate structure influence cell attachment (or not) or lifetime in circulation.

Despite having a portion of carbohydrates, the significant biological species DNA, RNA, ATP, cAMP, cGMP, NADH, and coenzyme A are not typically regarded as glycoconjugates. Covalently joining polysaccharides antigens with protein scaffolds results in glycoconjugates, which are intended to produce a sustained immunological response in the body [3]. Glycoconjugate-based immunisation successfully produced long-lasting immunological memory against carbohydrate antigens. Since their introduction in the 1990s, glycoconjugate vaccines have demonstrated efficacy against meningococcus and influenza. GlycoRNAs were discovered for the in 2021.

The entire biological study of carbohydrates is known as glycobiology [4, 5]. It is frequently necessary to attach carbohydrates to surfaces, tag them with fluorophores, or transform them into natural or artificial glycoconjugates, like glycopeptides or glycolipids, in order to comprehend the role and behaviour of complex carbohydrates. These glycoconjugates must be created using simple and reliable chemical techniques in order to support glycobiology and its "omics," glycomics. An overview of the quickly developing area of chemical reactions that specifically transform unguarded carbohydrates into glycoconjugates via the anomeric position is provided in this article. O-, N-, S-, and C-glycosides are included in the discussion as well as other anomeric bond types of the newly generated glycoconjugates [6–8].

The biosynthetic enzymes called glycosidases and glycosyltransferases catalyse the hydrolysis of interglycosidic connections and the biosynthesis of interglycosyltransferases. The variety of naturally occurring glycosyltransferases and glycosidases, each of which has a distinct substrate preference, reflects the diversity of natural glycans. Natural glycans are frequently found in varied forms and frequently formed in minuscule quantities, making it difficult to isolate and characterise them from natural sources. As a result, synthetic glycans are crucial to glycobiology, and glycan production methods have advanced significantly. Glycosyltransferases and glycosidases are advantageous biocatalysts for the synthesis of glycans because they are very effective under controlled conditions. In this chapter, we go over basic ideas in glycobiology and combine them with recent developments in comprehending the main functions of the glycome in health and illness. Glycans are saccharides or sugar chains that can be free or attached to proteins or lipids to form simple or complex glycoconjugates. We review how glycosylation patterns are altered in a variety of human diseases, including congenital disorders of glycosylation (CDGs) as well as autoimmune, infectious, and chronic inflammatory diseases.

Key points of Glycosylation [9, 10]:

- Development in the field of glycobiology during the past ten years has been fuelled by improvements in analytical techniques. Glycosylation is essential for both physiological and pathological cellular processes.

- Congenital abnormalities of glycosylation have shed light on the fundamental processes that link particular glycoconjugates to disease phenotypes.

- The glycosylation motifs of membrane bound glycoconjugates and their binding to sugar specific receptors control the interactions between immune cells that are mediated by cell surface molecules and propel cellular activation.

- Oncofetal phenotypes are frequently present in cancers and are mirrored in the structure of their glycoconjugates. These changes in glycosylation are responsible for the development of metastatic characteristics, the inhibition of apoptosis, and chemotherapy resistance.

- Abnormal O-linked N-acetylglucosamine-mediated signalling and enhanced glycation of numerous proteins are involved in the pathogenesis of many autoimmune diseases, including immunoglobulin A (IgA) nephropathy, systemic lupus erythematous, and inflammatory bowel disease.

- Abnormal O-linked N-acetylglucosamine-mediated signalling and increased glycation of numerous proteins are involved in the development of many autoimmune disorders, including immunoglobulin A (IgA) nephropathy, systemic lupus erythematous, and inflammatory bowel disease. • Immunoglobulin glycosylation regulates the effector actions of antibodies, opening new possibilities for their use in therapeutics.

There are five types of glycans produced [11, 12]:

1. Asparagine or arginine side-chain nitrogens are connected to N-linked glycans. Dolichol phosphate, a unique lipid, is required for N-linked glycosylation.

2. O-linked glycans that are joined to the hydroxyl oxygen on the side chains of serine, threonine, tyrosine, hydroxylysine, or hydroxyproline, or to the oxygen on lipids like ceramide.

3. phosphoglycans connected by a phosphoserine's phosphate.

4. C-linked glycans are an uncommon kind of glycosylation in which a sugar is bound to a carbon on a tryptophan side chain. One of the few naturally occurring materials is aloin.

5. Proteins and lipids are connected through glypiation, which is the attachment of a GPI anchor.

2. Humans' primary forms of glycosylation

2.1 N-linked glycosylation

A nitrogen atom of Asn residues at Asn-x-Ser/Thr motifs served as the connection point for the branched protein glycans. Many eukaryotic glycoproteins fold properly as a result of N-linked glycosylation, which is also crucial for cell-to-cell and cell-extracellular matrix adhesion. N-linked glycosylation occurs frequently in archaea and in the lumen of the endoplasmic reticulum of eukaryotes but extremely infrequently in bacteria. The N-linked glycans of a protein can affect a protein's activity, sometimes acting as an on/off switch, in addition to their role in protein folding and cellular attachment [13].

N-linked glycans are biosynthesized in three main steps [14–16]:

- Creation of a precursor oligosaccharide related to dolichol:

The production of dolichol-linked GlcNAc sugar is the first step in the N-linked glycosylation process. Dolichol is a lipid molecule made up of isoprene units that repeat. This molecule can be seen affixed to the ER membrane. The dolichol is joined to sugar molecules by a pyrophosphate bond (one phosphate was originally linked to dolichol, and the second phosphate came from the nucleotide sugar). The oligosaccharide chain is then lengthened by gradually adding different sugar molecules to create a precursor oligosaccharide.

- En bloc protein-to-precursor oligosaccharide transfer:

  The finished glycan is subsequently transported to the immature polypeptide in the lumen of the ER membrane after the precursor oligosaccharide has been produced. The energy generated when the pyrophosphate connection between the dolichol-glycan molecule is broken is what powers this reaction. A glycan must meet three requirements in order to be transferred to a developing polypeptide:

  - In the fundamental structure, asparagine must be situated in a particular consensus sequence (Asn–X–Ser or Asn–X–Thr or in rare instances Asn–X–Cys).

  - In the protein's three-dimensional structure, asparagine must be properly positioned (Sugars are polar molecules and thus need to be attached to asparagine located on the surface of the protein and not buried within the protein).

  - For N-linked glycosylation to begin, asparagine must be present on the endoplasmic reticulum's luminal side. Either secretory proteins or the transmembrane protein sections facing the lumen include target residues.

  The enzyme known as oligosaccharyltransferase is in charge of recognising the consensus sequence and transferring the precursor glycan to a polypeptide acceptor that is being translated in the lumen of the endoplasmic reticulum. Therefore, N-linked glycosylation is a co-translational process.

- The oligosaccharide's transformation:

  Two glucose residues from the structure are eliminated when the finished glycan is transferred onto the developing polypeptide. Some sugar residues are eliminated by the glycosidases enzyme group. By using a water molecule, these enzymes can dissolve glycosidic bonds. As exoglycosidases, these enzymes only digest monosaccharide residues found at the non-reducing end of glycans. This initial trimming step is believed to function in the ER as a quality control step to watch over protein folding.
  Glucosidase I and II take two glucose residues out of the protein once it has been correctly folded. The glycoprotein is prepared for transit from the ER to the cis-Golgi when the last third of the glucose residue is removed. This last glucose is eliminated via ER mannosidase. The glycoprotein cannot exit the endoplasmic reticulum, though, if the protein is improperly folded, leaving the glucose residues behind. To help with protein folding, a chaperone protein binds to the unfolded or partially folded protein. The following stage entails adding and removing additional sugar leftovers from the cis-Golgi. Glycosyltransferases and glycosidases, respectively, catalyse these changes. Four mannose residues in −1,2 linkages are eliminated

by a group of mannosidases in the cis-Golgi. High mannose, hybrid, and complex glycans are the three primary forms of glycans, whereas in the medial region of the Golgi, glycosyltransferases add sugar residues to the core glycan structure.

Functions of N-linked glycans [17, 18]:

- N-linked glycans serve both internal and external purposes.

Intrinsic:

- Provides the extracellular matrix and cell wall with structural elements.
- Modify the stability and solubility of proteins, among other qualities.

Extrinsic:

- Controls glycoprotein trafficking.
- Controls cell signalling (cell–cell and cell–matrix interactions).
- Clinical importance
    - Rheumatoid arthritis, type 1 diabetes, Crohn's disease, and malignancies have all been linked to changes in N-linked glycosylation.
    - Numerous disorders, the majority of which affect the nervous system, are caused by mutations in 18 genes involved in N-linked glycosylation.

2.2 O-linked glycosylation

The process of attaching a sugar molecule to a protein's serine (Ser) or threonine (Thr) residues is known as O-linked glycosylation. A post-translational alteration known as o-glycosylation takes place after the protein has been created. It happens in the cytoplasm of prokaryotes as well as the endoplasmic reticulum, Golgi apparatus, and occasionally the cytoplasm of eukaryotes. A variety of sugars can be added to serine or threonine, and they have an impact on the protein in many ways by altering protein stability and controlling protein activity. The body uses O-glycans, which are sugars attached to serine or threonine, for a variety of purposes, including immune system cell trafficking, recognising foreign objects, regulating cell metabolism, and preserving the flexibility of cartilage and tendons. Changes in O-glycosylation have a crucial role in a variety of disorders, including cancer, diabetes, and Alzheimer's, due to their wide range of functions. Eukaryotes, archaea, and a number of pathogenic bacteria, such as *Burkholderia cenocepacia*, *Neisseria gonorrhoeae*, and *Acinetobacter baumannii*, all exhibit O-glycosylation [19, 20].

- O-glycosylation types [21, 22]

1. O-N-acetylgalactosamine (O-GalNAc)

After the protein has folded, N-acetylgalactosamine (GalNAc) is added to a serine or threonine in the Golgi apparatus. GalNAc transferases (GALNTs), of which there are 20 different varieties, carry out the process. Other sugars or substances like methyl and acetyl groups may be added to the original O-GalNAc structure to change it. Eight core structures are produced as a result of these alterations. Because various cells contain different glycosyltransferases, or enzymes that can add more sugars, each cell's structure is unique. Galactose, N-acetylglucosamine, fucose, and sialic acid are often added sugars. Sulphates or acetyl groups can also be added to these sugars to change them.

O-GalNAc sugars are crucial for a number of functions, including as fertilisation, defence against invasive microorganisms, and leukocyte circulation during an immune response.

Membrane glycoproteins frequently contain O-GalNAc sugars, which improve the stiffness of the area near the membrane and enable the protein to stretch away from the membrane's surface. For instance, a region rigidified by O-glycans projects the low-density lipoprotein receptor (LDLR) from the surface of the cell.

2. O-N-acetylglucosamine (O-GlcNAc)

In contrast to O-GalNAc modifications, which often take place on proteins that will be secreted, N-acetylglucosamine (O-GlcNAc) addition to serine and threonine residues typically happens on cytoplasmic and nuclear proteins that remain in the cell. Although O-GlcNAc modifications are relatively new, the number of proteins that have these changes is growing quickly. It is the first instance of glycosylation occurring on a protein other than a secretory protein.

O-GlcNAcylation can also heighten the Warburg Effect, which is the alteration in the metabolism of cancer cells that promotes their proliferation. Both O-GlcNAcylation and phosphorylation are intriguing potential targets for cancer therapy because they both have the ability to modify particular residues and hence play crucial roles in controlling signalling cascades.

3. O-Mannose (O-Man)

O-mannosylation is the process by which a dolichol-P-mannose donor molecule transfers a mannose to a protein's serine or threonine residue. The donor molecule used in the majority of other O-glycosylation procedures is a sugar nucleotide. Another distinction between this O-glycosylation and others is that the process begins in the endoplasmic reticulum of the cell, not the Golgi apparatus. However, the Golgi is where further sugar addition takes place.

The process is present in all domains of life, including eukaryotes, (eu)bacteria, and archae(bacteria), despite recent claims to the contrary. The O-mannosylated human protein with the finest characterisation is -dystroglycan. Two domains of the protein that connect the extracellular and intracellular areas and anchor the cell in place are separated by O-Man sugars. In a sophisticated alteration, ribitol, xylose, and glucuronic acid can be added to this molecule to create a lengthy sugar chain. To stabilise the contact between -dystroglycan and the extracellular basement membrane, this is necessary. Without these adjustments, the glycoprotein cannot bind the cell, resulting in congenital muscular dystrophy (CMD), which is characterised by severe brain abnormalities.

4. O-Galactose (O-Gal)

Collagen contains lysine residues that are frequently modified to generate hydroxylysine, or O-galactose, by the addition of a hydroxyl group. Hydroxylysine can then undergo O-glycosylation modification as a result of this oxygen addition. The endoplasmic reticulum initiates the addition of a galactose to the hydroxyl group, which mostly takes place in the Golgi apparatus and only on certain sequences of hydroxylysine residues.

Although all collagens require this O-galactosylation for proper function, types IV and V of collagen are particularly prone to it. A glucose sugar may occasionally be combined with the primary galactose.

5. O-Fucose (O-Fuc)

An uncommon type of O-glycosylation known as O-Fucose (O-Fuc) occurs in the endoplasmic reticulum and is catalysed by two fucosyltransferases. Fucose sugars are added to serine and threonine residues. Both Toxoplasma gondii and Plasmodium falciparum have them, according to research.

The core fucose on the protein can be extended by a number of different enzymes, which allows for the addition of various sugars. Along with O-glucosylation, O-fucosylation is primarily observed on proteins' epidermal growth factor (EGF) domains. On EGF domains, O-fucosylation takes place between the second and third conserved cysteine residues. GlcNAc, galactose, and sialic acid are frequently added to extend O-fucose after the core sugar has been introduced.

6. O-Glucose (O-Glc)

O-glucosylation, like O-fucosylation, is a peculiar O-linked modification since it takes place in the endoplasmic reticulum, is catalysed by O-glucosyltransferases, and also necessitates the addition of a specific sequence to the protein. For instance, in clotting factors VII and IX, O-glucose is frequently bonded to serine residues between the first and second conserved cysteine residues of EGF domains. Additionally, it appears that O-glucosylation is required for the Notch protein's EGF domains to fold correctly.

Functions of O-linked glycans [23]:

The body has large amounts of all types of O-glycosylation, which are crucial for numerous cellular processes.

- Lewis epitopes are crucial for identifying blood types and for triggering an immune response in the event that we recognise alien organs. It's crucial to comprehend them before doing organ transplants.

- Immunoglobulins' hinge sections are heavily O-glycosylated in order to preserve their structural integrity, enable interactions with external antigens, and guard against proteolytic cleavage.

- O-glycosylation might be harmful to Alzheimer's patients. O-GlcNAc alterations are found in tau, the protein that builds up in Alzheimer's to produce neurodegeneration, and they may be related to the course of the illness.

- O-glycosylation alterations are very frequent in cancer. The ability of O-glycan structures, particularly the terminal Lewis epitopes, may facilitate tumour cell invasion into new tissues during metastasis.

2.3 C-mannosylation

In the sequence W-X-X-W, the initial tryptophan residue receives a mannose sugar (W indicates tryptophan; X is any amino acid). The first carbon of alpha-mannose and the second carbon of tryptophan combine to form a C-C bond. Not all sequences with this pattern are mannosylated, though. It has been determined that, in reality, only two thirds are, and that, in order for mannosylation to take place, it is clearly preferred that the second amino acid be one of the polar ones (Ser, Ala, Gly, and Thr). Recently, a breakthrough in the method for determining whether or not a sequence will contain a mannosylation site was made, with accuracy of 93% as opposed to 67% considering WXXW motif [24, 25].

One of the proteins that has this modification the most frequently is thrombospondin. Type I cytokine receptors are a different class of proteins that are subject to C-mannosylation. Because the sugar is connected to carbon rather than a reactive element like nitrogen or oxygen, c-mannosylation is unique. Human complement component 8 has the first crystal structure of a protein with this kind of glycosylation, which was established in 2011. It has been determined that C-mannosylation occurs on 18% of secreted and transmembrane human proteins [26]. Numerous studies have demonstrated that this activity is crucial for the secretion of proteins that include Trombospondin type 1, which are otherwise maintained in the endoplasmic reticulum.

2.4 Phosphoserine glycosylation

In the literature, Xylose, Fucose, Mannose, and GlcNAc Phosphoserine Glycans have all been documented. Only Dictyostelium discoideum, Leishmania mexicana, and Trypanosoma cruzi have been reported to contain fucose, xylose, and GlcNAc. On the cell-surface laminin receptor alpha dystroglycan, mannose has recently been discovered in a vertebrate, the mouse Mus musculus4. Since alpha dystroglycan is substantially conserved from lower vertebrates to mammals, it has been hypothesised that this unusual discovery may be related [27, 28].

2.5 GPI anchors (glypiation)

A GPI anchor is created during the process of glycosidation, a particular type of glycosylation. In this type of glycosylation, a glycan chain connects a protein to a lipid anchor.

For many cell-surface proteins, glycosylphosphatidylinositol (GPI) functions as a lipid anchor. The GPI anchor, which is widely utilised in eukaryotes and maybe in some Archaea but not in Eubacteria, is a posttranslational modification of proteins with a glycolipid. The majority of cell-surface proteins in protozoa are GPI-anchored proteins. Numerous GPI-anchored proteins in fungus eventually become a part of the cell wall. At least 150 GPI-anchored proteins have been found in humans, and they may play a number of different roles, including those of receptors, adhesion molecules, enzymes, transcytotic receptors and transporters, and protease inhibitors [29–31].

2.6 Glycosaminoglycans

The largest glycans produced by animal cells are known as glycosaminoglycans (GAG), which are often used to decorate proteins known as proteoglycans. In addition to their large length, GAG are distinctive for being highly sulphated. The names given to GAG chains, such as heparan sulphate, chondroitin sulphate, and dermatan sulphate, reflect this sulphation. Proteoglycans are a large family of different proteins that are often found tethered to cell membranes or stored in secretory granules, but they can also be secreted in the extracellular matrix. Proteoglycans typically have names ending in "can," such biglycan, versican, and aggrecan, but there are few exceptions because decorin, aggrin, and CD44 are all proteoglycans. From a single GAG chain on decorin to more than 100 chains on aggrecan, the number of GAG chains on proteoglycans varies substantially. Due to the presence of a Xyl residue that is b-linked to serine, GAG chains have a core structure that is distinct from other glycans. Additionally, there are two Gal units and a GlcA unit in the core. Keratan sulphates are the exception, since they lengthen the N-glycan and O-GalNAc cores, whereas the majority of GAG subclasses extend on this tetrasaccharide core [32–35].

Different GAG subclasses are defined by various core elongation kinds. Chondroitin sulphates and dermatan sulphates are made up of repeats of the disaccharide GlcA(b1–3)GalNAc, whereas heparan sulphates are characterised by repeats of the disaccharide GlcA(b1–4)GlcNAc(a1–4) (b1–4). The GAG backbone is polymerised during or following subsequent changes including epimerization and sulphation.

2.7 Glycolipids

In all spheres of life, glycolipids are a significant but frequently underappreciated portion of glycoconjugates. Glycolipids have an enormous range of structural variations, both at the glycan and lipid moiety levels. Animals, plants, and microorganisms all glycosylate various kinds of lipids. In the membranes of photosynthetic structures in plants, algae, and bacteria, glycerolipids are abundant as glycan-carriers. The most prevalent forms of these glycolipids are monogalactosyldiacylglycerol and digalactosyldiacylglycerol. A complex lipid structure known as lipid A in gram-negative bacteria transports a variety of heterogeneous and unique glycan chains to create lipopolysaccharides (see chapter on bacterial glycosylation). The class of glycosphingolipids, which is based on N-acyl sphingoid lipid, commonly known as ceramide, predominates in animals [36].

2.8 Glycosyltransferases

A set of enzymes known as glycosyltransferases catalyse the transfer of a sugar moiety from an active sugar onto acceptors that are either carbohydrates or other molecules. Glycosyltransferases, with the exception of hyaluronan synthase, lengthen glycans by attaching monosaccharides to the non-reducing ends of acceptor substrates. The product of the linkage-specific transfer reaction is fixed in a specific anomeric structure. Prokaryotic and eukaryotic genomes contain a large number of glycosyltransferase genes. Up to 5% of genomes contain genes involved in glycosylation when all transporters and enzymes necessary for substrate production and glycan breakdown are included. More than 30.000 glycosyltransferases have been identified to far worldwide [37, 38].

2.9 Hyaluronan

Hyaluronan, a polysaccharide with repeats of a disaccharide motif, differs from GAG in that it is not sulphated and has additional characteristics. First of all, it is secreted as a free polysaccharide and is not attached to any protein. Second, hyaluronan is extruded from the cell surface as a result of polymerisation of the molecule at the plasma membrane from its reducing end. The disaccharide GlcNAc(b1–4) GlcA can be repeated more than 10,000 times in the resultant polymers (b1–3).

The hydrophilic gel-like properties of hyaluronan are similar to those of a viscous lubricant due to its large molecular weight and negative charges. Hyaluronan can be produced by non-vertebrates as well [39].

In fact, many bacteria express hyaluronan as a component of their capsular structure, and even some enormous viruses do so. However, the function of the hyaluronan synthase gene is unknown. Three hyaluronan synthase (HAS) genes, with varying kinetic characteristics and end products, are present in the human genome. As evidenced by the severe cardiac and vascular abnormalities seen in Has2-knockout embryos, which pass away by mid-gestation, the HAS2 gene is crucial for mammalian development. On the other hand, mice lacking the Has1 or Has3 genes are viable and productive and develop normally.

2.10 Hybrid n-glycans

High-mannose glycans are known as high-mannose glycans, and hybrid glycans are known as having both unsubstituted terminal mannose residues and substituted mannose residues with a N-acetylglucosamine connection (as are present in complex glycans) [40].

2.11 Health and disease-related glycosylation

Numerous naturally occurring bioactive compounds are glycoconjugates; these chemicals' production, stability, action, and turnover in whole organisms can all be significantly impacted by the glycans that are connected to them. For instance, sulphated glycosaminoglycan heparin and its derivatives are among the most often prescribed medications in the world. Glycobiology and carbohydrate chemistry have grown in significance in contemporary biotechnology for this and many other reasons. Knowing a drug's glycan structure is necessary for patenting, getting FDA authorisation for usage, and keeping track of manufacture. Furthermore, with sales in the tens of billions of dollars yearly and an industry that is still expanding at an accelerating rate, glycoproteins -which include monoclonal antibodies, enzymes, and hormones -are currently the main products of the biotechnology sector. A number of human illness conditions are also defined by modifications in glycan production, which may be important for both diagnostic and therapeutic purposes [41].

2.11.1 Glycans in the pharmaceutical industry

On isolated or synthetic glycans or on substances that change their expression and recognition, several classes of profitable commercial goods are established. Many well-known small-molecule medications are natural substances that have glycans as part of their primary structure or as a sugar side chain. Examples include antibiotics and anticancer treatment medicines (i.e., a glycoside).

By producing different glycoconjugates, the glycocans that are expressed on the top surface of cells take part in a number of essential biological processes. Research into the therapeutic potential of complex glycoconjugates has been sparked by their identification as mediators of crucial biological processes. As glycoconjugates have become more readily available, they have been used extensively in the field of drug delivery. In order to widen the future therapeutic scope of drug delivery systems and provide effective cancer therapy, this review specifically discusses constitutive glycoconjugates of receptor-mediated binding of glycoprotein, glycolipids, and glycopeptides for cell-selective drug delivery [42, 43].

Synthetic glycoconjugates are presently employed to address a number of biological concerns relating to glycoconjugates and have produced new potential cancer, viral, and bacterial infection vaccines as well as novel biotechnological tools.

2.11.2 Opportunities and challenges: Research on synthetic glycoconjugates

More and more, synthetic oligosaccharides and glycoconjugates are used as biological research probes and as lead chemicals in the quest for new drugs and vaccines. However, the lack of universal techniques for the regular manufacture of this significant class of chemicals makes these efforts more difficult. The utilisation of unified monosaccharide building blocks, stereoselective glycosylation protocols, one-pot multi-step protecting group modifications, and convergent oligosaccharide assembly methodologies are just a few of the recent developments that are starting to address these issues. Additionally, chemo-enzymatic techniques that use various glycosyl transferases to alter a synthetic oligosaccharide precursor can speed up oligosaccharide synthesis. A lack of a variety of glycosyltransferases has been addressed by glycosynthases, which are mutant glycosidases that can easily create glycosidic bonds. The significance of carbohydrate chemistry is emphasised [44, 45].

3. Conclusion

Proteins and lipids are frequently modified by the non-template, dynamic process known as glycosylation. Glycans play a variety of important roles in how cells respond to environmental cues as well as how cells develop and differentiate. Particular variations in glycan composition are directly linked to a number of disorders. Our knowledge of the physiological and pathological processes that are controlled by glycans is improving as technological advancements start to overcome many of the obstacles provided by the complexity of glycoconjugates. Such initiatives are additionally aided by advancements in research instruments and training in the glycosciences, both of which promote the development of glycomedicine, in which glycobiology is used to create new treatments.

Conflict of interest

The authors declare no conflict of interest.

Author details

Smita Kumbhar[1*] and Manish Bhatia[2]

1 Department of Pharmaceutical Analysis, DSTS Mandal's College of Pharmacy, Solapur, India

2 Department of Pharmaceutical Chemistry, Bharati Vidyapeeth College of Pharmacy, Kolhapur, India

*Address all correspondence to: smitakumbharresearch@gmail.com

References

[1] Reily C, Stewart TJ, Renfrow MB, Novak J. Glycosylation in health and disease. Nature Reviews. Nephrology. 2019;**15**(6):346-366. DOI: 10.1038/s41581-019-0129-4

[2] Huang A, Kurhade SE, Ross P, et al. Disrupting N-glycosylation using type I mannosidase inhibitors alters B-cell receptor signaling. ACS Pharmacology & Translational Science. 2022;**5**(11):1062-1069. Published 2022 Oct 25. DOI: 10.1021/acsptsci.2c00153

[3] Wandall HH, Nielsen MAI, King-Smith S, de Haan N, Bagdonaite I. Global functions of O-glycosylation: Promises and challenges in O-glycobiology. The FEBS Journal. 2021;**288**(24):7183-7212. DOI: 10.1111/febs.16148

[4] Fu J, Yang J, Seeberger PH, Yin J. Glycoconjugates for glucose transporter-mediated cancer-specific targeting and treatment. Carbohydrate Research. 2020;**498**:108195. DOI: 10.1016/j.carres.2020.108195

[5] Chen N, Xie J. N-O linkage in carbohydrates and glycoconjugates. Organic & Biomolecular Chemistry. 2016;**14**(47):11028-11047. DOI: 10.1039/c6ob00120c

[6] Schnaar RL. Glycobiology simplified: Diverse roles of glycan recognition in inflammation. Journal of Leukocyte Biology. 2016;**99**(6):825-838. DOI: 10.1189/jlb.3RI0116-021R

[7] Schnaar RL. Glycans and glycan-binding proteins in immune regulation: A concise introduction to glycobiology for the allergist. The Journal of Allergy and Clinical Immunology. 2015;**135**(3):609-615. DOI: 10.1016/j.jaci.2014.10.057

[8] Alagesan K, Everest-Dass A, Kolarich D. Isomeric separation and characterisation of Glycoconjugates. Advances in Experimental Medicine and Biology. 2018;**1104**:77-99. DOI: 10.1007/978-981-13-2158-0_5

[9] Colombo C, Pitirollo O, Lay L. Recent advances in the synthesis of Glycoconjugates for vaccine development. Molecules. 2018;**23**(7):1712. Published 2018 Jul 13. DOI: 10.3390/molecules2307171

[10] Cheng S, Wantuch PL, Kizer ME, et al. Glycoconjugate synthesis using chemoselective ligation. Organic & Biomolecular Chemistry. 2019;**17**(10):2646-2650. DOI: 10.1039/c9ob00270g

[11] Dalziel M, Crispin M, Scanlan CN, Zitzmann N, Dwek RA. Emerging principles for the therapeutic exploitation of glycosylation. Science. 2014;**343**(6166):1235681. DOI: 10.1126/science.1235681

[12] Crispin M, Doores KJ. Targeting host-derived glycans on enveloped viruses for antibody-based vaccine design. Current Opinion in Virology. 2015;**11**:63-69. DOI: 10.1016/j.coviro.2015.02.002

[13] Crucho CI, Correia-da-Silva P, Petrova KT, Barros MT. Recent progress in the field of glycoconjugates. Carbohydrate Research. 2015;**402**:124-132. DOI: 10.1016/j.carres.2014.10.005

[14] Schachter H. The joys of HexNAc. The synthesis and function of N- and O-glycan branches. Glycoconjugate Journal. 2000;**17**(7-9):465-483. DOI: 10.1023/a:1011010206774

[15] Latxague L, Gaubert A, Barthélémy P. Recent advances in the chemistry of Glycoconjugate Amphiphiles. Molecules. 2018;**23**(1):89. Published 2018 Jan 2. DOI: 10.3390/molecules23010089

[16] Freeze HH, Aebi M. Altered glycan structures: The molecular basis of congenital disorders of glycosylation. Current Opinion in Structural Biology. 2005;**15**(5):490-498. DOI: 10.1016/j.sbi.2005.08.010

[17] Lowe JB, Marth JD. A genetic approach to mammalian glycan function. Annual Review of Biochemistry. 2003;**72**:643-691. DOI: 10.1146/annurev.biochem.72.121801.161809

[18] Hattrup CL, Gendler SJ. Structure and function of the cell surface (tethered) mucins. Annual Review of Physiology. 2008;**70**:431-457. DOI: 10.1146/annurev.physiol.70.113006.100659

[19] Wandall HH, Irazoqui F, Tarp MA, et al. The lectin domains of polypeptide GalNAc-transferases exhibit carbohydrate-binding specificity for GalNAc: Lectin binding to GalNAc-glycopeptide substrates is required for high density GalNAc-O-glycosylation. Glycobiology. 2007;**17**(4):374-387. DOI: 10.1093/glycob/cwl082

[20] Fukuda M. Roles of mucin-type O-glycans in cell adhesion. Biochimica et Biophysica Acta. 2002;**1573**(3):394-405. DOI: 10.1016/s0304-4165(02)00409-9

[21] Hakomori S. Structure, organization, and function of glycosphingolipids in membrane. Current Opinion in Hematology. 2003;**10**(1):16-24. DOI: 10.1097/00062752-200301000-00004

[22] Proia RL. Glycosphingolipid functions: Insights from engineered mouse models. Philosophical Transactions of the Royal Society of London. Series B, Biological Sciences. 2003;**358**(1433):879-883. DOI: 10.1098/rstb.2003.1268

[23] Schnaar RL. Glycolipid-mediated cell-cell recognition in inflammation and nerve regeneration. Archives of Biochemistry and Biophysics. 2004;**426**(2):163-172. DOI: 10.1016/j.abb.2004.02.019

[24] Sonnino S, Mauri L, Chigorno V, Prinetti A. Gangliosides as components of lipid membrane domains [published correction appears in Glycobiology. 2007 Oct;17(10):1030]. Glycobiology. 2007;**17**(1):1R-13R. DOI: 10.1093/glycob/cwl052

[25] Paulick MG, Bertozzi CR. The glycosylphosphatidylinositol anchor: A complex membrane-anchoring structure for proteins. Biochemistry. 2008;**47**(27):6991-7000. DOI: 10.1021/bi8006324

[26] Orlean P, Menon AK. Thematic review series: Lipid posttranslational modifications. GPI anchoring of protein in yeast and mammalian cells, or: How we learned to stop worrying and love glycophospholipids. Journal of Lipid Research. 2007;**48**(5):993-1011. DOI: 10.1194/jlr.R700002-JLR200

[27] De Macedo CS, Shams-Eldin H, Smith TK, Schwarz RT, Azzouz N. Inhibitors of glycosyl-phosphatidylinositol anchor biosynthesis. Biochimie. 2003;**85**(3-4):465-472. DOI: 10.1016/s0300-9084(03)00065-8

[28] Ward S, O'Sullivan JM, O'Donnell JS. The biological significance of von Willebrand factor O-linked glycosylation. Seminars in Thrombosis and Hemostasis. 2021;**47**(7):855-861. DOI: 10.1055/s-0041-1726373

[29] Paladino S, Lebreton S, Zurzolo C. Trafficking and membrane organization of GPI-anchored proteins in health and diseases. Current Topics in Membranes. 2015;**75**:269-303. DOI: 10.1016/bs.ctm.2015.03.006

[30] Maloney FP, Kuklewicz J, Corey RA, et al. Structure, substrate recognition and initiation of hyaluronan synthase. Nature. 2022;**604**(7904):195-201. DOI: 10.1038/s41586-022-04534-2

[31] Zhuo L, Hascall VC, Kimata K. Inter-alpha-trypsin inhibitor, a covalent protein-glycosaminoglycan-protein complex. The Journal of Biological Chemistry. 2004;**279**(37):38079-38082. DOI: 10.1074/jbc.R300039200

[32] Taylor KR, Gallo RL. Glycosaminoglycans and their proteoglycans: Host-associated molecular patterns for initiation and modulation of inflammation. The FASEB Journal. 2006;**20**(1):9-22. DOI: 10.1096/fj.05-4682rev

[33] Volpi N. Therapeutic applications of glycosaminoglycans. Current Medicinal Chemistry. 2006;**13**(15):1799-1810. DOI: 10.2174/092986706777452470

[34] Varki A. Nothing in glycobiology makes sense, except in the light of evolution. Cell. 2006;**126**(5):841-845. DOI: 10.1016/j.cell.2006.08.022

[35] Shivatare SS, Shivatare VS, Wong CH. Glycoconjugates: Synthesis, functional studies, and therapeutic developments. Chemical Reviews. 2022;**122**(20):15603-15671. DOI: 10.1021/acs.chemrev.1c01032

[36] Ohtsubo K, Marth JD. Glycosylation in cellular mechanisms of health and disease. Cell. 2006;**126**(5):855-867. DOI: 10.1016/j.cell.2006.08.019

[37] Dondoni A, Massi A. Design and synthesis of new classes of heterocyclic C-glycoconjugates and carbon-linked sugar and heterocyclic amino acids by asymmetric multicomponent reactions (AMCRs). Accounts of Chemical Research. 2006;**39**(7):451-463. DOI: 10.1021/ar068023r

[38] Raman R, Raguram S, Venkataraman G, Paulson JC, Sasisekharan R. Glycomics: An integrated systems approach to structure-function relationships of glycans. Nature Methods. 2005;**2**(11): 817-824. DOI: 10.1038/nmeth807

[39] Von Moos E, Ben RN. Recent advances in the synthesis of C-linked glycoconjugates. Current Topics in Medicinal Chemistry. 2005;**5**(14):1351-1361. DOI: 10.2174/156802605774643024

[40] Kinoshita T. Biosynthesis and biology of mammalian GPI-anchored proteins. Open Biology. 2020;**10**(3):190290. DOI: 10.1098/rsob.190290

[41] Mironov AA, Beznoussenko GV, Polishchuk RS, Trucco A. Intra-Golgi transport: A way to a new paradigm? Biochimica et Biophysica Acta. 2005;**1744**(3):340-350. DOI: 10.1016/j.bbamcr.2005.03.005

[42] Ding F, Zhang Y. Biomedical applications of Glycoconjugates. Mini Reviews in Medicinal Chemistry. 2018;**18**(18):1508-1523. DOI: 10.2174/1389557518666180518083427

[43] Ernst B, Magnani JL. From carbohydrate leads to glycomimetic drugs. Nature Reviews. Drug Discovery. 2009;**8**(8):661-677. DOI: 10.1038/nrd2852

[44] Boltje TJ, Buskas T, Boons GJ. Opportunities and challenges in synthetic oligosaccharide and glycoconjugate research. Nature

Chemistry. 2009;**1**(8):611-622. DOI: 10.1038/nchem.399

[45] Hettiarachchi IL, Meng S, Chahine M, Li X, Zhu J. Stereoselective β-Mannosylation via anomeric O-alkylation with L-sugar-derived electrophiles. European Journal of Organic Chemistry. 2021;**2021**(48):6682-6687. DOI: 10.1002/ejoc.202100903

Chapter 9

A Scientific Ethnomedical Study Using Microbes on Gaucher Disease: An *In-Silico* Analysis

Sreeram Sudhir and Amritha Pozhaiparambil Sasikumar

Abstract

Gaucher disease (GD) is an inherited metabolic disorder caused by the deficiency of enzyme acid β-Glucosidase resulting in the deposition of harmful quantities of lipids/fats. To date, enzyme replacement therapy (ERT) and substrate reduction therapy (SRT) are the only modes of treatment approved by the FDA for Gaucher disease. In this study, we evaluated the ability of microbial bioactive compounds as a drug candidate. The treatment based on molecular docking against selected protein targets plays a crucial role in the future treatment of this disease. Microbial compounds contain bioactive compounds in the form of alkaloids and others of natural origin. Through molecular docking the deep binding affinity of 10 selected compounds present in algae, bacteria, and fungi against the enzyme acid β-Glucosidase of GD using Maestro Schrodinger software, in addition, the ADMET properties are also predicted. Out of these compounds, Lipoxazolidinone C, Cinnamic acid, and Marinopyrrole A, have a sturdy interaction with the Gaucher disease target enzyme, and it can be considered as an effective drug target for Gaucher disease. Our findings reveal a novel discovery towards biology mainly pointing to microbes as a drug formulation. Further, these compounds could be analyzed for their stability through molecular dynamics techniques.

Keywords: Gaucher disease, *In-silico*, Ethnomedicine, acid β-glucosidase, microbes, bioactive compounds

1. Introduction

Ethnomedicine is the study of traditional medicine based on the bioactive compounds of plants and animals, the mother of all other systems of medicines- Ayurveda, Siddha, Unani, Naturopathy, and even modern medicine. These ethnomedicine have played a major role throughout the world in treating and preventing diseases. The various sources of natural medicinal products could be terrestrial plants, terrestrial microbes, marine microbes, and even vertebrates and invertebrates [1].

During the 'golden era' of antibiotic discovery, the generation time of pathogens varies from minutes to weeks, leading to the inevitability of resistance selection. This reinforced the need for new chemical entities. The two novel antibiotics that are approved by FDA for human use are linezolid and daptomycin. There is a need for the discovery of an alternative drug using natural medicinal products.

Microorganisms are ubiquitous interact with all other organisms and inhabit every environment on Earth. These are the leading producers of the useful natural products, indicating their excellency in drug formulation. Various portions of microbial genomes are devoted to production of secondary metabolites. Recently, scientists have begun to realize and discover their role in the medical community. These are an ample source of structurally diverse bioactive substances which have led to the discovery of drugs mainly penicillin, cephalosporins, polyketides, and tetracyclines [2]. A single microbe can produce several the secondary metabolites. They include antibiotics, anticancer agents, immunosuppressants, anthelmintics, and many more. With the development of Computer technology, in silico approaches have been widely used to elucidate the pharmacological use of plants and microbes in drug discovery [3]. Therefore the 'new era' of drug discovery is believed to prevent and control the consequence of disease and illness in a more rational way [4]. Generally, microorganisms are differentiated on the basis of their cellular organization as shown in **Figure 1**.

According to National Organization for Rare Diseases (NORD), Gaucher Disease (GD) is an orphan disease, an inherited metabolic disorder in which deficiency of the enzyme β- glucosidase results in the accumulation of harmful quantities of lipids/fats. Especially the glycolipid glucocerebroside, throughout the body especially within the bone marrow, spleen, and liver. Researchers have identified three distinct forms of GD: Type 1 - Non-neuronopathic GD, Type 2 - Acute neuronopathic GD, Type 3- Chronic neuronopathic GD [5]. The gene mutations lead to the replacement of amino acids in the enzyme β- glucosidase which reduces the protein stability and the catalytic activity. Personalized treatment is required depending on the type of GD.

The drug therapy options approved by FDA include (ERT) Enzyme Replacement Therapy and (SRT) Substrate Reduction Therapy [6, 7]. The cost of ERT and SRT are very high as for most orphan drugs. These kinds of treatment measures are not available for rural people as they are unaware due to the lack of facilities in hospitals. The ultimate aim of the study is the application of virtual screening and network pharmacology which enriches the active compounds among the candidates, thereby indicating the action mechanism of beneficial microbes, reducing the cost, and increasing the efficiency of the whole procedure, seeking an alternative solution for GD.

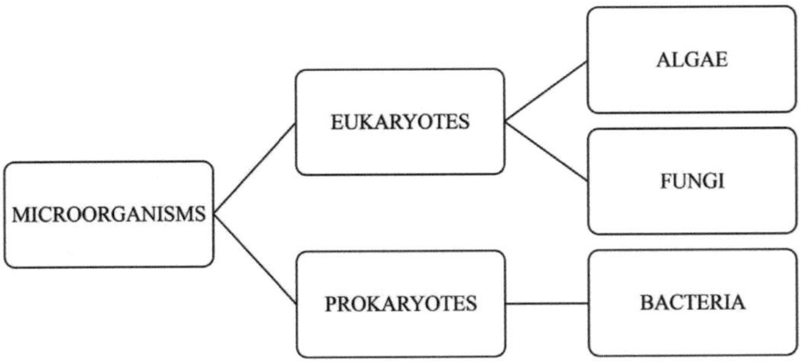

Figure 1.
Microbial classification based on cellular organization.

In our study, we construct the network of relationships among the medicinal microbes, their natural compounds, and the biological targets of the diseases. We hereby performed a deep virtual screening process through the molecular docking studies to test the binding efficiency of selected bioactive compounds from the microbes as a drug candidate. This is first in-silico work using the microbes as the core elements for the therapeutic studies against the GD, which brings out the novelty of the work carried out, attempting to find an alternative solution for GD.

2. Methodology

The structure-based drug designing was performed, which serves as a powerful tool in identifying new lead compounds in the process of drug discovery [8]. The sources of the chemicals from the microbes are purely based on the literature work done intensively during the whole work.

2.1 Databases

The 3D protein structure was retrieved from Protein Data Bank. All the corresponding ligand molecules were retrieved after intensive literature review from various online sources and the 2D structure of these bioactive compounds were retrieved from PubChem (https://pubchem.ncbi.nlm.nih.gov/).

2.2 Protein preparation

The proteins were assembled by removing the native auto inducer all water molecules. Hydrogen was re-added using the protein residue template in Maestro v10.2. This is a vital stage in the preparation of protein as any modification can be re-addressed like missing side chains, and updating the missing residues. To enhance the structure the water molecules were removed, increasing the entropy of the target molecule.

2.3 Ligand preparation

Initially the ligands were converted into 3D structure using the Ligprep tool in maestro Schrödinger v10.2. The ligand was geometrically optimized.

2.4 ADMET activity

An account of druggability is very essential while performing a docking study, the ligands were checked for Absorption, distribution, metabolism, excretion, and toxicity (ADMET) test. It is a preliminary step in drug preparation. The knowledge on drugs for Gaucher disease is very scanty, and it is very reasonable to make out more and reduce the cost of treatment as a lot of developing countries can rely on it. 12 compounds successfully scored well in all the ADMET parameters analyzed using Qikprop version 4.4. in the Schrodinger suite [9]. Some important parameters like CNS, Blood-barrier coefficient, human blood absorption, Lipinski's rule of three and five were analyzed. The bioactive phyto-compounds which displayed pragmatic result were chosen for the ADME and preferable docking poses has been tabbed for the rationale of docking [10].

2.5 Molecular docking

Molecular docking outlays the ligand's preferred orientation with the target molecule while interacting with each other in forming a highly stable complex. For this purpose, we have employed Maestro v10.2 to conduct the extra precision (XP) docking for speculating the binding affinity, analyzing the efficacy of the ligand, and inhibitory constant of ligand against the target. In this study, the entire ligand was docked with the target molecule flexibly using the Glide Xtra precision (XP) tool. As a result of successful docking, we have obtained better docking scores, poses with accurate hydrophobic contacts between target residues to ligand [11].

2.6 PyMOL

PyMOL is an open-source molecular visualization tool commercialized by Schrödinger, which can produce high-quality 3D images of small molecules, biological macromolecules like proteins. It is one of the most trusted tools for visualization in structural biology and it operates on Python language.

2.7 LigPlot

A computer program able to generate 2D schematic representation of protein-ligand interaction from the standard PDB input file. The interactions shown are basically of hydrogen bonds and hydrophobic contacts. In this hydrogen bonds are indicated by dashed lines between the atoms involved whereas hydrophobic interactions are represented by an arc with spokes facing towards the ligand atoms they come in contact with. The interacted atoms are represented by the spokes facing them back [12].

3. Result and discussion

3.1 ADMET analysis

The ADMET (Adsorption, Distribution, Metabolism, Excretion, and Toxicity) analysis was performed for evaluating the drug-likeness of 50 compounds from microorganisms. The prediction was performed using the Quikprop version 4.4 in the Schrodinger suite [8]. Drug likeness properties of the selected compounds were determined by Lipinski's rule of five, Jorgensen's rule of three, molecular weight, CNS activity, dipole movement, Volume, Total solvent accessible surface area (SASA), Brain/blood partition coefficient, metabolic reactions, Human oral absorption and Percent Human Oral Absorption. It is believed that ADME shows the toxicity of small molecules [13]. The drug-like property's prediction was then evaluated and the results were portrayed in **Table 1**.

ADME is an essential tool for analyzing the proposed molecule's oral bioavailability as possible drugs. Statistics estimate that almost half of the candidate drugs do not undergo clinical trials because they fail to meet the suitable levels of efficacy, toxic effect on the body, making it unsafe for human use [14]. According to the literature study, 50 compounds were selected for ADME Analysis, from which the prediction results were shown by the 10 compounds from different microorganisms, especially bacteria, fungi, and algae (**Figure 2**).

DOI: http://dx.doi.org/10.5772/intechopen.107545

Name of compound (PDB Id)	Molecular weight	Volume	Dipole movement	SASA	Donor HB	Accpt HB	#metab	QPlog BB	CNS	Human oral absorption	Percent human oral absorption	Rule of five	Rule of three
Lipoxazolidinone C (23642823)	307.432	1195.068	4.198	702.848	0	4.5	3	−1.204	−2	3	100	0	0
Cinnamic acid (444539)	148.161	568.531	6.693	369.072	1	2	0	−0.565	−1	3	79.474	0	0
Marinopyrrole A (24797083)	510.16	1230.393	5.425	639.808	1	3.5	2	−0.456	0	1	83.287	2	1
Chlorohydroaspyrone B (25016145)	220.652	699.441	3.611	421.719	1	5.4	2	−0.583	0	3	81.892	0	0
Chlorohydroaspyrone B (24900165)	341.409	1114.774	3.441	627.858	3	6.7	6	−1.239	−2	3	79.198	0	0
Racemosin A (155148)	288.299	882.289	8.137	495.888	0	4.75	2	−0.157	0	3	100	0	0
Apralactone A (102411411)	332.352	968.272	6.07	518.358	2	6.25	4	−0.852	−1	3	80.909	0	0
LBM-415 (9690139)	396.418	1245.941	4.227	697.146	2	10.7	3	−1.868	−2	2	58.058	0	0
Spirotryprostatin B (9928968)	363.415	1120.217	4.923	610.282	1	8.5	4	−0.829	−1	3	85.127	0	0
Dehydrocurvularin (6438143)	290.315	903.643	6.955	510.217	1	4.5	4	−1.03	−2	3	80.753	0	0

Table 1.
Analysis of ADMET properties for the microbial compounds.

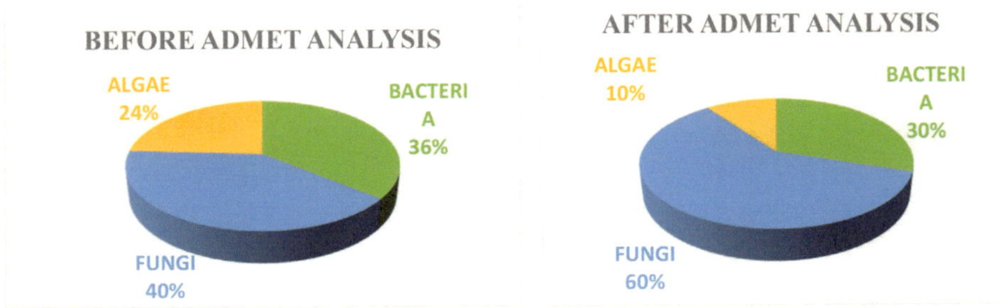

Figure 2.
Bioavailability of microbial compounds before and after ADMET analysis.

3.2 Molecular docking

Computational docking was implemented to predict binding of the 10 compounds (**Figure 3**) which represents alkaloids, antibacterial, antimicrobials from microorganisms mainly bacteria, fungi, and algae with acid β-glycosidase as the target protein.

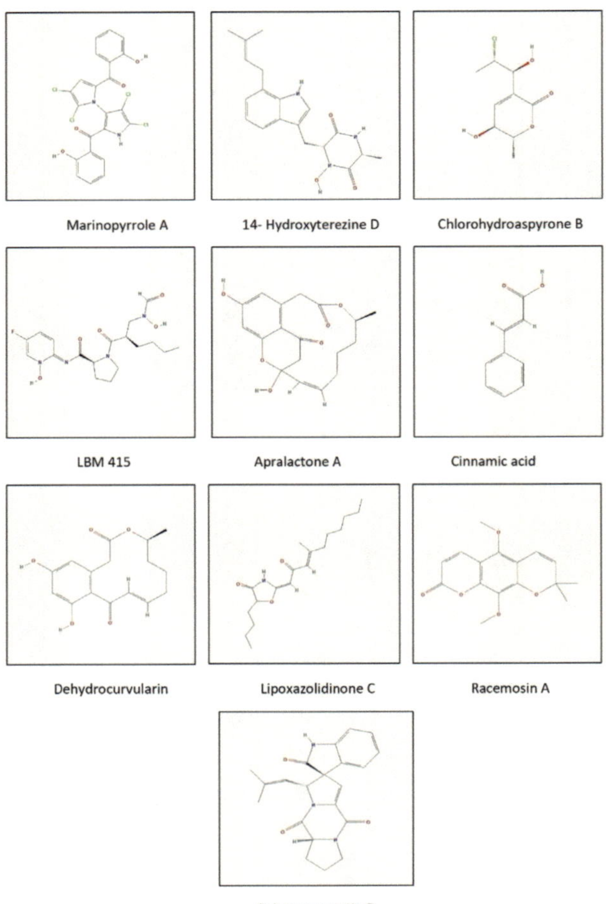

Figure 3.
2D chemical structures of the selected microbial bioactive compounds.

Glide Score is an empirical scoring function that approximates the ligand binding free energy, including force field (electrostatic, van der Waals) contributions It highlights docking accuracy, database enrichment, and binding affinity prediction. Glide approximates a complete systematic search of the conformational, orientational, and positional space of the docked ligand.

Out of 10 microbial bioactive compounds, Lipoxazolidinone C, Marinopyrrole A, LBM-415, were the promising bacterial compounds, Cinnamic acid, Chlorohydroaspyrone B, 14-hydroxyterezine D, Apralactone A, Spirotryprostatin B, and Dehydrocurvularin belongs to the fungal compounds, and Racemosin A is the only compound belonging to algae. The binding scores of each compound with the target protein acid β-glycosidase are depicted in **Table 2**.

Among the 10 ligands, the compound Lipoxazolidinone C from *Marinispora sp* (Bacteria) had the least Glide score of −10.56 Kcal/mol (**Table 2**). The binding mode for Lipoxazolidinone C to acid β-glycosidase was attributed to H-bond interaction with GLU 482 with a bond length of 2.1 Å, while amino acid residue ASN 377 was positioned at a distance of H-bond with a bond length of 2.0 Å with Cinnamic acid from *Cladosporium sp.* of fungi with a glide score of −10.33 Kcal/mol. The third

Name of the compound (PBD ID)	Microbe species	G. Score	Residues interacted	Bond length (Å)	Total number of bonds
Lipoxazolidinone C (23642823)	*Marinispora sp.*	−10.56	GLU-482 (H-O)	2.1	1
Cinnamic acid (444539)	*Cladosporium sp.*	−10.33	ASN-377 (O-H)	2	1
Marinopyrrole A (24797083)	*Strepttomyces saccurensis*	−9.6	SER-447 (O-H)	2.6	4
			GLU-446 (H-O)	1.9	
			ASN-377 (H-O)	2.3	
			ASN-377 (H-O)	2.3	
Chlorohydroaspyrone B (25016145)	*Exophiala sp.*	−9.17	SER-447 (O-H)	2.2	3
			ASN-262 (O-H)	2.1	
			ASN-377 (H-O)	1.7	
14-hydroxyterezine D (24900165)	*Aspergillus sydowi*	−8.82	ARG-444 (O-H)	2	1
Racemosin A (155148)	*Caulerpa racemosa*	−8.44	ASN-262 (O-H)	2.8	2
			(O-H)	1.9	
Apralactone A (102411411)	*Curvularia sp.*	−8.31	ASN-377 (H-O)	1.8	3
			GLY-379 (O-H)	2.1	
			GLU-446 (O-H)	2.5	
LBM-415 (9690139)	*Streptomyces sp.*	−7.77	GLU-446 (O-H)	2	2
			GLY-379 (O-H)	2.1	
Spirotryprostatin B (9928968)	*Aspergillus sydowi*	−7.4	GLU-446 (H-O)	2.1	1
Dehydrocurvularin (6438143)	*Curvularia sp.*	−6.06	ARG-252 (O-H)	1.9	3
			ASN-262 (O-H)	1.8	
			GLU-211 (H-O)	1.9	

Table 2.
Docking scores of β- glucosidase with microbial compounds.

docking scores were received by the ligand Marinopyrrole A from *Streptomyces saccurensis* (Bacteria) with a Glide score of −9.6 Kcal/mol. Marinopyrrol A interacts with SER 447, GLU 446, ASN 377 forming four H-bonds of length 2.6, 1.9, 2.3, 2.3 Å respectively. Followed by the Glide score of −9.17 Kcal/mol was Chlorohydroaspyrone B from the microbe *Exophiala sp*. (Fungi). The residues were SER 477, ASN 262, and ASN 377 forming three H-bonds with the bond lengths of 2.2, 2.1, and 1.7 Å respectively, while amino acid residues ARG 444 were positioned at a distance of 2.0 Å of H-bond with ligand 14-hydroxyterezine D from *Aspergillus sydowi* (Fungi) with a Glide score of −8.82 Kcal/mol (**Figure 4**).

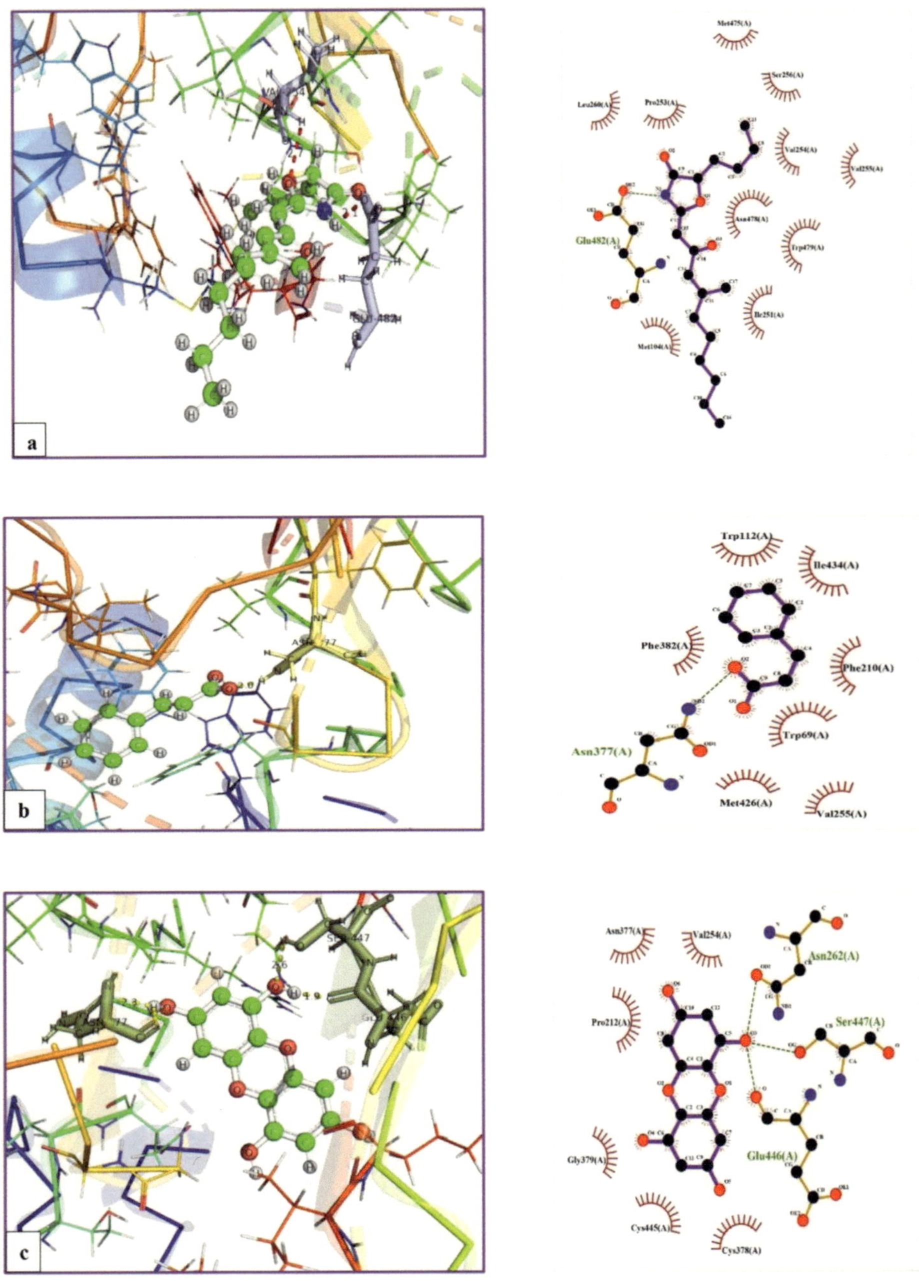

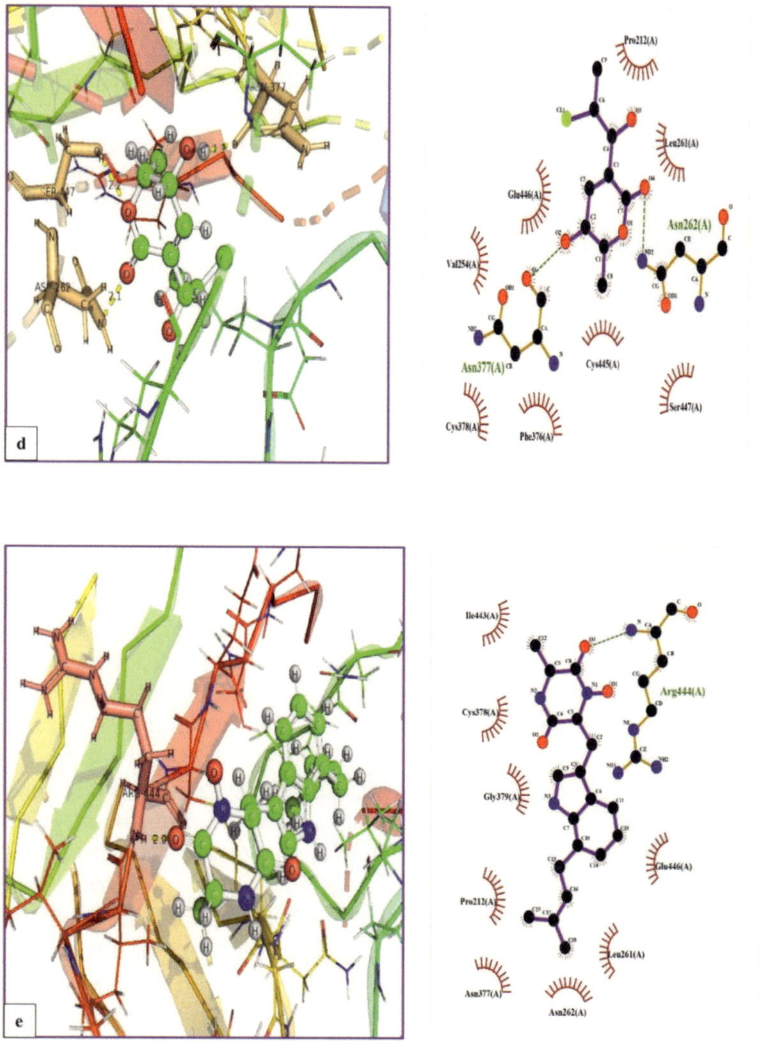

Figure 4.
The docking complex of (a) Lipoxazolidinone C, (b) Cinnamic acid, (c) Marinopyrrole a, (d) Chlorohydroaspyrone B, and (e) 14-hydroxyterezine D with the X-ray structure of acid β-glucosidase. 3D interaction (left) and 2D schematic diagram using Ligplot (right).

In addition, Racemosin A from *Caulerpa racemose* (Algae) interacts with ASN 262 with two H-bonds, while amino acid residues ASN 377, GLY 379, and GLU 446 are positioned at a distance of H-bond with Apralactone A which is obtained from *Curuvularia sp.* (Fungi). LBM-415 from *Streptomyces sp.* (Bacteria) interacts with GLU 446 and GLY 379 with two H-bonds, while amino acid residues GLU 446 are positioned at a distance of H-bond with Spirotryprostatin B from *Aspergillus sydowi* (Fungi). Last but not the least, the microbial ligand Dehydrocurvularin from *Curvularia sp*. (Fungi) interacted with the target protein with residues ARG 252, ASN 262, and GLU 211 forming three H-bonds. Taken together we propose the above indicated microbial bioactive compounds as a candidate for drug for GD, thus limiting viral maturation.

Secondary metabolites of microbial origin have been proven to be an important source for new pharmaceuticals and drug lead candidates like antibacterial agents like penicillin, an antifungal drug like echinocandin B, cholesterol-lowering agent lovastatin, and more [15].

In line with our findings, the bioactive compound Lipoxazolidinone C has unusual 4-oxazolidinone heterocycle at its core, representing a wide spectrum of antibacterial and anti-microbial activity similar to those of the commercial antibiotic linezolid (Zyvox) [16]. Another study suggests that 4-oxazolidinones are valuable scaffolds of antimicrobial development [17]. Cinnamic acid and its phenolic analogs are natural substances. Isopropyl 4-hydroxycinnamate and butyl 4-hydroxycinnamate were found to have almost similar antifungal activity as commercial fungicide iprobenfos against *Pythium sp.* [18]. For decades, cinnamic acid and its derivatives have attained huge attention for their anticancer as well as antitumor potentials [19]. Similarly, cinnamic, coumaric, ferulic, and sinapic acids show inhibitory activity against several Gram-positive and Gram-negative bacteria [20] and have been found to be potential natural antifouling agents inhibiting larval settlement of *Balanus neritina* [21]. The marine natural product, marinopyrrole A has been shown to have potent antibiotic activity against Gram-positive pathogens [22]. According to the data of ChEBI, the biological roles of marinopyrrole A are marine, bacterial metabolite, as well as antimicrobial, antibacterial, and antineoplastic agents. Due to the antibiotic and cytotoxicity, marinopyrrole A and its derivatives are possible for SAR studies [23]. The cultural broth of marine fungal strain from genus *Exophiala* produced new aspyrone derivatives called Chloroaspyrones A and B. Both the compounds displayed moderate to weak antibacterial activity when tested against *S. aureus* [24]. 14-hydroxyterezine is a type of diketopiperazine alkaloids, isolated from ethyl acetate of *Aspergillus sydowi*, exhibits weak cytotoxicity against human alveolar basal carcinoma A-549 cells [25]. Racemosin A is a unique bisindole alkaloid possessing a structure derived from a green alga. Studies suggest that Racemosin A significantly attenuates the $A\beta_{25\text{-}35}$ induced SH-SY5Y cell damage with an increase in cell viability in a neuro-protective assay [26] and shows anti-cancer activity exhibiting a strong inhibitor against human breast cancer cell lines [27]. Apralactone A has shown moderate concentration-dependent cytotoxicity in 36 cancer cell line panels, playing an important role in the development of anticancer drugs [28]. In vitro drug susceptibilities tests and in vivo characterization in an animal model showed that LBM-415 had a good antimicrobial activity that is equivalent to the marketed antibiotic agents [29]. LBM 415 is the first peptide deformylase (PDF) inhibitor class being developed for clinical trials for oral and parenteral treatment for the respiratory tract, and skin structure infections caused by susceptible gram-positive and gram-negative organisms [30]. In an experiment, scientists isolated a novel compound named Spirotryprostatin B which inhibited the cell cycle progression of tsFT210 cells at the G2/M phase, in addition, they show cytotoxic activity on the growth of human chronic myelogenous leukemia K562 cells and human promyelocytic leukemia HL-60 cells [31]. In a recent study, Dehydrocurvularin (DCV) was revealed to have a potent irreversible inhibitor of ATP-citrate lyase (ACLY) through classical chemoproteomic profiling indicating the anti-cancer mode of action of DCV [32]. Similarly, dehydrocurvularin was found to be a fungal metabolite during the screening of fungal metabolites inhibiting TGF-β dependent signaling [33].

4. Conclusion

The present molecular docking analysis of microbial compounds against Gaucher disease (GD) target protein acid beta-glucosidase has prominent favorable compounds of natural origin with good binding to the Gaucher disease target.

Lipoxazolidinone C, Cinnamic acid, and Marinopyrrole A are the most prominent compounds on the Gaucher enzyme target sites. These bioactive compounds were also found to display good antibacterial, antimicrobial, antibiotic, and antifungal activity against various human pathogens. In summary and from the theoretical evidence based on previous in-vitro confirmatory studies, we recommend further in-vivo investigation assessment to analyze the predicted affinity of the selected bioactive compounds against the Gaucher Disease.

Acknowledgements

The authors hereby acknowledge heartfelt gratitude to Dr. R. Sathishkumar for providing timely assistance for the successful completion of this work.

Author's contribution

Amritha P S and Sreeram S have drafted the manuscript, and collected the articles. Sreeram. S has done the PyMOL visualizations and Amritha P.S. reviewed the manuscript.

Funding

No funding was received for conducting this study.

Conflicts of interest

The authors hereby declare no competing interest.

Ethics approval

This article does not contain any studies involving animals performed by any of the authors. This article does not contain any human participants involving performed by any of the authors.

Consent for participation

Not applicable as no clinical trials were involved in this study.

Availability of data and material

All data generated or analyzed during this study are included in this published article.

Author details

Sreeram Sudhir[1] and Amritha Pozhaiparambil Sasikumar[2*]

1 Department of Botany, PSG College of Arts and Science, Coimbatore, TN, India

2 Department of Zoology, PSGR Krishnammal College for Women, Coimbatore, TN, India

*Address all correspondence to: amritha3097@gmail.com

References

[1] Chin YW, Balunas MJ, Chai HB, Kinghorn AD. Drug discovery from natural sources. The AAPS Journal. 2006;**8**(2):E239-E253. DOI: 10.1007/BF02854894

[2] Dewick PM. Medicinal Natural Products: A Biosynthetic Approach. 2nd ed. Chichester, UK: John Wiley & Sons; 2002

[3] Yi F, Li L, Xu LJ, Meng H, Dong YM, Liu HB, et al. In silico approach in reveal traditional medicine plants pharmacological material basis. Chinese Medicine. 2018;**13**(1):1-20. DOI: 10.1186/s13020-018-0190-0

[4] Ballabh B, Chaurasia OP. Traditional medicinal plants of cold desert Ladakh—Used in treatment of cold, cough and fever. Journal of Ethnopharmacology. 2007;**112**(2):341-349. DOI: 10.1016/j.jep.2007.03.020

[5] Khan M et al. Gaucher's disease: Prenatal and post Natal diagnostic dilemma and biochemical aid – Case series and review of literature. British Journal of Medicine and Medical Research. 2017;**19**(5):1-11. DOI: 10.9734/BJMMR/2017/29680

[6] Substrate Reduction Therapy (Oral Medication) for Gaucher Disease. National Gaucher Foundation. Available from: www.gaucherdisease.org/gaucher-diagnosis treatment/treatment/substrate-reduction/; [Accessed: September 10, 2018]

[7] Enzyme Replacement Therapy for Gaucher Disease. National Gaucher Foundation. Available from: www.gaucherdisease.org/gaucher-diagnosis treatment/treatment/enzyme-replacement-therapy/; [Accessed September 10, 2018]

[8] Anderson AC. The process of structure-based drug design. Chemistry & Biology. 2003;**10**(9):787-797. DOI: 10.1016/j.chembiol.2003.09.002

[9] Quikprop, module 4.4. New York: Schrodinger Suite; 2012

[10] Vijayakumar S et al. Novel ligand-based docking; molecular dynamic simulations; and absorption, distribution, metabolism, and excretion approach to analyzing potential acetylcholinesterase inhibitors for Alzheimer's disease. Journal of Pharmaceutical Analysis. 2018;**8**(6):413-420. DOI: 10.1016/j.jpha.2017.07.006

[11] Maniam GP et al. Homology modeling and molecular docking studies on type II diabetes complications reduced PPARγ receptor with various ligand molecules homology modeling and molecular docking studies on type II diabetes complications reduced PPARg receptor with various ligand molecule. Biomedicine & Pharmacotherapy. 2017;**92**:528-535. DOI: 10.1016/j.biopha.2017.05.077

[12] Wallace AC, Laskowski RA, Thornton JM. LIGPLOT: A program to generate schematic diagrams of protein-ligand interactions. Protein Engineering, Design & Selection. 1995;**8**(2):127-134. DOI: 10.1093/protein/8.2.127

[13] Pajouhesh H, Lenz GR. Medicinal chemical properties of successful central nervous system drugs. NeuroRx. 2005;**2**(4):541-553. DOI: 10.1602/neurorx.2.4.541

[14] Pellegatti M. Preclinical in vivo ADME studies in drug development: A critical review. Expert Opinion

on Drug Metabolism & Toxicology. 2012;**8**(2):161-172

[15] Misiek M, Hoffmeister D. Fungal genetics, genomics, and secondary metabolites in pharmaceutical sciences. Planta Medica. 2007;**73**(02):103-115. DOI: 10.1055/s-2007-967104

[16] Barbachyn MR, Ford CW. Oxazolidinone structure–activity relationships leading to linezolid. Angewandte Chemie, International Edition. 2003;**42**(18):2010-2023. DOI: 10.1002/anie.200200528

[17] Mills JJ, Robinson KR, Zehnder TE, Pierce JG. Synthesis and biological evaluation of the antimicrobial natural product lipoxazolidinone a. Angewandte Chemie. 2018;**130**(28): 8818-8822. DOI: 10.1002/ange.201805078

[18] Tawata S, Taira S, Kobamoto N, Zhu J, Ishihara M, Toyama S. Synthesis and antifungal activity of cinnamic acid esters. Bioscience, Biotechnology, and Biochemistry. 1996;**60**(5):909-910. DOI: 10.1271/bbb.60.909

[19] De P, Baltas M, Bedos-Belval F. Cinnamic acid derivatives as anticancer agents-a review. Current Medicinal Chemistry. 2011;**18**(11):1672-1703. DOI: 10.2174/092986711795471347

[20] Sova M. Antioxidant and antimicrobial activities of cinnamic acid derivatives. Mini Reviews in Medicinal Chemistry. 2012;**12**(8):749-767. DOI: 10.2174/138955712801264792

[21] Qi SH, Xu Y, Xiong HR, Qian PY, Zhang S. Antifouling and antibacterial compounds from a marine fungus *Cladosporium* sp. F14. World Journal of Microbiology and Biotechnology. 2009;**25**:399-406. DOI: 10.1007/s11274-008-9904-2

[22] Hughes CC, Prieto-Davo A, Jensen PR, Fenical W. The marinopyrroles, antibiotics of an unprecedented structure class from a marine *Streptomyces* sp. Organic Letters. 2008;**10**:629-631. DOI: 10.1021/ol702952n

[23] Cheng C, Pan L, Chen Y, Song H, Qin Y, Li R. Total synthesis of (±)-marinopyrrole a and its library as potential antibiotic and anticancer agents. Journal of Combinatorial Chemistry. 2010;**12**(4):541-547. DOI: 10.1021/cc100052j

[24] Zhang D, Yang X, Kang JS, Choi HD, Son BW. Chlorohydroaspyrones a and B, antibacterial aspyrone derivatives from the marine-derived fungus *Exophiala* sp. Journal of Natural Products. 2008a;**71**:1458-1460. DOI: 10.1021/np800107c

[25] Zhang M, Wang WL, Fang YC, Zhu TJ, Gu QQ, Zhu WM. Cytotoxic alkaloids and antibiotic nordammarane triterpenoids from the marine-derived fungus aspergillus sydowi. Journal of Natural Products. 2008;**71**(6):985-989. DOI: 10.1021/np700737g

[26] Liu DQ, Mao SC, Zhang HY, Yu XQ, Feng MT, Wang B, et al. Racemosins a and B, two novel bisindole alkaloids from the green alga Caulerpa racemosa. Fitoterapia. 2013;**91**:15-20. DOI: 10.1016/j.fitote.2013.08.014

[27] Xiao X, Xu M, Yang C, Yao Y, Liang LN, Chung PE, et al. Novel racemosin B derivatives as new therapeutic agents for aggressive breast cancer. Bioorganic & Medicinal Chemistry. 2018;**26**(23-24):6096-6104. DOI: 10.1016/j.bmc.2018.11.014

[28] Greve H, Schupp PJ, Eguerva E, Kehraus S, Kelter G, Maier A, et al. Apralactone a and a new stereochemical class of curvularins from the marine

fungus *Curvularia* sp. European Journal of Organic Chemistry. 2008;**30**:5085-5050. DOI: 10.1002%2Fejoc.200800522

[29] Osborne CS, Neckermann G, Fischer E, Pecanka R, Yu DH, Manni K, et al. In vivo characterization of the peptide deformylase inhibitor LBM415 in murine infection models. Antimicrobial Agents and Chemotherapy. 2009;**53**(9):3777-3781. DOI: 10.1128/AAC.00026-09

[30] Bowker KE, Noel AR, McGowan AP. In vitro activities of nine peptide deformylase inhibitors and five comparator agents against respiratory and skin pathogens. International Journal of Antimicrobial Agents. 2003;**22**(6):557-561. DOI: 10.1016/S0924-8579(03)00246-2

[31] Cui CB, Kakeya H, Osada H. Spirotryprostatin B, a novel mammalian cell cycle inhibitor produced by aspergillus fumigatus. The Journal of Antibiotics. 1996;**49**(8):832-835. DOI: 10.7164/antibiotics.49.832

[32] Deng Z, Wong NK, Guo Z, Zou K, Xiao Y, Zhou Y. Dehydrocurvularin is a potent antineoplastic agent irreversibly blocking ATP-citrate lyase: Evidence from chemoproteomics. Chemical Communications. 2019;**55**(29):4194-4197. DOI: 10.1039/C9CC00256A

[33] Rudolph K, Serwe A, Erkel G. Inhibition of TGF-β signaling by the fungal lactones (S)-curvularin, dehydrocurvularin, oxacyclododecindione and galiellalactone. Cytokine. 2013;**61**(1):285-296. DOI: 10.1016/j.cyto.2012.10.011

Chapter 10

Spectrophotometric/Titrimetric Drug Analysis

Nagib Qarah and Ezzouhra El-Maaiden

Abstract

The importance of pharmaceuticals comes from their direct connection to human life. Therefore, many analysis techniques such as chromatography, spectroscopic methods, and others have been developed for one goal, which is to ensure that the drug reaches humans with high quality. Spectrophotometric and titrimetric methods have been in general use for the last 40 years and over this period have become the most important analytical instrument in the modern-day laboratory. In many applications, other techniques could be employed in pharmaceutical analysis, but none rival UV–visible spectrometry as well as titrimetry, for their simplicity, versatility, speed, accuracy, and cost-effectiveness. This chapter highlights the spectroscopic methods in the ultraviolet and visible regions, as well as the titration methods that are still widely used in the field of pharmaceutical analysis. The types of titrations, as well as the most important reactions used in spectrophotometric methods, are presented. Examples of the most important applications in the field of pharmaceutical analysis are also presented.

Keywords: analysis, spectrophotometric, titrimetric, pharmaceutical, electromagnetic radiation

1. Introduction

The majority of the methods currently available used in pharmaceutical analysis are high-performance liquid chromatography (HPLC), ultra-performance liquid chromatography (UPLC), high-performance thin layer chromatography (HPTLC), gas chromatography (GC), gas chromatography/mass spectrometry (GC/MS), liquid chromatography/mass spectrometry (LC/MS), capillary electrophoresis (CE), voltammetry, HPLC/NMR, etc., all require highly sophisticated instruments which are very expensive, involve tedious multiple extraction steps and are time-consuming. Therefore, there is a constant need for developing analytical methods, such as titrimetry and spectrophotometry that are simple, sensitive, rapid, accurate, precise, and inexpensive and that can be easily adapted by the pharmaceutical industry. In recent years, the assay methods in the monographs including titrimetric and spectrometric analytical methods can be seen in the literature for pharmaceutical analysis.

Titrimetric methods have maintained their great value as an analytical tool despite the steadily growing resort to purely physical methods which often necessitate very sophisticated and expensive instrumentation.

The titrimetric techniques are still widely used in the analysis for the assay of bulk drug materials and their share in the European Pharmacopeia (EP) is almost 70%. Also, in the United States Pharmacopeia (USP) more than 40% of low molecular weight organic compounds are determined by aqueous or non-aqueous titration [1]. In fact, titrimetric methods are still as widely used as ever in pharmaceutical analysis, especially since the development of physicochemical assays of measurement, as well as spreading of non-aqueous titration method and potentiometric end point detection, expanding and improving the field of application of titrimetric methods, especially in the pharmaceutical analysis. The European and United States Pharmacopeias are adopting many analytical methods to ensure the quality of the drug, such as titration, spectrometry, chromatography, and others. These methods and their respective proportions are included in **Table 1** according to the edition of European (The European Pharmacopeia and Council of Europe, 2002) and US (United States Pharmacopeia, 2004) pharmacopeias [2, 3]. It is noted from the table that spectroscopic and titration methods are still widely used in the pharmaceutical analysis. To name a few, in the literature survey, titrimetric methods have been used for the determination of terbinafine [4–8], ethionamide [9–13], and Amoxicillin [14–20] in pharmaceutical formulations. In addition to many drug formulations that were estimated using titration methods.

Further, among the various instrumental methods available for trace analysis, UV–visible spectrophotometry continues to be one of the most popular, because of its simplicity and cost-effectiveness. UV–visible spectrophotometry is one of the most widespread techniques were used in analytical chemistry for drug analysis, capable of producing accurate and precise results. For these reasons, procedures using this technique are found in analytical, pharmaceutical, and research laboratories. Specially, in the field of pharmaceutical analysis, spectrophotometric offers the best detection sensitivity, accuracy, and reproducibility of drug analysis in the bath of drug research, development, and laboratories quality control testing of marketed drug products.

In the United States Pharmacopeia (USP), UV–visible spectrophotometric methods still provide the majority of the spectrophotometric procedures, there are still over 200 specific monographs containing UV–visible spectrophotometric measurements in the current version of (USP36-NF31). As well as, the number of UV–visible spectrophotometric assays used in the pharmaceutical analysis is increasing more than other spectrophotometric techniques, such as IR and fluorescence.

If we follow the international refereed journals that are concerned with publishing scientific research in the field of drug analysis, we will find that the majority of

USP	European Pharmacopeia	Method
44	16	HPLC
41	70	Titration
9	10	UV–visible spectrophotometry
6	4	Other

Table 1.
Proportion of titrimetric/spectrophotometric methods used for the assay of bulk drug according to European and Unites States pharmacopeias [00,000].

published research has used the spectrophotometric technique in analysis, directly or indirectly. To name a few, in the estimation of some anti-infective agents in pharmaceuticals, we will find that most of the published research about it used spectroscopic methods [21–30]. We also find that browsing through the majority of pharmaceutical analysis books finds that all of them give more space in that books to talk about spectrophotometric techniques and their various applications, especially in the field of drug analysis.

The above proves beyond any doubt that titrimetric and spectrophotometric methods are considered to present and future as the most important methods used in the analysis of pharmaceutical formulations with their accuracy in measurements.

2. Titrimetric techniques and their applications in pharmaceutical analysis

Although about 200 years have elapsed since the publication of the first papers dealing with titrimetric analysis [31], the technique is still as widely used as ever in pharmaceutical analysis because of its robustness, cheapness, and capability for high precision, with also many advantages associated with these methods which include saving time and labor, and no need of using reference standards. In fact, titrimetric methods to these days are still widely used in pharmaceutical analysis simultaneously with the development of physicochemical methods for different measurements, as well as the spreading of non-aqueous titration method and potentiometric end point detection, expanding and improving the field of application of titrimetric methods, especially in the pharmaceutical analysis.

Titrimetry is the volumetric procedure for the determination of the concentration of the drug sample by adding a known concentration of the standard drug substance. This reacts quantitatively with the sample solution. Then a chemical reagent is used to detect the endpoint by the color change, the precipitate, or complex formation at the equivalent point of the titration. This reagent is known as the indicator.

2.1 Types of titrations commonly used in the pharmaceutical analysis

- Acid-base reactions: These reactions are based upon the titrations of the acidic or basic compounds by the consequent acids or bases. In addition, many drugs can be classified as acids or bases based on the presence of some functional group in the drug and these drugs can be analyzed using this type of reaction. In this type of reaction, H^+ reacts with OH^- to form H_2O as in the following examples: These reactions are mainly based upon the reactions of the hydrogen ion and hydroxide ion to form water.

$$H^+ + OH^- \rightarrow H_2O \tag{1}$$

A classic application of this type of titration is the determination of aspirin (acetylsalicylic acid) [32].

- Complexometric reactions: These types of titrations are based on the complexation reactions by using the complexing agent such as ethylenediaminetetraacetic acid (EDTA). these reactions are carried out by complex formation by combining ions by using complexing agents like EDTA. The endpoint is detected by using metal ion detectors.

- Precipitation reactions: These titrations are based on the precipitate formation.

Example: AgCl titrations: these reactions are carried out by the formation of the precipitate by combining the ions by using the precipitating reagents.

A precipitation reaction is a titration in which the reaction between the analyte and the titrants forms an insoluble precipitate. Most precipitation titrations involve standard Ag^+ as a titrant and Cl^-, SCN^- as an analyte. An example is a titration of chloride ions with silver nitrate solution to form a silver chloride precipitate. This type of reaction is used in pharmaceutical assays of many drugs, especially the drugs that are found as chloride salts such as bupropion hydrochloride (antidepressant drug) [33].

- Redox reactions: Redox reactions are more widely used in titrimetric pharmaceutical analysis than other types of reactions. The ions may exist in different oxidation states resulting in the possibility of a very large number of redox reactions. Many of these reactions satisfy the requirements for use in titrimetric analysis and applications are numerous. These reactions also are important for some basic functions of life, such as photosynthesis [34].

A good example of a redox reaction is the thermite reaction, in which iron atoms in ferric oxide lose (or give up) O atoms to Al atoms, producing Al_2O_3 [3].

$$Fe_2O_{3(s)} + 2Al_{(s)} \rightarrow Al_2O_{3(s)} + 2Fe_{(l)} \quad (2)$$

The successful application of a redox reaction to titrimetric analysis requires, among other things, the means for detecting the equivalence point. Therefore, it is worth examining the changes that occur in variations that are most pronounced in the region of the equivalence point.

In the pharmaceutical formulation, a common application of this type of titration involves iodine I_2, potassium permanganate $KMnO_4$, and cerium (VI). The direct titration method against iodine (sometimes termed iodimetry) refers to titrations with a standard solution of iodine.

($I_2 + 2e^- \rightarrow 2I^-$ iodine is oxidizing agent)

Iodine has low solubility in water but the complex I_3^-, is very soluble. So, in the most direct titrations with iodine (iodimetry) iodine solutions are prepared by dissolving I_2 in a concentrated solution of KI (potassium iodide). This type of titration (iodimetry) can be used in the assay of many pharmaceutical compounds such as ascorbic acid (vitamin C), benzylpenicillin, ampicillin, cloxacillin, methicillin, carbenicillin, cefazolin, cephalothin, cephaloglycin, cephalexin, cephalosporin C, 7-aminocephalosporanic acid, and cefoxitin [35, 36].

- The titrant is (I_2 + KI) solution.

  (that can be standardized against $Na_2S_2O_6$; sodium thiosulfate).

- The analyte is ascorbic acid solution, for example.

- The indicator is a starch; the endpoint is the appearance of the blue color.

While the indirect titration method (sometimes termed iodometry) deals with the titration of iodine liberated in chemical reactions.

($2I^- \rightarrow I_2 + 2e^-$ iodine is reducing agent)

The second method (Iodometry) called indirect or back titration that involves an excess of KI being added, reducing the analyte and liberating I_2. The amount of I_2 produced is then determined by a back titration using $Na_2S_2O_3$ as a reducing titrant. The iodometry titration can be used in the assay of many pharmaceutical compounds such as amoxicillin and diethylcarbamazine citrate [14, 37–39].

The titrant is a thiosulfate solution,

- The titration flask contains the analyte and iodide in an acid medium.
- The liberated I_2 is then titrated with thiosulfate using a starch indicator.
- The endpoint is the disappearance of the blue color.

Potassium permanganate ($KMnO_4$) and cerium (IV) also are widely used as an oxidizing titrant in the assay of pharmaceutical compounds such as famotidine citrate, diethylcarbamazine citrate, minoxidil, hydrogen peroxide and Pantoprazole [40–44], Vitamin C, Ofloxacin, and ketotifen [45–47], respectively.

- Non-aqueous reactions: These reactions are based upon the titrations by using the non-aqueous titrants. Non-aqueous titrations are titrations carried out in the absence of water. In potentiometric titrations, absolute potentials or potentials concerning standard half-cells are not usually required, and measurements are made while the titration is in progress. The equivalence point of the reaction will be revealed by a sudden change in the potential in the plot of e.m.f. reading against the volume of the titration solution, and we can determine the end-point graphically. The graphical method (the differential method) involves a plot of the change in potential per unit change in the volume of reagent (ΔE/ΔV) as a function of the average volume of the reagent added. The end-point is taken as the maximum in the curve and is obtained by extrapolation of the experimental points (**Figure 1**).

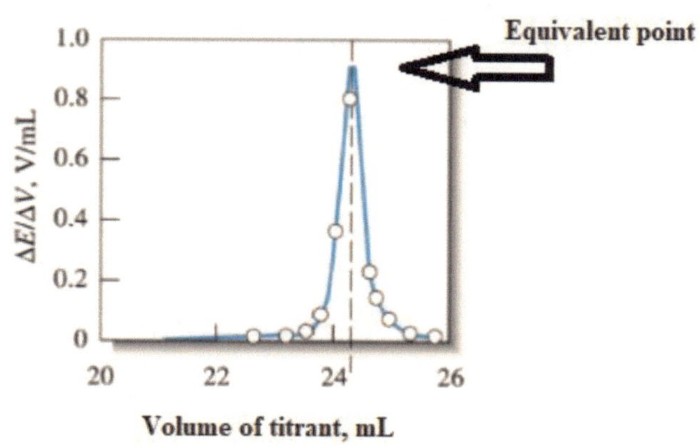

Figure 1.
Potentiometric titration curve.

Non-aqueous titration is the most common titrimetric procedure used in the pharmaceutical assays of many drugs [7, 15, 27]. Non-aqueous titrations are widely used in Volumes I and II of the British Pharmacopeia for the assay of drug substances. A large number of drugs are either weakly acidic or weak base. The weak acids are usually titrated with tetrabutylammonium hydroxide (Bu_4NOH) or potassium methoxide (CH_3OK) in dimethyl formamide (DMF) as a solvent. Weak bases are dissolved in glacial acetic acid and titrated with perchloric acid ($HClO_4$). For weak bases, the titration medium usually used for non-aqueous titration of bases is perchloric acid in acetic acid. However, perchloric acid is not a primary standard substance, so it can be standardized using potassium hydrogen phthalate ($KHC_8H_4O_4$) in a glacial acetic acid, and acetous crystal violet as an indicator.

The overall reactions with drug base occurring as follows:

$$HClO_4 + \text{basic drug} \rightarrow \text{basic drug } H^+ + ClO_4^- \quad (3)$$

That is, the perchloric acid acts as a monoprotic acid and 1 mole of perchloric acid is equivalent to 1 mole of the basic drug. British Pharmacopeia (BP) recommends a non-aqueous titration as a reference method for the assay of methyldopa which is a cardiovascular drug using 0.1 M perchloric acid as titrant and crystal violet solution as indicator. In general, the reaction taking place between a primary amine and perchloric acid may be expressed as follows:

$$RNH_2 + HClO_4 \rightarrow [RNH_3]^+ + ClO_4^- \quad (4)$$

Also, several drugs are weakly acidic. Such substances can be titrated against strong bases like potassium methoxide and sodium methoxide, in solvents like toluene-methanol. The principle is similar to the titration of weak bases against perchloric acid. Potassium methoxide and sodium methoxide are not primary standard substances. So, they can be standardized by dimethylformamide (DMF, $H - CON(CH_3)_2$) and benzoic acid using methanolic thymol blue as an indicator. Ethosuximide, for example, is an antiepileptic drug and can be assayed by non-aqueous titration. The drug can be prepared in DMF. The titration can be done with sodium methoxide using azo-violet as an indicator.

3. Spectrophotometric techniques fundamentals, important, and its applications in pharmaceutical analysis

3.1 Fundamentals of spectrophotometric techniques

Ultraviolet–visible spectrophotometry indicates the absorption spectrum in the region between 200 and 800 nm. The absorption in the ultraviolet and visible region depended on the molecules that contain π electrons and non-bonding electrons pairs, which can absorb the energy of ultraviolet or visible light to rise to a higher anti-bonding molecular orbital. The more easily excited the electrons, the longer the wavelength of light they can absorb.

This technique is one of the spectroscopic methods based on the interaction of electromagnetic radiation with the material. Electromagnetic radiation (**Figure 2**) is considered as waves of energy propagated from a source in space and consists of oscillating electric and magnetic fields at right angles to each other. Each

DOI: http://dx.doi.org/10.5772/intechopen.109364

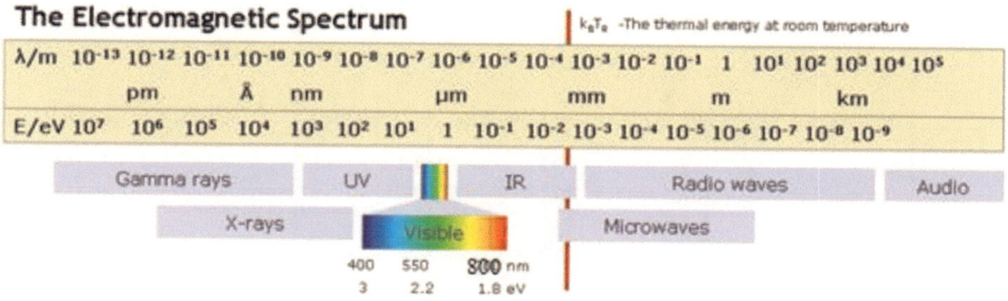

Figure 2.
Electromagnetic spectrum.

Electromagnetic radiation has characteristics of wavelength (λ), frequency (ν), or wave number, ν $[\frac{1}{\lambda}]$. Molecule or ion may absorb energy from Electromagnetic radiation of suitable wavelength (or frequency) resulting in: (a) Electronic excitation caused by absorption of UV–visible radiation leading to UV–visible spectroscopy. (b) Molecular rotation by absorption of microwave radiation leading to microwave. (c) Vibrational excitation is caused by the absorption of infrared radiation leading to infrared spectroscopy.

The UV–visible spectral method involves UV–visible spectroscopy. This arises due to the absorption of ultraviolet (UV) or visible radiation with the sample resulting in an electronic transition within the molecule or ion. The relationship between the energy absorbed in an electronic transition, the frequency (ν), wavelength (λ), and wave number (ν) of radiation-producing transition is:

$$\Delta E = hv = h\,\frac{c}{\lambda} = hvc \tag{5}$$

where h is Planck's constant, c is the velocity of light. ΔE is the energy absorbed during an electronic transition in a molecule or ion from a lower-energy state (E1) (ground state) to a high-energy state (E2) (excited state). The energy absorbed is given by

$$\Delta E = E2 - E1 = hv \tag{6}$$

Potentially, three types of ground state orbitals may be involved: (i) σ (bonding) molecular as in C – C, (ii) π (bonding) molecular orbital as in C = C, and (iii) n (non-bonding) atomic orbital as in C – Br, C – OH. In addition, two types of antibonding orbitals may be involved in the transition, σ^* (sigma star) orbital and π^* (pi star) orbital. A transition in which a bonding σ electron is excited to an antibonding σ orbital is referred to as $\sigma - \sigma^*$ transition. In the same way, $\pi - \pi^*$ represents the transition of one electron of a lone pair (non-bonding electron pair) to an antibonding π orbital. Thus the following electronic transitions can occur by the absorption of ultraviolet and visible light: $\sigma - \sigma^*$, $n - \sigma^*$, $n - \pi^*$, $\pi - \pi^*$. The energy required for various transitions (**Figure 3**) obeys the following order: $\sigma - \sigma^* > n - \sigma^* > \pi - \pi^* > n - \pi^*$.

$\sigma - \sigma^*$ transition: This transition can occur in compounds in which all the electrons are involved in the formation of single bonds (σ-bond only) and there is no lone pair of an electron, such as saturated hydrocarbon like methane, ethane, etc. which requires radiation of high energy with short wavelength (less than 150 nm). The usual

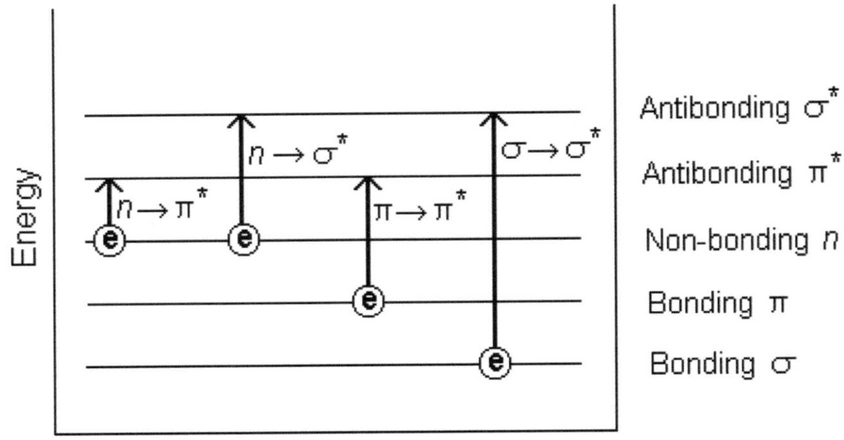

Figure 3.
The types of the transition electrons.

measurement cannot be done below 200 nm. Thus the region of transition below 200 nm is called the vacuum ultraviolet region. Methane which contains only C – H, σ-bond can undergo $\sigma - \sigma^*$ transition exhibiting absorption peak at 125 nm. Ethane has an absorption peak at 135 nm which also must arise from the same type of transition but here electrons of C – C bond appear to be involved. Since the strength of the C – C bond is less than that of C – H bond, less energy is required for excitation, as a result, absorption occurs at a lower wavelength. Thus organic molecules in which all the valence shell electrons are involved in the formation of σ-bonds do not show absorption in the normal ultraviolet region, that is, 180–400 nm. $n - \sigma^*$ transition: This type of transition takes place in a saturated compound containing one hetero atom with unshared pair of electrons. Examples of such transitions are saturated alkyl halides, alcohols, ethers, amines, etc. which are commonly used as a solvent because they start to absorb at 260 nm. However, these solvents cannot be used when measurements are to be made in 200–260 nm. In such cases saturated hydrocarbons which only give rise to $\sigma - \sigma^*$ transition must be used. However, the drawback is that these are poor solvating agents. $\pi - \pi^*$ transition: This transition is available in compounds with unsaturated centers of the molecules. Examples of such transitions are alkenes, alkynes, aromatics, carbonyl compounds, etc. this transition requires lesser energy, and hence, the transition of this type occurs at a longer wavelength within the region of the UV-spectrophotometer. In unconjugated alkenes, the absorption band is around 170–190 nm. In carbonyl compounds, the band due to $\pi - \pi^*$ transition appears at 180 nm and is more intense, that is, the value of the molar extinction coefficient is high. The introduction of the alkyl group to the olefinic linkage shifts the position of the band to a longer wavelength by 3–5 nm per alkyl group. The shift depends on the type of the alkyl group and the stereochemistry of the double bond. $n - \pi^*$ transition: This type of transition occurs in unsaturated bonds containing at least one hetero atom like O, N, S, and halogen with n electron. Examples of such transitions are aldehydes and ketones, etc. Saturated aldehydes (C = O) show both types of transitions, that is, low energy $n - \pi^*$ and high energy $\pi - \pi^*$ occurring around 290 and 180 nm, respectively. In aldehydes and ketones $n - \pi^*$ transition arises from the excitation of a lone pair of electrons in a 2p orbital of an oxygen atom with the anti-bonding π orbital of the carbonyl group. When hydrogen is replaced by an alkyl group as in ketone, this results in the shift of the band to a shorter wavelength. Besides the above transition, high energy but quite intense $\pi - \pi^*$ transition also occurs in carbonyl compounds. However, the molar extinction coefficient (ε) values associated with $n - \pi^*$ transition are generally low and range from 10 to 100 while values for $\pi - \pi^*$ transition, on the other hand, normally fall in the range between 1000 and 10,000.

The quantitative analysis using UV–visible spectrophotometry is based mainly on the Beer-Lambert law, which explains the relationship between the absorbance of analyte under analysis and its concentration:

$$A = \log I_0/I = \varepsilon Cx \tag{7}$$

where ε is molar absorptivity, x is the path length, and C is the concentration of analyte.

3.2 Important and application of spectrophotometric in the pharmaceutical analysis

The basis of spectrophotometric methods is the simple relationship between the absorption of radiation by a solution and the concentration of the colored species in the solution [48]. A molecule or ion exhibits absorption in the visible or UV region when the radiation (photons) causes an electronic transition in the molecule or ion containing one or more chromophoric groups (**Table 2**). The functional groups on drug molecules are targeted for quantitative analysis of pharmaceutical formulations using UV–visible spectrophotometry techniques. The quantitative analysis using UV–visible spectrophotometry is based mainly on the Beer-Lambert law, which explains the relationship between the absorbance of the analyte under analysis and its concentration:

$$A = \log I_0/I = \varepsilon Cx \tag{8}$$

where ε is molar absorptivity, x is the path length, and C is the concentration of the analyte.

Methods usually are based on ion-pair, charge-transfer complex formation reactions, and redox-complexation reactions, which formed the backbone of

Chromophore	λ_{max} (nm)	ε_{max} (l mol^{-1} cm^{-1})	Transition
H2C = CH2	171	15,530	$\pi - \pi^*$
H2C = CH – CH = CH2	217	20,900	$\pi - \pi^*$
CH3 – C = O	180 290	10,000 17	$\pi - \pi^*$ $n - \pi^*$
H2C = CH – CH = O	218 320 208	18,000 30	$\pi - \pi^*$ $n - \pi^*$ $n - \pi^*$
CH3 – COH = O	208	32	$\pi - \pi^*$
H2C = CH – COOH	206 242	13,500 250	$\pi - \pi^*$

Table 2.
Examples of some common chromophoric groups.

spectrophotometric methods. The developed methods were applied to dosage forms, including tablets, injections, syrup, capsules, and also spiked human urine wherever possible [7, 14, 17, 19, 21–30, 33, 37, 44, 47]. The details of those important reactions and more examples for each application are given.

3.2.1 Ion-pair complex

Ion-pair formation results from electrostatic according to Coulomb attraction law without the formation of a covalent bond [49]. The formation of an ion-pair complex between the drug and the choice dye followed by its extraction into an organic solvent for absorbance measurement is a widely used reaction as the basis of spectrophotometric assays for pharmaceutical formulations. These are the simplest of the spectrophotometric methods ever developed since they involve mere mixing of drug and dye solutions in an organic solvent before measuring the absorbance of the colored species. However, these methods require the drug to be present in the base or acid forms for complexation. For example, typical, some methods based on extractive spectrophotometric are used for the determination of some formulations after selecting the optimum conditions by preliminary experiments, such as pH, buffer, and solvent; at the wavelength of maximum absorption; (a) bromocresol purple used for terbinafine [21, 24], nifedipine [50], sulfadimidine, sulfaguanidine, sulfametrole, sulfaquinoxaline, and sulfamethoxazole [51], hydroxyzine dihydrochloride [52], lercanidipine [53], oxomemazine hydrochloride [54], and atorvastatin [55].

The widely used spectrophotometric methods in trace analysis are based on the possibility of converting the constituent to be determined into a substance whose solution is strongly colored. Such a solution shows differential absorption to light of different wavelengths (**Table 3**).

3.2.2 Redox-complexation (oxidation:reduction reactions)

These reactions involve a transfer of electrons between two species and a change in the oxidation number of species by gaining or losing an electron, generating a colored species. Many scientific published papers indicated oxidation-reduction reactions, that include; valganciclovir hydrochloride with iron (III) and $KMnO_4$ [30], amoxycillin, ampicillin, and cloxacillin with iodate [17], Olanzapine with N-Bromosuccinimide and Cerium (IV) sulfate [56], captopril with a mixture of $KBrO_3$ and KBr [57], to name a few.

Ultraviolet	<400 nm
Violet	400–450 nm
Blue	450–500 nm
Green	500–570 nm
Yellow	570–590 nm
Orange	590–620 nm
Red	620–800 nm
Infrared	>800 nm

Table 3.
The wavelengths of the visible and ultraviolet regions.

3.2.3 Charge-transfer complexation

The charge-transfer complex is formed from a combination of two molecules, one of which acts as an electron donor and the other as an electron acceptor. Based on the charge-transfer complexation, albendazole with picric acid [58] (**Figure 4**), chloranilic with tyrosine [59], carvedilol with iodine [60] to name a few, were determinates using spectrophotometric techniques.

4. The general methodology for the development of spectrophotometric methods

To develop a quantitative method for an unknown concentration substance using spectroscopic methods, the first step is by chooses the appropriate wavelength that corresponds to the highest absorbance. We can also choose the appropriate wavelength from the literature.

4.1 Step 1: method development

4.1.1 Optimization conditions

Several experimental variables such as the pH of the buffer system, choice of organic solvent, the volume of dye, and shaking time for the extraction of the ion-pair complex were tested with respect to their effect on complex formation.

For the development of spectroscopic methods, oxidation and reduction reactions, and complex formation are considered the backbone of these methods. These types of reactions produce colored products whose absorbance is measured. The sensitivity of the method and the degree of color stability are studied through several variables, the most important of which is the acid concentration/pH reagent concentration, nature of solvent, temperature, etc. until we reach the optimum conditions for the method. Before all that, the wavelengths of the colored products are scanned until the maximum wavelength (λ_{max}) is obtained. The range at which the attainment of maximum color and stability occurs in the color species formation is termed as an optimum condition of each parameter.

4.2 Study of the composition of the complex (stoichiometry)

Job's method of continuous variation [61] was followed for finding out the composition of the ion-association complex formed between the studied drugs and selected dyes.

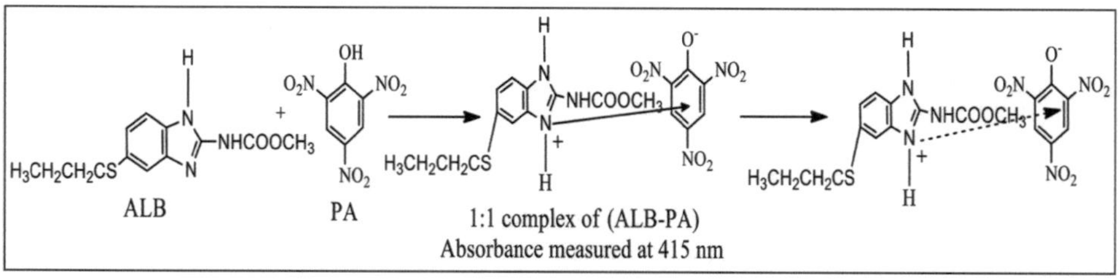

Figure 4.
Reaction pathway for the formation of electron donor-acceptor complex due to Albendazole and picric acid interaction [58].

4.3 Chemistry of the colored species formed

The chemistry of the colored species formed in each method is ascertained either through probability with the existing experimental evidence or through analogy with the literature methods.

5. Method validation (validation of analytical results)

After optimizing the experimental variables for maximum complex formation and extraction, some analytical performance characteristics such as linearity, limits of detection (LOD) and quantification (LOQ), accuracy and precision, robustness and ruggedness, and selectivity were investigated using standard solutions of drugs under study.

5.1 A calibration curve (linearity)

In quantitative analyzes using spectroscopic methods, the standard curve is always needed. Where the active substance of the pure drug is subjected to the same optimal conditions for the samples under study and the absorbance was measured at the maximum length. This is followed by plotting the absorbance measurements against the concentrations of the samples. A straight line passing through the origin is obtained if Beer's law is obeyed. This curve may then be used in the subsequent determination of the constituent under the same conditions.

5.2 Sensitivity of the method (LOD and LOQ)

Knowledge of the sensitivity of the color is important and the following terms are commonly employed for expressing the sensitivity. For more sensitive spectrophotometric methods, ε is $^{>} 1 \times 10^4$ L. mol^{-1}. cm^{-1} and values of ε $^{<} 1 \times 10^3$ l. mol^{-1}. cm^{-1} correspond to less sensitive methods. Sandell's sensitivity [62] refers to the number of μg of the constituent determined, converted to the colored product, which is a column solution of cross section 1 cm^2, shows an absorbance of 0.001 (expressed as μg/cm^2). Limits of detection LOD and LOQ are the smallest amount of an analyte that can be determined and quantified by a particular method. The LOD and LOQ values were calculated using the formulae:

$$\text{LOD} = \frac{3.3S}{m} \text{ and LOQ} = \frac{10S}{m} \tag{9}$$

where S is the standard deviation of replicate (n = 7) absorbance of blanks and m is the slope of the calibration curve.

5.3 Precision and accuracy

The purpose of carrying out a determination is to obtain a valid estimate of a true value. When one considers the criteria according to which an analytical procedure is selected, precision and accuracy are usually the first to come to mind. Precision and accuracy together determine the error of an individual determination. They are among the most important criteria for judging the results generated by the analytical procedure.

To evaluate the precision and accuracy of the methods, standard drug solution at three concentration levels was subjected to analysis on the same day (intra-day) in seven replicates and on five consecutive day (inter-day) by preparing all solutions afresh each day. Mean (×) and standard deviations (SD) were obtained by back-calculated drug concentration at each level. Accuracy and precision were evaluated in terms of relative error (RE) and relative standard deviation (RSD), respectively.

5.4 Robustness and ruggedness

Robustness is the measure of its capacity to remain unaffected by small, but deliberate, variations in parameters of the method and indicates its reliability during normal usage, while ruggedness represents the degree of reproducibility of examined results, found by analyzing the same samples under condition variables. The assay procedure was repeated after making a small incremental variation in the optimized condition such as the pH of buffer and reagent volume, and the effect of these variations was investigated to assess the robustness of the method. To evaluate ruggedness, the determination was performed by a single analyst using three instruments in the same laboratory and also by three analysts using a single instrument. Each study was performed on three levels of analyte.

5.4.1 Selectivity

It can be defined as the degree to which a method can quantity the analyte accurately in the presence of interferes. The selectivity of the developed methods was examined using placebo blank and synthetic mixture analyses. To a certain amount (mg) of the placebo blank (talc, starch, sucrose, lactose, and other compounds) prepared, accurately known amount (mg) of pure drug was added, mixed thoroughly and the mixture extract was prepared as usual; and then steps described under the procedure for dosage forms were followed. The % recovery of pure drug in the mixture was computed, which is taken as a measure of selectivity.

5.5 Accuracy by recovery experiments (standard-addition method)

Accuracy by recovery experiments: To ascertain the accuracy of the proposed methods, recovery experiments were performed *via* the standard addition technique. If the % of recovery calculated using the formula given below is satisfactory, confidence in the accuracy of the procedure is enhanced.

$$\%recovery = \frac{\sum XY - \sum X \sum Y}{\sum X^2 - \left(\sum X\right)^2} \tag{10}$$

where X = amount of the constituent added in μg (spectrophotometry) or mg (titrimetry), Y = amount of the constituent found, μg or mg.

5.6 Evaluation of accuracy and precision by comparison of two methods

To evaluate the accuracy and precision of the method, one often compares the method being developed or the "test method" with an existing method called the reference, standard or official method [63]. Student's t-test (comparison of two means); suppose that a sample is analyzed by two different methods, each repeated several times and that the mean values obtained are different, student's t-test will tell, with a given probability, whether it is worthwhile to seek an assignable cause for the difference between the two means. The test gives a yes or no answer to the correctness of the null hypothesis with a certain confidence, such as 95% or 99%. The procedure is as follows: suppose that sample has been analyzed by two different methods (test and reference methods) yielding means X_1 and X_2 and standard deviations S_1 and S_2, n_1 and n_2 is the number of individual results obtained by two methods, t is calculated using the following formula:

$$t = \frac{X_1 - X_2}{S}\sqrt{\frac{n_1 n_2}{n_1 + n_2}} \tag{11}$$

Here, it is presupposed that S_1 and S_2 are the same. If S_1 and S_2 are different, S is calculated using the following formula:

$$S = \sqrt{\frac{\Sigma(X_1 - X_1)^2 + \Sigma(X_2 - X_2)^2}{n_1 + n_2 - 2}} \tag{12}$$

F-test (comparison of two standard deviations); using the formula:
$F = S^2_T/S^2_R$.
where S^2_T is the variance of the test method, S^2_R is the variance of the reference method.

F-test uses for the calculation of F-ratio (larger variance/smaller variance). If the calculated F-value is in the table [64, 65], one can conclude that the methods are not significantly different in precision at a given confidence level.

6. Conclusion

Realizing the importance and usefulness of these two techniques; titrimetry and spectrophotometry and valuing their unique features, the author has attempted to explain of applications these simple and inexpensive techniques for the determination of different pharmaceutical formulations. The advantages and superior performances of these two techniques; titrimetry and spectrophotometry compared with the existing techniques are rapidly, simplicity, sensitivity, and use of inexpensive reagents and chemicals.

Modern methods of analysis (LCMS, GCMS, NMR, and Mass) involve sophisticated and costly equipment and pose problems of maintenance. Hence, they may not be within the reach of most of the laboratories and small-scale industries, which produce bulk drugs and pharmaceutical formulations. Among various techniques, titrimetry and spectrophotometry, still enjoy a significant role in the assay of several classes of drugs at macro, semi-micro (titrimetry), micro, or nanogram (spectrophotometry) levels. They are simple, economically viable, and easy to carry out. Visible spectrophotometry is the simplest of the spectrophotometric techniques and it is in wide use in the quantitative analysis of active substances. The spectrophotometric procedure is also recommended in Pharmacopoeial monographs such as Indian Pharmacopeia, British Pharmacopeia, USP, EP, etc. Hence, spectrophotometry is generally preferred in small-scale industries and most laboratories for routine quality assurance because of its overwhelming advantages, such as speed, simplicity, cost-effectiveness, specificity/selectivity, and sensitivity. Titration is also a simple technique giving accurate and precise results. The non-aqueous titration with visual or potentiometric end point detection has maintained its importance in pharmaceutical analysis and has been accepted by a majority of modern pharmacopeias as an official analytical method.

Conflicts of interest

There are no conflicts of interest to declare.

Author details

Nagib Qarah[1]* and Ezzouhra El-Maaiden[2]

1 Hodeidah University, Hodeidah, Yemen

2 University Hassan I, Settat, Morocco

*Address all correspondence to: nagib2015qarah@gmail.com

References

[1] Gorog S. The changing of pharmaceutical analysis. TrAC Trends in Analytical Chemistry. 2007;**26**:12-17. DOI: 10.1016/J.TRAC.2006.07.011

[2] The European pharmacopoeia. 4 th ed. Strasbourg: Council of Europe; 2002. p.55. (Chapter 2.2.40)

[3] United States Pharmacopoeia. 27th ed. Rockville, MD: The USP Convention Inc.; 2004

[4] Japanese Pharmacopoeia. Ministry Of Health, Labour And Welfare; Vol. 17. Tokyo, Japan: Chiyoda-ku; 2016. pp. 910-911

[5] The European Pharmacopeia (EP). European Directorate for the Quality of Medicines & Health Care (EDQM). 7th ed. Strasbourg, France: Council of Europe; 2011. pp. 3047-3048

[6] The British Pharmacopoeia (BP). European Directorate for the Quality of Medicines & Health Care (EDQM). London: Her Majesty's Stationery Office; 2012. pp. 2112-2113

[7] Cardoso SG, Schapoval ES. UV spectrophotometry and nonaqueous determination of terbinafine hydrochloride in dosage forms. Journal of AOAC International. 1999;**82**(4):830-833

[8] Ali TA, Abdelsabour SM, Eldessouky H, Mohamed GG, Elsayed YS. Potentiometric determination of terbinafine hydrochloride antifungal drug in pharmaceutical and biological fluids using ion selective electrodes. Journal of Basic and Environmental Sciences. 2018; **5**:80-92

[9] British Pharmacopoeia Volume I & II Monographs: Medicinal and pharmaceutical substances. Ethionamide. London, UK: European Directorate for the Quality of Medicines & Health Care (EDQM); 2009

[10] Reddy BS, Krishna RR, Sastry CSP. Titrimetric determination of some 353 antitubercular drugs by sodium nitrite and N-bromosuccinimide (NBS) using internal 354 indicators. Indian Drugs. 1982;**20**:28-29

[11] Ciesielski W, Krenc A, Zlobinska U. Potentiometric Titration of Thioamides and 356 Mercaptoacids with Iodine in Alkaline Medium. Vol. 50. Warsaw, Poland: Chemia Analityczna; 2005. pp. 397-405

[12] Obtemperanskaya SI, Buzlanova MM, Karandki IV. Potentiometric determination 359 of some drugs and other physiologically active substances using a silver sulfide ion-360 selective electrode. Journal of Analytical Chemistry. 1996;**51**:419-423

[13] Basavaiah K, Qarah NAS, Abdulrahman SAM. Application of cerium (IV) as an oxidimetric agent for the determination of ethionamide in pharmaceutical formulations. Journal of Pharmaceutics. Vol. 2016. 2016. Article ID: 5410573. DOI: 10.1155/2016/5410573

[14] Qarah NAS, Abdulrahman SAM, Algethami FK, Basavaiah K, El-Maaiden E. New applications for amoxicillin determination in pure form and pharmaceuticals based on iodateiodide mixture: Titrimetry and spectroscopy studies. Quimica Nova. 2020;**43**:44-49. DOI: 10.21577/0100-4042.20170455

[15] Kilic E, Koseoglu F, Akay MA. The non-aqueous titrimetric assay of selected antibiotics using tetra-N-

butylammonium hydroxide as titrant. Journal of Pharmaceutical and Biomedical Analysis. 1994;**12**:347-352

[16] Belal F, EL-Brashy A, Ibrahim F. Titrimetric determination of some penicillins using 2-iodoxybenzoate. Journal of Association of Official Analytical Chemistry. 1990;**73**:896-901. DOI: 10.1093/jaoac/73.6.896

[17] Qureshi SZ, Qayoom T, Helalet MI. Simultaneous spectrophotometric and volumetric determinations of amoxycillin, ampicillin and cloxacillin in drug formulations: Reaction mechanism in the base catalysed hydrolysis followed by oxidation with iodate in dilute acid solution. Journal of Pharmaceutical and Biomedical Analysis. 1999;**21**:473-482. DOI: 10.1016/s0731-7085(99)00205-8

[18] Shukla IC, Vinod K, Brijesh S. Application of ammonium hexanitratocerate (IV) for the determination of some antibiotics. Journal of the Indian Chemical Society. 2011;**88**:1383-1388. DOI: 10.5281/zonodo.5787917

[19] Chaudhary S, Ali SK, Singh YP. Spectrophotometric and titrimetric methods for the determination of gentamycin and amoxycillin. Oriental Journal of Chemistry. 2010;**26**:75-80

[20] Hasan HM, Habib IH, Omar SK. Mercurimetric titration of some beta lactam antibiotics in bulk and pharmaceutical products. Der Pharmacia Sinica. 2012;**3**:327-331

[21] Qarah NAS, Basavaiah K. Assay of terbinafine hydrochloride by extractive-spectrophotometry with alizarin red S-A modified approach. Eurasian Journal of Analytical Chemistry. 2015;**10**:34-45

[22] Patel HD, Patel MM. Development and validation of UV-spectrophotometric method for simultaneous estimation of terbinafine HCl and mometasone furoate in combined dosage form. Asian Journal of Research in Chemistry. 2013;**6**(1):29-34

[23] Jain PS, Chaudhari AJ, Patel S, Patel Z, Patel D. Development and validation of the UV-spectrophotometric method for determination of terbinafine hydrochloride in bulk and in formulation. Pharmaceutical Methods. 2011;**2**:198-202. DOI: 10.4103/2229-4708.90364

[24] Qarah NAS, Basavaiah K, Swamy N. Ion-pair extractive spectrophotometric assay of terbinafine hydrochloride in pharmaceuticals and spiked urine using bromocresol purple. Journal of Applied Spectroscopy. 2016;**83**:694-702. DOI: 10.1007/s10812-016-0350-x

[25] Qarah NAS, Basavaiah K, Abdulrahman SAM. Spectrophotometric determination of ethionamide in pharmaceuticals using Folin–Ciocalteu reagent and iron(III)-ferricyanide as chromogenic agents. Journal of Taibah University for Science. 2017;**11**:718-728. DOI: 10.1016/j.jtusci.2016.07.002

[26] Raghu MS, Basavaiah K, Abdulrahaman SAM, Prashanth KN, Vinay KB. Sensitive and selective spectrophotometric methods for the determination of pheniramine maleate in bulk drug and in its formulations using sodium hypochlorite. Journal of Analytical Chemistry. 2013;**68**:969-976. DOI: 10.1134/S1061934813110129

[27] Abdulrahmana SAM, Algethami FK, Qarah NAS, Basavaiahd K, El-Maaiden E. Development of non-aqueous titrimetric and spectrophotometric methods for the determination of valganciclovir hydrochloride in bulk

drug and tablets. Annales Pharmaceutiques Françaises. 2021;**79**: 489-499. DOI: 10.1016/j.pharma.2021.01.010

[28] Abdulrahman SAM, Devi OZ, Basavaiah K, Vinay KB. Use of picric acid and iodine as electron acceptors for spectrophotometric determination of lansoprazole through a charge-transfer complexation reaction. Journal of Taibah University for Science. 2016;**10**:80-91. DOI: 10.1016/j.jtusci.2015.05.001

[29] Konidala SK, Silpa NYS, Samrajyam K, Devi OTD, Srinivasan R. Development and validation of new spectroscopic method for the estimation of valganciclovir HCl in bulk and pharmaceutic dosage form. World Journal of Pharmaceutical Research. 2014;**3**:4773-4782. DOI: 10.14419/ijac.v8i2.30926

[30] Qarah NAS, Basavaiah K, Abdulrahman SAM. Application of redox reactions for the determination of valganciclovir hydrochloride in pharmaceuticals. Brazilian Journal of Pharmaceutical Sciences. 2020;**56**: e17784. DOI: 10.1590/s2175-9790 2019000317784

[31] Beckurts H. The Methods of Mass Analysis. Braunschweig: Vieweg; 1913

[32] Robert DB. The titrimetric determination of acetylsalicylic acid in analgesic tablets. Journal of Chemical Education. 1985;**62**:811-812. DOI: 10.1021/ed062p811

[33] Abdulaziz SMA, Basavaiah K, Vinay KB. Titrimetric and spectrophotometric assay of bupropion hydrochloride in pharmaceuticals using mercury(ii) nitrate. Ecletica Quimica. 2010;**35**:9-16. DOI: 10.1590/S0100-46702010000300001

[34] Brown TE, LeMay HE, Bursten BE, Murphy C, Woodward P. Chemistry: The Central Science. A Text Book. 12th ed. USA: Pearson; 2012. pp. 131-135

[35] Silva CR, Simoni JA, Collins CH. Ascorbic acid as a standard for iodometric titrations. An analytical experiment for general chemistry. Journal of Chemical Education. 1999;**76**: 1421. DOI: 10.1021/ed076p1421-1422

[36] Sawai T, Takahashi I, Yamagishi S. Iodometric assay method for beta-lactamase with various beta-lactam antibiotics as substrates. Antimicrobial Agents and Chemotherapy. 1978;**13**: 910-913

[37] Swamy N, Prashanth KN, Basavaiah K. Titrimetric and spectrophotometric assay of diethylcarbamazine citrate in formulations using iodate and iodide mixture as reagents. Brazilian Journal of Pharmaceutical Sciences. 2015;**51**:43-52. DOI: 10.1590/S1984-82502015000100005

[38] Attih EE, Essien EE, Eseyin OA, Oladimeji HO, Igboasoiyi AC. Assay of dihydroartemisinin by iodometric titration. Nigerian Journal of Pharmaceutical and Applied Science Research. 2012;**1**:74-82

[39] Umesha KB, Chandramouli M, Basavanna V, Ningaiah S. Simple and reliable method for the estimation of albendazole in antiparasitic drug formulations. Letters in Applied Nanobioscience. 2021;**10**:2202-2206. DOI: 10.33263/LIANBS102.22022206

[40] Basavaiah K, Devi OZ. Application of oxidizing properties of permanganate to the determination of famotidine in pharmaceutical formulations. Journal of the Mexican Chemical Society. 2010; **54**(4):182-191

[41] Qarah NAS, Basavaiah K. Titrimetric and spectrophotometric assay of diethylcarbamazine citrate in pharmaceuticals using permanganate as oxidant. International Journal of MediPharm Research. 2017;**3**:210-222

[42] de Sousa RA, Semaan FS, Baio JAF, Cavalheiro ETG. Fast determination of minoxidil by photometric flow titration. Ecletica Química. 2005;**30**:79-84. DOI: 10.1590/S0100-467020050 00300010

[43] Norman VK, David M, Heather CEM. H_2O_2 determination by the I^{3-} method and by $KMnO_4$ titration. Analytical Chemistry. 1994;**66**: 2921-2925. DOI: 10.1021/ac00090a020

[44] Basavaiah K, Rajendraprasad N, Tharpa K, Anilkumar UR, Hiriyanna SG, Vinay KB. Titrimetric and spectrophotometric assay of pantoprazole in pharmaceuticals using permanganate. Journal of the Mexican Chemical Society. 2009;**53**:34-40

[45] SM AL-G, AM AL-o. Differential electrolytic potentiometric titration of vitamin C in pharmaceutical preparations. Journal of Food and Drug Analysis. 2005;**13**:295-300. DOI: 10.38212/2224-6614.2574

[46] Ramesh PJ, Basavaiah K, Devi OZ, Rajendraprasad N, Vinay KB. Titrimetric assay of ofloxacin in pharmaceuticals using cerium (IV) sulphate as an oxidimetric reagent. Journal of Analytical Chemistry. 2012;**67**: 595-599. DOI: 10.1134/S10619348 12060135

[47] Raghu MS, Basavaiah K, Prashanth KN, Vinay KB. Titrimetric and spectrophotometric methods for the assay of ketotifen using cerium (IV) and two reagents. International Journal of Analytical Chemistry. 2013;**2013**:697651, 9 pages. DOI: 10.1155/2013/697651

[48] Norman J. Color and chemical constitution. Journal of Chemical Education. 1962;**39**:596. DOI: 10.1021/ ed039p596

[49] Florea M, Ilie M. Ion-pair spectrophotometry in pharmaceutical and biomedical analysis: Challenges and perspectives. In: Sharmin E, Zafar F, editors. Spectroscopic Analyses - Developments and Applications. Rijeka: IntechOpen; 2017. pp. 173-191. DOI: 10.5772/intechopen.69778.ch8

[50] Rahman N, Khan NA, SNH A. Extractive spectrophotometric methods for the determination of nifedipine in pharmaceutical formulations using bromocresol green, bromophenol blue, bromothymol blue and eriochrome black T. II FARMACO. 2004;**59**:47-54. DOI: 10.1016/j.farmac.2003.10.001

[51] Nour El-Diena FA, Mohamed GG, Khaledb E, Frag EYZ. Extractive spectrophotometric determination of sulphonamide drugs in pure and pharmaceutical preparations through ion-pair formation with molybdenum(V) thiocyanate in acidic medium. Journal of Advanced Research. 2010;**1**:215-220. DOI: 10.1016/ j.jare.2010.05.005

[52] Rajendraprasad N, Basavaiah K, Vinay KB, Revanasiddappa HD. Sensitive and selective extractive spectrophotometric method for the determination of hydroxyzine dihydrochloride in pharmaceuticals. Journal of the Mexican Chemical Society. 2010;**54**:233-239. DOI: 10.29356/jmcs. v54i4.918

[53] Erk N. Extractive spectrophotometric methods for

determination of lercanidipine. Pharmazie. 2003;**58**:801-803

[54] El-Didamony AM. Extractive spectrophotometric methods for the determination of oxomemazine hydrochloride in bulk and pharmaceutical formulations using bromocresol green, bromocresol purple and bromophenol blue. Archiv der Pharmazie - Chemistry in Life Sciences. 2005;**338**:190-197. DOI: 10.1002/ardp.200400947

[55] Erk N. Extractive spectrophotometric methods for determination of atorvastatin in bulk and pharmaceutical formulations. Analytical Letters. 2011;**36**:2699-2711. DOI: 10.1081/AL-120024645

[56] Anna K, Barbara S, Helena PU, Joanna İLED. Spectrophotometric determination of olanzapine by its oxidation with N-bromosuccinimide and cerium (IV) sulfate. Analytical Sciences. 2006;**22**:829-833

[57] El-Didamony AM, Erfan EAH. Utilization of oxidation reactions for the spectrophotometric determination of captopril using brominating agents. Spectrochimica Acta Part A: Molecular and Biomolecular Spectroscopy. 2010;**75**: 1138-1145. DOI: 10.1016/j.saa.2009.12.075

[58] Swamy N, Basavaiah K. Simple and rapid spectrophotometric assay of albendazole in pharmaceuticals using iodine and picric acid as CT complexing agents. Brazilian Journal of Pharmaceutical Sciences. 2014;**50**: 839-850. DOI: 10.1590/S1984-82502014000400019

[59] Darwish IA, Khalil NY, Darwish HW, Alzoman NZ, Al-Hossaini AM. Spectrophotometric and computational investigations of charge transfer complexes of chloranilic acid with tyrosine kinase inhibitors and application to development of novel universal 96-microwell assay for their determination in pharmaceutical formulations. Spectrochimica Acta Part A: Molecular and Biomolecular Spectroscopy. 2021;**252**:119482. DOI: 10.1016/j.saa.2021.119482

[60] Cardoso SG, Ieggli CVS, Pomblum SCG. Spectrophotometric determination of carvedilol in pharmaceutical formulations through charge-transfer and ion-pair complexation reactions. Pharmazie. 2007;**62**:34-37. DOI: 10.1691/ph.2007.1.6075

[61] Willard HH, Merritt LL, Dean JA, Seatle FA. Instrumental Methods of Analysis. 6th ed. New Delhi, India: CBS Publishers; 1986. p. 941

[62] Sandell EB. Colorimetric determination of trace of metals. Journal of Physical Chemistry. 1945;**49**:263-264. DOI: 10.1021/j150441a012

[63] Massart DL, Vandeginste BGM, Dewing SN, Michotte Y, Kaufman L. Chemometric: A Text Book. Amsterdam: Elsevier; 1988

[64] Day RA, Underwood AL. Quantitative Analysis. 6th ed. New Jersey, USA: Prentice-Hall; 1993. p. 250

[65] Bassett J, Denney RC, Jaffery GH, Mendham J. Vogel's Text Book of Quantitative Inorganic Analysis. 4th ed. New York, NY: John Wiley and Sons; 1987. p. 906

Section 4

Cocrystal Engineering

Chapter 11

Chemistry and Modern Techniques of Characterization of Co-Crystals

Akbar Ali, Aleksey Kuznetsov, Muhammad Ibrahim, Azhar Abbas, Nadia Akram, Tahir Maqbool and Ushna

Abstract

Co-crystals are multicomponent molecular materials held together through non-covalent interactions that have recently attracted the attention of supramolecular scientists. They are the monophasic homogeneous materials where a naturally occurring pharmaceutical active ingredient (API) and a pharmaceutically acceptable co-crystal former are bonded together in a 1:1 *via* non-covalent forces such as H-bonds, π–π, and van der Waals forces. Co-crystallization is a promising research field, especially for the pharmaceutical industry, due to the enormous potential of improved solubility and bioavailability. Co-crystals are not the only multicomponent molecular materials, as there are many other forms of multicomponent molecular solids such as salts, hydrates, solvates, and eutectics. The formation of co-crystals can roughly be predicted by the value of ΔpK_a, that is, if the ΔpK_a is more than 3, then this monophasic homogeneous material usually falls in the category of salts, whereas if the ΔpK_a is less than 2, then co-crystals are usually observed. A number of methods are available for the co-crystal formation, broadly classified into two classes established on state of formation, that is, solution-based and solid-based co-crystal formation. Similarly, a number of techniques are available for the characterization of co-crystals such as Fourier transforms-infrared spectroscopy, single-crystal and powder X-ray diffraction, etc. In this chapter, we will discuss the available methods for co-crystallization and its characterization.

Keywords: co-crystallization, non-covalent interactions, co-crystallization techniques, SC-XRD, FT-IR

1. Introduction

Co-crystals are crystalline complexes containing neutral molecular components combined by non-covalent forces forming a crystal framework [1]. Co-crystals are also defined as the combination of ionic or molecular pharmaceutical active ingredient (API) and co-crystal former that are solid at room temperature [2]. A comparison can also be drawn about the selection of salt. In this instance, the pK_a controversy concerns the selection the acid-base duos that combine to form salts. Study displays that a pK_a variance of minimum two digits (in base and acid) is essential to generate a salt that is solid in H_2O. The formation of co-crystals can roughly be predicted by the value of ΔpK_a; that is, if

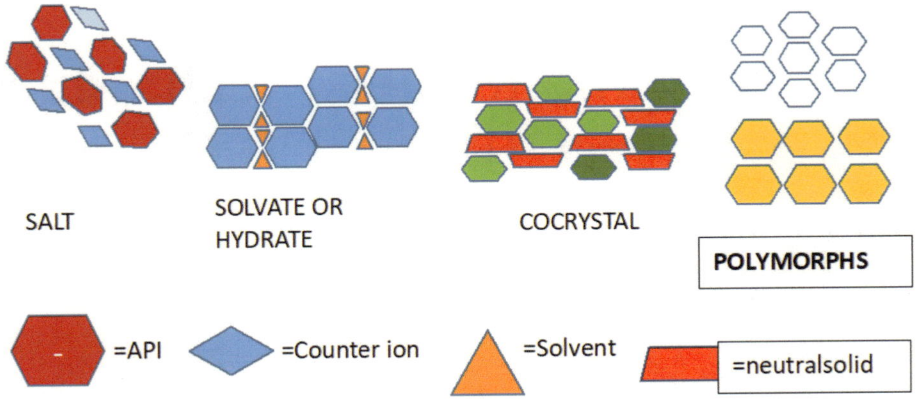

Figure 1.
Common solid-state systems and their respective components.

the ΔpK_a is more than 3, then this monophasic homogeneous material usually falls in the category of salts, whereas if the ΔpK_a is less than 2, then co-crystals are usually observed [3]. Accordingly, solvates hydrates, clathrates, or inclusion compounds (host and guest molecules), and pseudopolymorphs are excluded from the definition of co-crystals because all the mentioned species contain a liquid or gas component under ambient conditions, whereas a co-crystal contains only the solid constituents at room temperature. A general representation of various solid-state systems is given in **Figure 1** [1].

Synthesis of co-crystals is a formidable task due to numerous constrictions like the nature of a solvent, the reactants, (1:1) equivalent of the co-crystal former and API, stirring, pH, heat, sort of glassware, etc., which are the effective variables associated with the mechanism of co-crystallization. The question here is how the neutral molecules interact to form a single state of same union (co-crystal) rather than a collection of untainted crystals [4]. The answer to this question is that the force responsible for co-crystal formation is electrostatic in nature; that is, it involves the attraction affinity of negative charge for positive charge. Intermolecular forces like X···X interactions (X = F, Cl, Br, I), hydrogen bonding, π···π stacking, and van der Waal interactions are involved for the development of co-crystals [5]. Thus, non-covalent interactions are the key factor in designing of co-crystal systems.

Many methods are available for the co-crystal production in which grinding is the pioneer one that was used the first time in 1893 when equal molarities of p-benzoquinone and hydroquinone produced quinhydrone co-crystals [6]. In the interim, numerous new well-defined co-crystals have been formed by both wet grinding and neat methods.

In this chapter, co-crystallization techniques and co-crystallization characterization techniques such as SC-XRD and powder X-ray diffractometry (P-XRD) which are two techniques extensively used for the structure determination of solids having single large crystal and solid in the powder form, respectively, density functional theory (DFT), spectroscopic analysis (UV/IR/FTIR), and morphological (PXRD, SEM, SXRD) and thermal analysis (DSC, TGA) are reviewed.

2. Techniques of co-crystallization

Various methods for co-crystal formation are currently employed, which may be broadly categorized into two classes established on the state of formation:

solution-based and solid-based methods [7]. The solution-based techniques utilize large amounts of solvents, which require the separation of solvents after crystallization; on the other hand, solid-based route requires no or limited amount of a solvent [8]. The solution co-crystallization has several advantages over solid-state processes comprising better regulation of crystal properties, higher purity, and greater industrial scale. Solution co-crystallization can completely remove impurities from the crystallized product, helping to restrain challenges to achieve selective polymorphic crystallization. It is also a useful strategy for manufacturing co-crystals on an industrial level as the tools essential for extensive fabrication have been previously widely used in the pharmaceutical, food, and agrochemical manufacturing units. Solution co-crystallization has potential applications in various steps of co-crystal production, from initial screening to scale-up for commercial fabrication [9]. Though the solution co-crystallization is beneficial, solid-state co-crystallization is important from the green chemistry perspective.

2.1 Solution-based co-crystallization of nutraceuticals

Nutraceuticals which are a novel category of mixtures with recognized best-ever protection that can be used as attainable contenders are naturally arising for crystallization in the pharmaceutical industry. In 1989, Nutraceuticals, a terminology devised by DeFelice could be demarcated as a diet (or portion of a diet) that offers health or medical assistance, containing the preclusion or cure of a syndrome. Common types of nutraceuticals comprise polyphenols (e.g., phenolic acids, coumarins, stilbenes, and flavonoids) and vitamins [10]. There exist well-recognized approaches for the preparation of co-crystals, which result in crystals with desirable properties that help to evaluate crystal habit and other characteristics [11]. Isothermal ternary phase diagrams (**Figure 2**) show co-crystallization stability area when different components of the co-crystal are dissolved in solvents having similar and dissimilar solubility [12].

2.1.1 Evaporative co-crystallization

Co-crystallization is an ordinary evaporation technique for spawning co-crystals, archetypally implemented for procurement of single-crystal co-crystals appropriate for diffraction studies to explicate the co-crystal structure. The procedure embroils the cloud seeding and development of a co-crystal from a solution of equally API and co-crystal former in a solvent, with super-saturation as long as by elimination of the solvent from the solution through vaporization. Distinct co-crystals, or the main part of the crystal sample, are garnered prior the solution vanish to aridness to certify the retrieval of an unsoiled crystal(s). A low degree of desiccation is customarily sought to make sure the development of a large number of minor crystals is disproportionate to an insignificant number of larger crystals. As crystal structure identification is a necessary step in the discovery of novel co-crystal forms, evaporative co-crystallization is evident in the majority of the co-crystal related research papers, and there are countless examples of it in the literature [13].

2.1.2 Cooling co-crystallization

It is performed by decreasing the temperature of the solution. A mixture of components and a solvent is heated to obtain a clear saturated solution and then, the temperature is decreased to get a supersaturated solution, and finally, co-crystals are

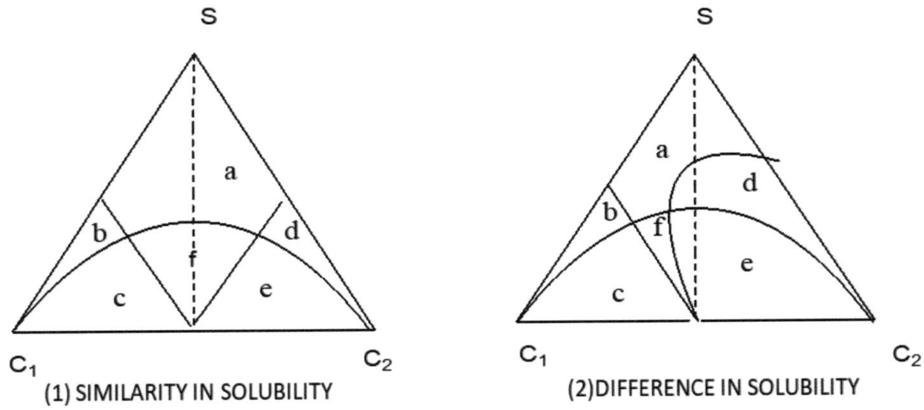

Figure 2.
Ternary phase diagrams with unlike solubility of components C_1 plus C_2 in the solvent S. Area "a" is for solution; "b" is for the component C_1 and solvent; "c" is for the component C_1 and co-crystal; "d" is for the component C_2 and solvent; "e" is for the component C_2 and co-crystal, and "f" is for the co-crystal.

precipitated out [14]. Cooling of crystals technique was used to formulate co-crystals of nicotinamide:carbamazepine using ethyl alcohol in an excess to create an accessible solution co-crystallization approach. Solvent miscellany, desupersaturation kinetics, and requirement of the thermodynamically stable co-crystal functioning series were used in the design of the procedure, which was displayed throughout to have at 1 L gauge the 90% yield. An analogous methodology was used by Holaň et al. in the formation of citric acid:agomelatine co-crystals, and the effect of freezing level and seed quantity on the crystal proportion dissemination in the concluding yield was evaluated [15].

2.1.3 Reaction co-crystallization

This method is based on the above **Figure 2** for components having different solubility in a solvent. A component C_1 is added to the solution of a component C_2 near its saturation to obtain co-crystals [16]. The reaction co-crystallization is used to harvest co-crystals of carbamazepine:saccharin by mixing different starting solutions of both of the preparatory components. The technique was systematized by the ternary stage illustration and demonstrated a resilient functioning series for the co-crystal development and validated the predictable connection in induction period and supersaturation. Nicotinamide:carbamazepine co-crystal production was also implemented by the reaction co-crystallization using open-air conditions [17].

2.1.4 Isothermal slurry conversion

In this methodology, slurry is obtained with the conversion time depending on various factors such as nucleation, growth kinetics, relative concentration of co-former and API, and the resultant solubility [18]. This methodology implicates the formation of the mixture of the API and co-crystal former, generally in a stoichiometric ratio, in a solvent with a compact portion of deposit incessantly enduring in excess of a solvent. Technique, the addition of the API to a mixture of co-crystal former in a solvent, can be also adjusted in functional terms. However, this is a solution-based process, which does not entail the production of an immaculate (completely dissolved) preliminary solution, as is the situation of prior approaches pronounced above. The degree at which the slurry transformation transpires will diverge centered on the solubility, driving force, the comparative amount of the API and co-crystal former, and the cloud seeding and evolutionary kinetics of the system. A kinetic description of the isothermal slurry transformation of arbitrary co-crystals is inadequate. Zhang et al. scrutinized the adaptation time for theophylline to transform into a stoichiometric ratio glutaric acid co-crystal. While the slurry transformation process usually required a more quantity of starting components and will experience some material damage owing to enduring solubility in the solvent, it is considered as one of the best auspicious screening methodologies owing to its extraordinary proficiency [19].

2.2 Solid state co-crystallization

These methods of co-crystallization involve limited or no use of solvent and are therefore regarded as environment friendly, green, and economically viable. Following procedures are adopted in these methods.

2.2.1 Grinding

Grinding may be either neat grinding, that is, dry grinding or solvent-assisted grinding [20]. In dry or neat grinding method, stoichiometric amounts of selected solids for co-crystallization are mechanically (using mechanical force to create supramolecular synthons, that is, involving mechanochemistry, which is considered as eco-friendly route as it avoids the use of solvents) or manually mixed at high pressure while avoiding their melting [21]. A major disadvantage of the dry grinding is the absence of heating stage involved in co-crystallization, which is shown by many studies to be important in the co-crystallization process [22]. On the other hand in the liquid-assisted milling the above shortcoming is overtaken through adding little amount of liquid to the solids for the co-crystallization. The little quantity of solvent performs as a catalyst for the co-crystal development; better results have been obtained through this method [23]. Two carboxylic acid:sulfathiazole co-crystals were formed by milling stoichiometric proportions of sulfathiazole and the needed carboxylic acid in a Retsch blender grind at a frequency of 25 Hz and a temperature not exceeding 37°C for 90 min and it was done [22]. Compared with solution-based approaches, solid milling is associated with higher performance because no product is lost due to its solubility in a solvent. Problems with dry milling can comprise impossibility to form a co-crystal, inadequate modifications to the co-crystal, and crystalline flaws with the presence of possible several amorphous compounds [24].

2.2.2 Contact formation

Co-crystals have been prepared through mixing without using any mechanical force; however, this process requires controlled conditions of temperature and pressure. Various factors affect the formation of co-crystals such as pre-milling, moisture, and size of premixed materials [25, 26]. The extemporaneous production of co-crystals by intermixing an uncontaminated target molecule and co-crystal former using organized conditions has been stated. During co-crystallization, no mechanical forces are employed in this technique. However, in various circumstances, slight milling of untainted constituents separately afore intermixing has been completed. The impact on the co-crystallization rate of pre-milling of the elementary constituents carbamazepine and nicotinamide was described by Rodriguez-Hornedo et al. It was shown that the co-crystallization rate can be increased by using milled components as compared to unmilled components (12 vs. 80 days, correspondingly). Furthermore, the greater co-crystallization degree has been described for the indistinguishable arrangement at maximum temperatures and comparative dampness, nevertheless of the mechanical stimulation [20]. The formation of an isoniazid benzoic acid co-crystal *via* spontaneous co-crystallization was reported as well [24]. We found that a higher frequency of pre-grinding of uncontaminated components significantly improved the reaction rate [27].

2.2.3 Twin screw extrusion

In twin screw extrusion (TSE) technique, the mixing of materials is carried out in a device known as a twin screw extruder in which milling of the starting materials is carried out below their melting points. Proficient intermixing and high surface interaction and consequently enhanced co-crystal formation are achieved without using the solvent provided by this method [25, 26]. The two co-/counter-rotating screws are accompanied by twin screw units in a solitary barrel. Screw activity offers immediate intermixing and mobility of components sideways the span of the barrel. The materialization of four model co-crystals consumes a 16 mm TSE with four manageable temperature regions as reported by Daurio et al. Theophylline:citric acid, carbamazepine:saccharin, nicotinamide:cinnamic acid, and caffeine:oxalic acid co-crystals were formed by slight grinds of the dry fine particles of both starting components *via* the extruder. The effect of heat on the alteration to a co-crystal was specific to the co-crystal arrangement described, with no ostensive temperature effect on the co-crystal of carbamazepine:saccharin and robust temperature effect on the co-crystal of cinnamic acid: nicotinamide. In a different investigation, the same authors reported a saccharin:AMG-157 co-crystal formed from twin screw extrusion and solution crystallization. Co-crystals from TSE were presented to have augmented bulk density, surface region, and movement characteristics compared to those prepared from solution crystallization.

2.2.4 Hot melt extrusion (HME)

Hot melt extrusion is a comparatively modern addition to the co-crystal grounding options. Using a warmed screw extruder, this special technique achieves simultaneous softening and combining of the API and co-crystal former. Usually, the initial components are combined in the definite stoichiometric ratio and supplied to the warmed extruder. The complete intermixing of the starting components in the stoichiometric ratio occurs by melting. The co-crystal nucleates amenably in the melt and the uncontaminated co-crystal extrudate is separated from the extruder constantly. The benefits of the technique are as follows: the purging using organic solvents, rapid working times, improved adaptation compared with the solution-based techniques, reduced leftover, and the tools offering itself well to the constant drug manufacturing [8]. Co-crystal formation of carbamazepine:cinnamic acid by a single screw and twin screw extruder is reported by Moradiya et al. Co-crystals prepared by the twin screw extruder presented improved suspension characteristics as compared with those gained *via* single screw/solution-based procedures. Extrusion melt as an incessant engineering performance was applied to harvest indomethacin:saccharin co-crystals. Their studies demonstrated the three critical process parameters (CPP): temperature profile, screw speed, and forage rate, which are desired in the engineering of good-quality co-crystals. Furthermore, the rate of dissolution of co-crystals is not affected by temperature. However, as was established on Rietveld investigation the co-crystal uniform crystallinity is affected by temperature. It has been shown that in the conditions of unevenness in the crystal-form quality because of the process temperature, the dissolution degree will be affected successively. Moreover, the dissolution profile can be affected by the unit size of co-crystals.

This method helps in avoiding solvents and saves time due to the increased conversion to co-crystals. Besides other benefits of HME, this method falls within the requirement of US FDA practice analytical expertise for controlling, analyzing, and designing the engineering of pharmaceuticals. For example, drugs such as Rezulin, Kaletra, and Norvir have been prepared through this method and got FDA approval [28]. Other benefits include scaling-up of production to an industrial scale and being more economical because it is a continuous process.

2.3 Miscellaneous methods of co-crystal preparation

2.3.1 Heat-induced co-crystallization

Co-crystallization method using heat is a novel method to form co-crystals. It has several advantages compared with the solvent evaporation method such as it does not need any organic solvent and can be used without drug coformer solubility determination that is a time-consuming and laborious work [29].

2.3.2 Spray drying method

Spray drying is an instant and incessant method for solid manufacturing, generating dry fine particles from precursor *via* a warm air torrent [30, 31]. For drug-coformer different solubility systems, where an uncontaminated co-crystal cannot be designed by the solvent evaporation technique, co-crystallization *via* spray drying process can be used as an alternative process. Theophylline: nicotinamide, carbamazepine:glutaric acid, caffeine:glutaric acid, and succinic acid:urea co-crystals, as instances of different schemes, their untainted co-crystals cannot be produced by the solvent evaporation process; however, when spray drying process is employed, it efficaciously produces uncontaminated co-crystals. Patil et al. reported the co-crystallization *via* the spray drying process using carbamazepine and nicotinamide as drug and coformer models respectively in a stoichiometric ratio. Accidentally, nicotinamide:carbamazepine co-crystal produced by the spray drying methodology has an analogous characteristic with a co-crystal produced by the liquid facilitating grinding [32].

2.3.3 Supercritical fluid technology

Materials that have pressure and temperature greater than their critical state (P_c and T_c) are supercritical fluids. The leading objective of supercritical fluid technology is to regulate cloud seeding and crystal development courses. The most conspicuous supercritical fluid used in the pharmaceutical arena is carbon dioxide, with critical temperature and pressure of 31.0°C and 7.39 atm, respectively, because of its non-toxicity, non-flammability, and low-cost properties [22, 33]. Numerous approaches of employing the supercritical fluid carbon dioxide to produce co-crystals are as follows: (1) where CO_2 is used as an anti-solvent known as gas anti-solvent crystallization (GAS). As an example, the SAS (supercritical anti-solvent crystallization) and AAS (atomization and anti-solvent crystallization) methods of supercritical fluid technology were successfully used in the formation of the indomethacin:saccharin co-crystal, (2) where the carbon dioxide is used as a liquid and molecular movement enhancer called co-crystallization with the supercritical solvent (CSS), (3) where CO_2 is utilized as a solvent and molecular movement enhancer called supercritical anti-solvent crystallization (SAS), (4) where CO_2 is used as corsage enhancer or anti-solvent called atomization and anti-solvent crystallization (AAS), (5) where CO_2 is used as corsage enhancer or anti-solvent called supercritical fluid improved atomization (SEA), and (6) where CO_2 is used as a solvent known as rapid expansion of supercritical solutions (RESS) [34].

2.3.4 Laser irradiation

A current technique for co-crystallization described by Titapiwatanakun et al. uses carbon dioxide irradiation treatment for the production of a malonic acid:caffeine (1:2) and oxalic acid:caffeine (1:2) co-crystals. The energy given to the unit throughout irradiation spawns a quick escalation in heat in a short period, triggering the softening of the crystalline compound, monitored by material intermixing, and next prompts recrystallization upon freezing. In this scheme, requirements for a co-crystal former component that can be used for this process are that a co-crystal former is necessarily sublimable, to accelerate a cloud seeding method by the vapor phase [35].

2.3.5 Electrochemically induced co-crystallization

Urbanus et al. reported the perspective of using co-crystallization in combination with electrochemistry to exclude *in situ* products of acids in formation of a co-crystal system of 3-nitrobenzamide and cinnamic acid. Their results show that electrochemistry is used to attain neutral carboxylic acids by locally altering the pH and inducing limited dynamics of co-crystallization [36].

2.3.6 Acoustic resonant mixing

Acoustic resonant mixing (RAM) is used to combine the API and co-crystal former in the existence of a solvent to produce a co-crystal without any milling media. The supply of mechanical energy into a wet powder mixture is performed acoustically, promoting the complete intermixing of the constituents. Utilizing a laboratory RAM resonant acoustic blender operating at 80–100G and 60 Hz, a series of carbamazepine co-crystals have been efficaciously formed. The co-crystal product has been separated at a wide array of gauges from the lab, 100 mg, 1.5 g, and 22 g, and the equipment seems to hold itself up to scale [37].

2.3.7 Freeze-drying

Freeze drying, in principle recognized as lyophilization, has primarily been employed as dispensing scheme for a range of products, including foodstuff and drugs. The procedure functions to sublimate the component directly from the solid phase to the gas phase by decreasing the ambient pressure to cause the freezing of

H_2O within the component also known as sublimation. It has also recently emerged as a viable process for preparing novel solid-state forms of co-crystals. Eddleston et al. reported the preparation of new theophylline:oxalic acid co-crystals by lyophilization. Co-crystallization occurs through an amorphous state that is produced as solvent sublimes throughout lyophilization [38].

2.3.8 Electrospray technology

Electrospray is a method that uses an electric field to create and charge droplets at the same time. In this method, the solutes (substances to be dissolved) are carried by a solution that flows out of a capillary nozzle at a high potential and is subjected to an electric field, which causes the droplets of solution to elongate and create a jet. After the solution jet has been dried, the resulting particles can be collected using a powder collector that has already been loaded with material. Co-crystals of carbamazepine and itraconazole with a variety of coformers were reported as a possible outcome of this procedure by Patil et al. [39].

2.4 Nano co-crystallization

Pharmaceutical nano co-crystals can considerably enhance the delivery qualities of ailing decipherable medicines, which have long posed a considerable issue for the pharmaceutical business. The investigation is into the production of nano co-crystals with high commercial value. Methods such as precipitation, media grinding, and high-pressure homogenization can be used to manufacture nanocrystals on a large scale. When delivered orally, intravenously, pulmonaryly, ocularly, or topically, nanocrystals exhibited the promising therapeutic utility. In addition, nanostructured medicinal molecules can be targeted to specific locations. Usually formation process for the nano-crystals comprising top-down flow process is a ball grinding technique that uses shear forces to produce high-pressure homogeneous nano-size particles. Precipitation is one of the bottom-up procedures that includes the growth [40].

3. Co-crystal characterization

The determination of physicochemical properties of co-crystals is an important part of the research, and therefore, the combination of techniques is employed for the co-crystal characterization, as no single method can fully elucidate their structure and properties [41]. The following characterization techniques for the structure determination are outlined and represented diagrammatically in **Figure 3** [30].

3.1 Analyzing structure through XRD

Powder-XRD and SC-XRD are two techniques extensively used for the structure determination of solids having single large crystal and solid in the powder form, respectively. The SC-XRD elucidates the structural properties such as lattice parameters, unit cell, space group, and intermolecular interactions and is the most reliable technique [31]. However, the drawback of the method is that obtaining single crystals is a difficult task and PXRD cannot differentiate between co-crystal and additional solid states such as polymorph, solvate, and hydrate [33].

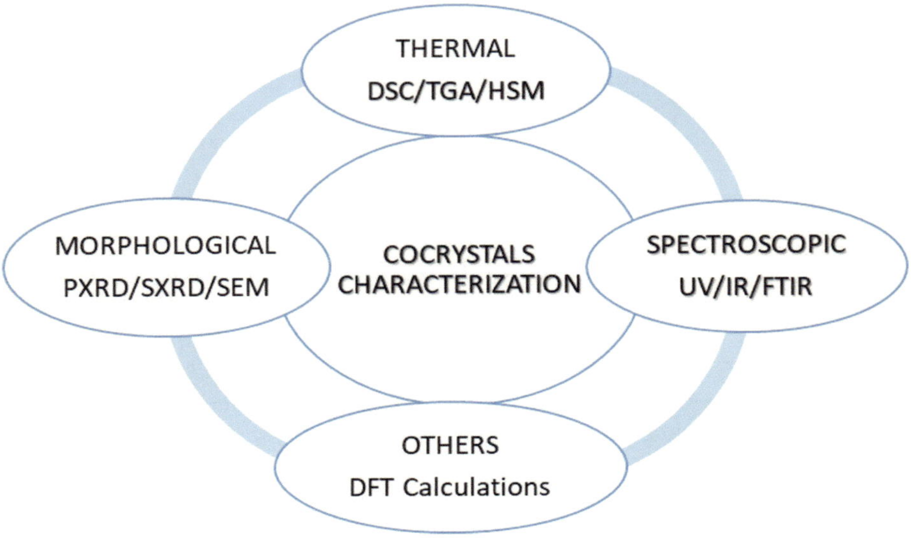

Figure 3.
Techniques for characterization of co-crystals.

3.2 Thermal analysis

Differential scanning calorimetry (DSC) is a frequently used technique for gaining thermal information such as enthalpy of melting and other melting data and is used for screening of co-crystals [22]. The type of solid formed can be identified from DSC thermogram. For example, a physical mixture has two endotherms indicating the melting points of components with no intermolecular forces between them [42], and a eutectic system has a particular endotherm having latent heat, not more than the corresponding components [43], while a co-crystal has a particular endotherm having latent heat lesser, higher, or in the middle of the parent components [44].

3.3 Spectroscopic methods

Various spectroscopic techniques such as Raman, nuclear magnetic reso¬nance (NMR), Fourier transform (FT-IR) infra-red spectroscopies, terahertz (THz) spectroscopic imaging, and various advanced applications of these methods are in practice to investigate the structure of co-crystals and find out the intermolecular forces between the components of co-crystals [45, 46].

3.4 Morphological analysis

The morphology of co-crystals is characterized by techniques such as fluorescence microscopy, scanning electron microscopy (SEM), and polarized optical microscopy [26, 47].

4. Conclusions

Co-crystallization is an effective tool and suggests one of the best auspicious routes to modify the physicochemical characteristics of the merging components.

DOI: http://dx.doi.org/10.5772/intechopen.108694

There are several methods for preparing co-crystals, extending from ordinary lab-size production to possibly large-scale unremitting fabrication. In this chapter, we have described the established and emerging approaches to co-crystal prepara-tion. Moreover, insights into the mechanisms of formation and techniques of characterization of co-crystals have also been presented.

Conflicts of interest

No conflicts of interest were declared by the authors.

Author details

Akbar Ali[1*], Aleksey Kuznetsov[2*], Muhammad Ibrahim[3], Azhar Abbas[4], Nadia Akram[1], Tahir Maqbool[1] and Ushna[1]

1 Department of Chemistry, Government College University Faisalabad, Faisalabad, Pakistan

2 Department of Chemistry, Technical University Federico Santa Maria, Santiago, Chile

3 Department of Applied Chemistry, Government College University Faisalabad, Pakistan

4 Department of Chemistry, University of Sargodha, Sargodha, Pakistan

*Address all correspondence to: akbarali@gcuf.edu.pk; akbarchm@gmail.com and aleksey.kuznetsov@usm.cl

References

[1] Schulthesisx N, Newman A. Pharmaceutical co-crystals and their physicochemical properties. Crystal Growth & Design. 2009;**9**(6):2950-2967

[2] Vishweshwar P, McMahon JA, Bis JA, Zaworotko MJ. Pharmaceutical co-crystals. Journal of Pharmaceutical Sciences. 2006;**95**(3):499-516

[3] Yadav AV, Shete AS, Dabke AP, Kulkarni PV, Sakhare SS. Co-crystals: A novel approach to modify physicochemical properties of active pharmaceutical ingredients. Indian Journal of Pharmaceutical Sciences. 2009;**71**(4):359

[4] Maruyoshi K, Iuga D, Antzutkin ON, Alhalaweh A, Velaga SP, Brown SP. Identifying the intermolecular hydrogen-bonding supramolecular synthons in an indomethacin–nicotinamide cocrystal by solid-state NMR. Chemical Communications. 2012;**48**(88):10844-10846

[5] Gao Y, Gao J, Liu Z, Kan H, Zu H, Sun W, et al. Coformer selection based on degradation pathway of drugs: A case study of adefovir dipivoxil–saccharin and adefovir dipivoxil–nicotinamide cocrystals. International Journal of Pharmaceutics. 2012;**438**(1-2):327-335

[6] Zhu W, Dong H, Zhen Y, Hu W. Challenges of organic "cocrystals". Science China Materials. 2015;**58**(11):854-859

[7] He G, Jacob C, Guo L, Chow PS, Tan RB. Screening for co-crystallization tendency: The role of intermolecular interactions. The Journal of Physical Chemistry. B. 2008;**112**(32):9890-9895

[8] Karimi-Jafari M, Padrela L, Walker GM, Croker DM. Creating cocrystals: A review of pharmaceutical cocrystal preparation routes and applications. Crystal Growth & Design. 2018;**18**(10):6370-6387

[9] Sopyan I, Fudholi A, Muchtaridi M, Sari P. Co-crystallization: A tool to enhance solubility and dissolution rate of simvastatin. Journal of Young Pharmacists. 2017, 1;**9**(2)

[10] Sinha AS, Maguire AR, Lawrence SE. Cocrystallization of nutraceuticals. Crystal Growth & Design. 2015;**15**(2):984-1009

[11] Trask AV, Jones W. Crystal engineering of organic cocrystals by the solid-state grinding approach. In: Organic Solid-State Reactions. Berlin, Heidelberg: Springer; 2005. pp. 41-70

[12] Ainouz A, Authelin JR, Billot P, Lieberman H. Modeling and prediction of co-crystal phase diagrams. International Journal of Pharmaceutics. 2009;**374**(1-2):82-89

[13] Wang IC, Lee MJ, Sim SJ, Kim WS, Chun NH, Choi GL. Anti-solvent co-crystallization of carbamazepine and saccharin. International Journal of Pharmaceutics. 2013;**450**(1-2):311-322

[14] McNamara DP, Childs SL, Giordano J, Iarriccio A, Cassidy J, Shet MS, et al. Use of a glutaric acid cocrystal to improve oral bioavailability of a low solubility API. Pharmaceutical Research. 2006;**23**(8):1888-1897

[15] Gröls JR, Castro-Dominguez B. Mechanochemical co-crystallization: Insights and predictions. Computers & Chemical Engineering. 2021;**153**:107416

[16] Childs SL, Rodríguez-Hornedo N, Reddy LS, Jayasankar A, Maheshwari C,

McCausland L, et al. Screening strategies based on solubility and solution composition generate pharmaceutically acceptable cocrystals of carbamazepine. CrystEngComm. 2008;**10**(7):856-864

[17] Zata Lini F, Pratama DE, Lee T. Co-crystallization kinetics of 2:1 benzoic acid–sodium benzoate Co-crystal: The effect of templating molecules in a solution. Crystals. 2021;**11**(7):812

[18] Jayasankar A, Reddy LS, Bethune SJ, Rodríguez-Hornedo N. Role of cocrystal and solution chemistry on the formation and stability of cocrystals with different stoichiometry. Crystal Growth & Design. 2009;**9**(2):889-897

[19] Jia Q, Wang J, Zhang S, Zhang J, Liu N, Kou K. Investigation of the solid–liquid ternary phase diagrams of 2HNIW• HMX cocrystal. RSC Advances. 2021;**11**(16):9542-9549

[20] Braga D, Giaffreda SL, Grepioni F, Pettersen A, Maini L, Curzi M, et al. Mechanochemical preparation of molecular and supramolecular organometallic materials and coordination networks. Dalton Transactions. 2006;**10**:1249-1263

[21] Friscic T, Jones W. Recent advances in understanding the mechanism of co-crystal formation via grinding. Crystal Growth & Design. 2009;**9**(3):1621-1637

[22] Mohammad AA, Velaga S. International Journal of Pharmaceutics. 2011;**407**:63-71

[23] Padrela L, de Azevedo EG, Velaga SP. Powder X-ray diffraction method for the quantification of cocrystals in the crystallization mixture. Drug Development and Industrial Pharmacy. 2012;**38**(8):923-929

[24] Chaudhari KR, Savjani JK, Savjani KT, Shah H. Improved pharmaceutical properties of ritonavir through co-crystallization approach with liquid-assisted grinding method. Drug Development and Industrial Pharmacy. 2022;**23**:1-0

[25] Ervasti T, Ketolainen J, Altonen JA. Spontaneous formation of theophylline–nicotinamide co-crystals. Scientia Pharmaceutica. 2010;**78**(3):622

[26] Nartowski KP, Khimyak YZ, Berry DJ. Tuning the spontaneous formation kinetics of caffeine: Malonic acid co-crystals. CrystEngComm. 2016;**18**(15):2617-2620

[27] Bairagi KM, Ingle KS, Bhowal R, Mohurle SA, Hasija A, Alwassil OI, et al. Interplay of halogen and hydrogen bonding through co–crystallization in pharmacologically active dihydropyrimidines: Insights from crystal structure and energy framework. ChemPlusChem. 2021;**86**(8):1167-1176

[28] Shan N, Toda F, Jones W. Mechanochemistry and co-crystal formation: Effect of solvent on reaction kinetics. Chemical Communications. 2002;**20**:2372-2373

[29] Kshirsagar SM, Chatale BC, Amin PD. Comparative evaluation of ibuprofen co-crystals prepared by solvent evaporation and hot melt extrusion technology. Journal of Drug Delivery Science and Technology. 2022;**1**(67):103003

[30] Healy AM, Worku ZA, Kumar D, Madi AM. Pharmaceutical solvates, hydrates and amorphous forms: A special emphasis on cocrystals. Advanced Drug Delivery Reviews. 2017;**117**:25-46

[31] Sathisaran I, Dalvi SV. Engineering cocrystals of poorly water-soluble drugs to enhance dissolution in aqueous medium. Pharmaceutics. 2018;**10**(3):108

[32] Tzatsi P, Goula AM. Encapsulation of extract from unused chokeberries by spray drying, co-crystallization, and ionic gelation. Waste and Biomass Valorization. 2021 Aug;**12**(8):4567-4585

[33] Miroshnyk I, Mirza S, Sandler N. Pharmaceutical co-crystals–An opportunity for drug product enhancement. Expert Opinion on Drug Delivery. 2009;**6**(4):333-341

[34] Obaidat R, Al-Ghzawi B, Al-Taani B, Al-Shari N. Co-crystallization of amoxicillin trihydrate and potassium clavulanate provides a promising approach for preparation of sustained-release microspheres. AAPS PharmSciTech. 2022;**23**(5):1-4

[35] Tsuchida S, Umemura H, Murata S, Miyabe A, Satoh M, Matsushita K, et al. Effect of humidity during sample preparation on bacterial identification using matrix-assisted laser desorption/ionization time-of-flight mass spectrometry. Journal of Chromatography B. 2021;**30**(1176):122780

[36] Wang Z, Li R, Zhao K, Yu F, Zhao J, Zhen Y, et al. A co-crystallization strategy toward high-performance n-type organic semiconductors through charge transport switching from p-type planar azaacene derivatives. Journal of Materials Chemistry C. 2022;**10**(7):2757-2762

[37] Ngilirabanga JB, Samsodien H. Pharmaceutical co-crystals: An alternative strategy for enhanced physicochemical properties and drug synergy. Nano Select. 2021;**2**(3):512-526

[38] Si-yu LI, Chen-guang ZH, Ming-xing ZH. Hot aerosol extinguishing agent based on freeze-drying co-crystallization process. Fire Science and Technology. 2021, 15;**40**(1):64

[39] Ngilirabanga JB, Samsodien H. Pharmaceutical co-crystal: An alternative strategy for enhanced physicochemical properties and drug synergy. Nano Select. 2021;**2**(3):512-526

[40] Peltonen L. Practical guidelines for the characterization and quality control of pure drug nanoparticles and nano-cocrystals in the pharmaceutical industry. Advanced Drug Delivery Reviews. 2018;**131**:101-115. DOI: 10.1016/j.addr.2018.06.009

[41] Li N, Qiao MW, Schlindwein N, Malek AD, Trappitt G. Pharmaceutical co-crystals: An overview. International Journal of Pharmaceutics. 2011;**419**(1-2):1-11

[42] Cherukuvada S, Nangia A. Eutectics as improved pharmaceutical materials: Design, properties and characterization. Chemical Communications. 2014;**50**(8):906-923

[43] Yamashita H, Hirakura Y, Yuda M, Terada K. Coformer screening using thermal analysis based on binary phase diagrams. Pharmaceutical Research. 2014;**31**(8):1946-1957

[44] Schultheiss N, Newman A. Pharmaceutical cocrystals and their physicochemical properties. Crystal Growth & Design. 2009;**9**(6): 2950-2967

[45] Chi Z, Wang M, Yang L, Li X, Cong X, Liu S, et al. Fourier transform near-infrared spectroscopy used for purity determination of rhein-L-arginine cocrystal (argirein). Analytical Sciences. 2013;**29**(6):661-664

[46] Vogt FG, Clawson JS, Strohmeier M, Edwards AJ, Pham TN, Watson SA. Solid-state NMR analysis of organic cocrystals and complexes. Crystal Growth & Design. 2009;**9**(2):921-937

[47] Rodríguez-Hornedo N, Nehm SJ, Seefeldt KF, Pagan-Torres Y, Falkiewicz CJ. Reaction crystallization of pharmaceutical molecular complexes. Molecular Pharmaceutics. 2006;**3**(3):362-367

Chapter 12

Modification of Physicochemical Properties of Active Pharmaceutical Ingredient by Pharmaceutical Co-Crystals

Raju Thenge, Vaibhav Adhao, Gautam Mehetre, Nishant Chopade, Pavan Chinchole, Ritesh Popat, Rahul Darakhe, Prashant Deshmukh, Nikesh Tekade, Bhaskar Mohite, Nandu Kayande, Nilesh Mahajan and Rakesh Patel

Abstract

The oral drug delivery is widely used and accepted routes of administration, but it fails to provide the therapeutic effectiveness of drugs due to low solubility, poor compression and oral bioavailability. Crystal engineering is the branch where the modification of API is of great importance. Co-crystallization of API using a co-former is a hopeful and emerging approach to improve the performance of pharmaceuticals, such as micromeritic properties, solubility, dissolution profile, pharmacokinetics and stability. Pharmaceutical co-crystals are multicomponent systems in which one component is an active pharmaceutical ingredient and the others are pharmaceutically acceptable ingredients that are of GRAS category. In multidrug co-crystals one drug acts as API and other drug acts as coformer. This chapter illustrates the guidance for more efficient design and manufacture of pharmaceutical co-crystals with the desired physicochemical properties and applications.

Keywords: co-crystals, physicochemical properties, characterization, evaluation, drug delivery

1. Introduction

A drug compound is classified using the biopharmaceutical categorization system according to its permeability and solubility in water [1]. When making decisions on the discovery and early development of new drugs, the Biopharmaceutical Classification System is a helpful resource. By categorizing drug compounds into four classes backed by their solubility associated with dose and intestinal permeability in combination with the dissolution properties of the dosage form, it enables the prediction of *in vivo* pharmacokinetics of oral immediate-release (IR) medicinal products [2]. The US Food and Drug Administration (FDA) guidelines for the Biopharmaceutical Classification System (BCS) were made available to increase the effectiveness of the drug product development process [3]. The Biopharmaceutical Classification Technique is a system for categorizing medicines according to their permeability and solubility. The US Food and Drug Administration has supplied it as a forecasting tool for intestinal drug absorption.

Oral administration is the most suitable and commonly employed route of drug delivery thanks to its simple administration, patient acceptability, cost efficiency, least sterility maintenance, and flexibility in the design of a dosage form. However, the main disadvantage with the formulating of oral drug delivery system lies with their poor oral bioavailability. The oral bioavailability of drug substances lies on several parameters including water solubility, drug permeability across biological membrane, dissolution rate, pre-systemic metabolism [4].

It is a factor that the poor water solubility and dissolution profile of drugs in GI fluid often causes the poor bioavailability. The oral bioavailability of drugs may be improved by increasing the aqueous solubility and dissolution profile of the drug substance in the GI fluids. As far as considering the BCS Class II drugs, the rate-limiting step is the drug release from the formulation in GI fluid and not the absorption from biological membrane; therefore, increase in the solubility may increase the bioavailability of BCS Class II drugs [5–8].

Only 1% of medication compounds entered the market in the pharmaceutical sector, and this is always due to inadequate biopharmaceutical qualities rather than toxicity or a lack of therapeutic efficacy [9–12]. Solubility is one of these biopharmaceutical qualities that is a big problem, because of their weak solubility, medications are always useless during production that can be sold. Increasing the solubility of medication ingredients is currently one of the pharmaceutical company's biggest concerns. Particle size reduction is one of the techniques that have been utilized to increase the water solubility of pharmaceuticals [5, 6]. Creating salt [7], emulsification [8, 9], co-solvent solubilizations [10], and employing polymers to transport medications that are not highly water soluble [11] are some examples. Even though it has been demonstrated that these techniques increase oral bioavailability, their effectiveness depends on the particular physicochemical characteristics of the medications under investigation [13, 14]. Pharmaceutical co-crystal formulation has been increasing interest over the past few years as a potential means of enhancing the bioavailability of medications with poor water solubility. Co-crystal and pharmaceutical co-crystal are two terms that must first be understood. There are several ways to define co-crystals [15]. Co-crystals are defined as structurally homogeneous/heterogeneous crystalline solids that include drug and coformer in specific stoichiometric proportions. The discrete neutral molecular reactants that make up co-crystals are solids at room temperature. According to this definition of co-crystals, a pharmaceutical co-crystal is a mixture in which one of the co-crystals' elements serves as an active medicinal ingredient and the other elements serve as coformers. An active drug hydrate is not a co-crystal, as is evident from the statement, but a solid-state drug hydrate is co-crystalline with a coformer to produce a co-crystal. [16]. The pharmaceutical sector currently places a lot of attention on co-crystal methods. Pharmaceutical co-crystals can successfully enhance the drug substance's solubility, dissolving profile, bioavailability and physical stability, in addition to other crucial features such as flowability, chemical stability, compressibility and hygroscopicity [17].

Because of the ability to tailor the physicochemical properties of the solid while preserving the chemical integrity of the medicine, co-crystals have sparked a great deal of interest in pharmaceutical research and development. Co-crystals are a subset of a larger category of multicomponent crystals, which are made up of two or more molecules that form a uniform crystalline lattice in a stoichiometric ratio that is clearly specified (often referred to as the drug and coformer). The drug and coformer are solid at higher temperatures than other types of multicomponent crystals like salt and solvates, and the intermolecular relationships in co-crystals are non-ionic in nature. Through co-crystallization, the variety of solid forms that can be produced from a medicine significantly expands; the physicochemical properties of co-crystals

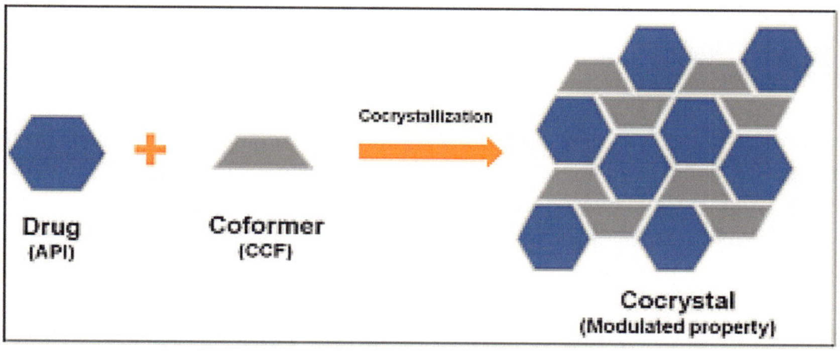

Figure 1.
Formations of co-crystals [18].

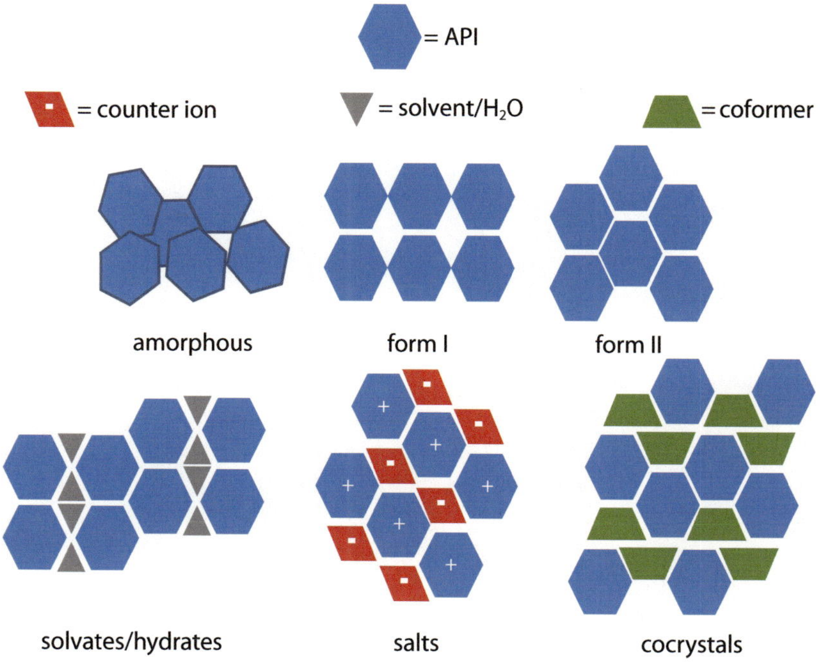

Figure 2.
Crystalline forms exist in different forms: Amorphous form, polymorph of pure API, solvates/hydrate forms, salt form and pharmaceutical co-crystals [19].

can change based on the properties of constituent molecules. Solubility, dissolution, moisture uptake, chemical stability, mechanical characteristics, and bioavailability are just a few of the pharmaceutically significant features that can change by co-crystallization. The most frequently praised property in literature is solubility [18]. The solubility restrictions of poorly soluble medicinal chemicals may be overcome through co-crystals (**Figures 1** and 2).

1.1 Crystal engineering and supramolecular chemistry in co-crystals formation

Crystal engineering can be used to create pharmaceutical co-crystals with the goal of enhancing an API's solid-state characteristics without changing its fundamental structure. A model for the quick development of medicinal co-crystals was created through crystal engineering. It can be described as an application of supramolecular chemistry concepts to solid states, with a focus on the notion that crystalline solids are real-world examples of self-assembly [20, 21] Co-crystals are created through intermolecular interactions such as hydrogen bonds, stacking interactions, and van der Waals contact forces. By changing the intermolecular interactions that regulate the breaking and formation of non-covalent bonds, such as hydrogen bonding, van der Waals force, stacking, electrostatic interactions, and halogen bonding, crystal engineering involves changing the crystal packing of a solid material [22, 23]. In the study of co-crystals, the term supramolecular synthon is widely employed. It is referred to as structural units inside supramolecular that can be created by known hypothetical synthetic procedures involving intermolecular interactions. This guarantees generality, which subsequently results in the predictability of one-, two- and three-dimensional patterns produced by intermolecular interactions. Supramolecular chemistry is nothing more than non-covalent molecular bonding that is recognized as a lock and key principle in biological processes through the concept of complementarity and selectivity. Carboxylic acids,

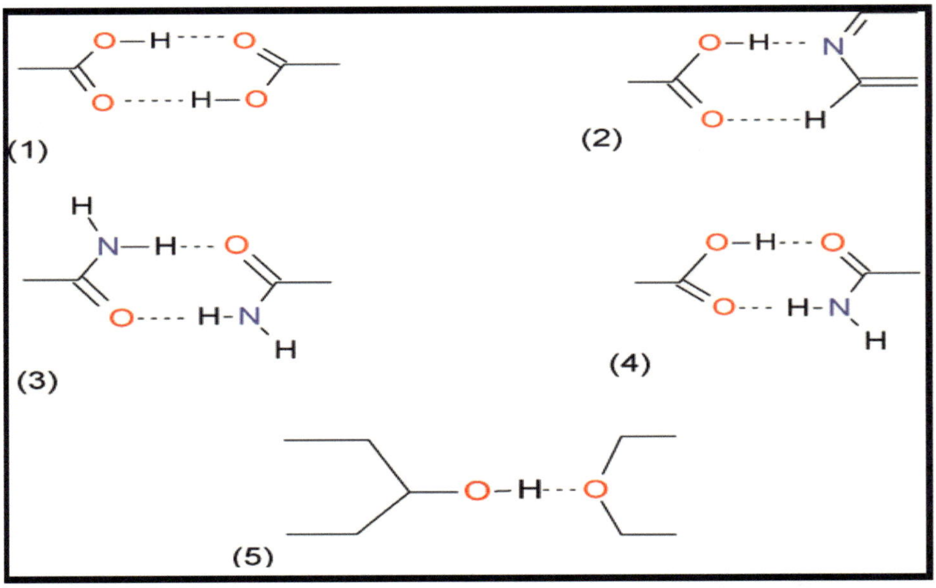

Figure 3.
Typical hydrogen bond utilized in crystal engineering [24].

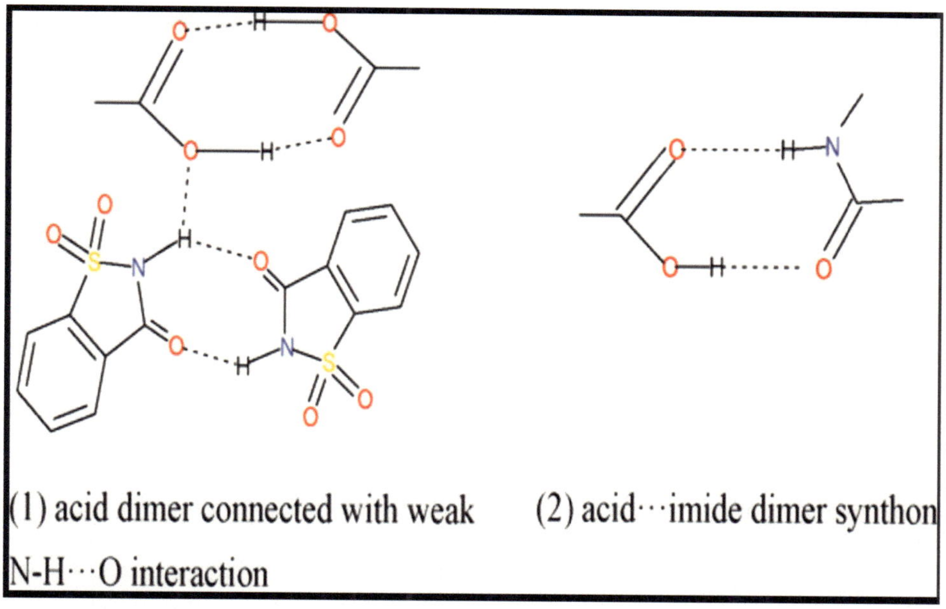

Figure 4.
Indomethacin: Saccharine co-crystal structure [33].

amides, carbohydrates, alcohols and amino acids are good examples of pharmaceutically approved crystallizers that can be combined with APIs. **Figure 3** depicts the most prevalent supramolecular synthon used in pharmaceutical co-crystals.

The carboxylic acid functional group, which is present in many medications, has been extensively researched in the field of pharmaceutical co-crystals. The synthesis of carboxylic acid homosynthon through the C=O···H−O hydrogen bond is highly frequent when the hydrogen bond donor and acceptor are self-complementary [25]. A second popularly researched homosynthon is the amide homodimer, which forms co-crystals *via* the CO···H−N hydrogen bond.

A part from homosynthons, some favourable heterosynthons are carboxylic acid-pyridine, carboxylic-amide and alcohol-ether. Recently, studies of hydrogen bonds competition have attracted increasing interest from a number of researchers [26, 27]. Heterosynthons are stronger than homosynthons; for example, the acid-amide heterosynthons favoured over both carboxylic acid and amide homodimer [28]. Through analysis of the Cambridge Structural Database (CSD) [29], it is discovered that the competitive hydroxyl-hydroxyl homosynthon is substantially favoured over the hydroxyl-pyridine and hydroxyl-cyano heterosynthons. One of the most popular heterosynthons, carboxylic acid-pyridine heterosynthons, contains an O−H···N hydrogen bond, which is generated when the carboxylic acid reacts with a suitable N-containing heterocycle [30, 31]. In contrast to carboxylic acid homodimer, carboxylic acid-pyridine heterosynthons were preferred, according to the CSD study [32]. These empirical findings about the hierarchy of supramolecular synthons are very helpful for designing co-crystals. Reality, however, does not always support this. The structure of the indomethacin and saccharin (IND-SAC) co-crystals revealed that, contrary to the more advantageous indomethacin carboxylic acid saccharin imide heterosynthons predicted by empirical rules, the indomethacin carboxylic acid dimer interacts with the saccharin imide dimer synthon through a weak N−H···O bond in **Figure 4** [33].

1.2 Physicochemical properties of co-crystals

For the creation of APIs, co-crystals' physicochemical characteristics are crucial. Adjusting the physicochemical parameters of pharmaceutical co-crystals during drug development improves the stability and efficacy of the dosage form [34]. Numerous studies have been conducted on physicochemical characteristics such as solubility, dissolution, crystallinity, melting point, bioavailability, and stability. The following list summarizes some important physicochemical characteristics of pharmaceutical co-crystals [35].

1.2.1 Melting point

The temperature at which the solid and liquid phases are in balance determines the melting point, which is a fundamental physical characteristic. The value is calculated using the ratio of the change in fusion enthalpy over the change in fusion entropy because melting point is a thermodynamic process where the free energy of transition is equal to zero [35]. Over a conventional melting point apparatus or the Kofler method, DSC is the preferred approach for getting precise melting point data because it allows for the determination of additional thermal data, such as the enthalpy of fusion [35]. It is a common practice to determine a compound's melting point in order to characterize or identify its purity. However, in the field of pharmaceutical sciences, the melting point also has significant value because of its relationships with water solubility and vapour pressure [21]. Although it was necessary to make assumptions about the entropy of fusion, the melting point has actually been directly connected to the log of solubility [36]. In order to tune an API's aqueous solubility towards a specific purpose, it would be highly helpful to know the melting point of that API before it was synthesized.

1.2.2 Stability

Stability has the great importance during the development of new chemical entity. For the evaluation parameters of pharmaceutical co-crystals, stability also plays an important role. A newly produced co-stability crystal is often tested under four conditions: relative humidity (RH) stress, temperature stress, chemical stability and solution stability. Because the amount of water in the co-crystals might cause quality degradation, the relative humidity stress is used to determine the ideal storage conditions for the product. During investigations involving the sorption and desorption of water, it was discovered that co-crystals performed better [37]. Thermal stress and chemical stability are relatively less studied areas about co-crystals properties. Very few reports were discovered, and the few research conducted demonstrated that thermal stress investigations can be a useful tool for learning more about physicochemical stability [38]. When creating these materials, it is critical to evaluate the co-crystals' chemical stability. According to Schultheiss and Newman, solubility stability is the capacity of the co-crystals' constituents to remain in solution and not rapidly crystallize. Solution stability is a crucial factor in the creation of new drugs. To understand how co-crystals behave in release media, stability tests are conducted in addition to solubility or dissolution experiments [39].

1.2.3 Solubility

An important factor in determining pharmaceutical qualities of co-crystal is its solubility. Salt generation, solid dispersion and particle size reduction are a few traditional techniques for improving weakly aqueous medication solubility [40]. With these strategies, there are limitations in practice. Using pharmaceutical co-crystals is a novel way to alter the physicochemical characteristics of medicinal molecules, such as their solubility and dissolution. Researcher interest in solubility is high [40].

1.2.4 Intrinsic dissolution

It assesses the intrinsic qualities of the drug as a function of the dissolution medium, such as pH, ionic strength, and counter ions, and is independent of formulation effects [40]. Intrinsic dissolution measures the rate of dissolution of a pure pharmacological component from a constant surface area. When the sample is squeezed into a disc or pellet for the intrinsic dissolution test, there should not be any shape changes and the disc needs to stay intact throughout the experiment. The majority of the APIs investigated for co-crystallization are categorized as class II pharmaceuticals under the Biopharmaceutics Classification System (BCS), which have high permeability and low solubility. Therefore, intrinsic dissolution rate is a reliable predictor of API *in vivo* performance. Even if the intrinsic dissolution rate is a crucial factor to research, it can get trickier with co-crystals. In order to collect and correctly interpret intrinsic dissolution data on co-crystals, a number of aspects must be taken into account, and additional experiments may be required [41].

1.2.5 Bioavailability

Bioavailability is a determination of rate and extent of drugs that reaches to the systemic circulation [42] . The bioavailability of newly formed moiety is determined with the help of animal experimentation. The ultimate goal for co-crystal investigation is to improve bioavailability of an APIs. Animal bioavailability is important for a newly prepared compound. The limited numbers of animal bioavailability studies are available on co-crystals [43].

1.3 Pharmaceutical co-crystal design strategies

A pharmaceutical co-crystals have rapidly emerged as a new class of Active Pharmaceutical Ingedients. In order to get co-crystals first step is to study the structure of target drug and find out the functional group present in drug molecule, which can interact between molecules when a suitable coformer is present. The next step is to pick a coformer. The primary requirement for a coformer is that it must be suitable and acceptable for use in pharmaceutical products, such as pharmaceutical excipients and substances that have been designated as generally recognized as safe (GRAS) for use as food additives. Co-crystal design must start with the choice of coformer. There is a wealth of useful empirical and theoretical guidance available during the synthesis of co-crystals, including the Cambridge Structural Database, hydrogen bonds and intermolecular interactions. A useful tool for examining intermolecular interactions in crystals is the Cambridge Structural Database. By referring to the structural property relationships present in classes of recognized crystal structures found in the Cambridge Structural Database, it can be used to study the outline of stable hydrogen bonds. Based on data from Cambridge Structural Database, a supramolecular library of coformers has been created [44, 45].

When determining the intermolecular interactions between an API and a coformer molecule in the majority of pharmaceutical co-crystal structures, hydrogen bonds are a key factor [42]. To facilitate the design of hydrogen bonded solids, the following

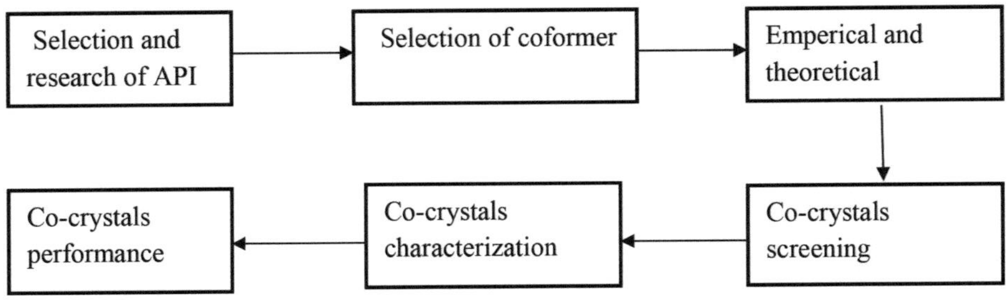

Figure 5.
Steps for co-crystal design and screening [49].

guidelines were put forth [46]. (1) All good proton donors and acceptors are used in hydrogen bonding; (2) if six-membered rings can form intermolecular hydrogen bonds, they will frequently do so with a preference for doing so; and (3) the best proton donors and acceptor are left over after intermolecular hydrogen bonds have formed, from intermolecular hydrogen bonds to one another. The next step is screening of co-crystals, which is an experimental process to determine if the selected coformer candidate is able to crystallize with targeted API molecule. Various screening methods of co-crystals are solution method [47], hot stage thermal microscopy [48] and computed crystal energy landscape method [48]. The aim of co-crystals characterization includes the chemical structural confirmation and crystallographic analysis of newly formed supramolecular synthon, its thermal features, solubility and stability. The final step is performance of newly formed co-crystals that include both *In vivo* and *In vitro* tests. *In vitro* test comprises the dissolution and intrinsic dissolution rate and *in vivo* test refers to animal oral bioavailability measurements, the measurement of rate and extent of drug that reaches to the systemic circulation [49] (**Figure 5**).

1.3.1 Selection of coformer

Pharmaceutical co-crystals are formed by incorporating a certain stoichiometric ratio of given API with pharmaceutically acceptable coformer molecule in the crystal lattice. Greater diversity is possible with co-crystal solid forms because of numerous choices of pharmaceutically acceptable coformers, including pharmaceutical excipients, food additives as well as other generally regarded as safe (GRAS) APIs. Since different physicochemical natures of coformers result in different physicochemical properties and *in vivo* behaviours of the produced co-crystal coformer selection become a crucial step for pharmaceutical co-crystal design, an ineffective and time-consuming initial method for choosing a coformer involved trying to co-crystallize a specific API with different pharmaceutically acceptable ingredients. Later, after the Cambridge Structure Database (CSD) was built, the "supramolecular synthon approach" was used to successfully screen coformer for the development of co-crystals [50].

There were two types of supramolecular synthons, including homosynthon and heterosynthon. In general, supramolecular heterosynthon represented more robust hydrogen bond than homosynthon and was the most reliable and rational channel to form co-crystals. Although the "supramolecular synthon approach" with computer assistance significantly accelerated the design of co-crystals, the physicochemical characteristics and *in vivo* behaviours of the resulting co-crystals could still not be predicted from chosen coformers because the main objective of such an approach was to determine whether hydrogen bonds could exist between APIs and coformers.

When selecting coformers for pharmaceutical co-crystal design, little attention is currently paid to the physicochemical (i.e. stability and its degradation pathway) and biopharmaceutical (i.e. intestinal absorption mechanism and metabolic pathway) properties of coformers and APIs. However, some coformers, particularly GRAS APIs, may accelerate drug degradation and may also inhibit efflux/influx transporters and metabolic enzymes involved in drug absorption and metabolism. Aspirin, for instance, was regarded as a GRAS API and used as a coformer in pharmaceutical co-crystals.

1.4 Co-crystal formation methods

Till date a number of techniques are used for the formulation of co-crystals. The most general method is based on solution method and grinding method [51]. The solution method is of great significance for synthesis of co-crystals, which qualify for single X-ray diffraction testing can only be prepared through this method. Solution methods include evaporation of heterometric solution method, reaction crystallization method and cooling crystallization. Grinding method comprises solvent drop grinding and neat grinding. Apart from these methods, there are also lots of recently promising techniques, such as hot stage microscopy, ultrasound-assisted co-crystallization and co-crystallization using supercritical fluid [52].

1.4.1 Solution methods

Based on these two approaches, solution crystallization can occur [52]. In order to reach the crystal stability region in solvents that are not congruently saturated, either (1) use solvents or solvent mixtures where the co-crystals are congruently saturated and the components have similar solubilities, or (2) use non-equivalent reactant concentrations. When the two co-crystal components are equally soluble in solvent and solution, strategy one is used. The 1:1 co-crystals will form through co-crystallization with equimolar components using the solvent evaporation method. When the components of co-crystals have non-equivalent solubility, strategy two is used. A single-component crystal or a combination of individual component and co-crystals may form during co-crystallization as a result of the evaporation of an equimolar solution. For this circumstance, the reaction co-crystallization approach has been used. In RC experiments, the more soluble reactant is dissolved in a saturated or nearly saturated solution of the less soluble reactant, which causes the solution to supersaturate in terms of co-crystals. Another solution method called cooling crystallization is varying the temperature of the crystallization system, which has great potential for large scale of production of co-crystals. In a reactor, particularly a jacketed vessel, substantial amounts of solvent and reactants are first combined. The system is then heated to a higher temperature to ensure that all solutes are completely dissolved in the solvent and is then cooled. When the solution becomes supersaturated with respect to co-crystals as the temperature decreases, co-crystals will form [53].

1.4.2 Grinding methods

There are two distinct methods for producing co-crystals through grinding [51, 54, 55]. The first technique, known as neat grinding or dry grinding, entails mixing the drug and coformer components together and then physically pounding them into powder using a mortar and pestle, a ball mill or a vibratory mill (mechanically). The second method for creating co-crystals through grinding involves adding small amounts of a suitable solvent. This method is known as liquid-assisted grinding, also known as solvent drop, or wet co-grinding. By adding small amounts of a suitable solvent, the kinetics of co-crystal formation by grinding can be significantly increased [56].

1.4.3 Hot melt extrusion

Extrusion is a helpful technique for producing co-crystals because it involves improved surface contacts and highly effective mixing without the need for solvent. The compound's thermodynamic stability is the main factor that determines whether this method should be used. Four co-crystal formation models were used to study this method. Utilizing the solvent drop extrusion technique, the process was optimized and made more adaptable. The benefit of using the solvent drop extrusion technique is the ability to run the process at a lower temperature. The synthesis of carbamazepine-nicotinamide co-crystals with polymer as former was done using the hot melt extrusion method. Co-former, API and continuous co-crystallization were poured into the twin extruder. The temperature of the barrel also rises as a result of the mixture being added continuously [57].

1.4.4 Sonocrystallization method

Organic co-crystals of finite size have been prepared using a sonochemical technique that has been developed. The creation of nanocrystals was the primary motivation behind this technique. The preparation of caffeine-maleic acid co-crystals began with the application of the ultrasound technique. The comparison of the sonochemical method and the solvent drop grinding method for producing caffeine, theophylline, and L-tartaric acid as API and co-formers has begun. The methods produced consistent results, demonstrating the importance of the sonocrystallization method [58].

1.4.5 Supercritical fluid atomization technique

In the supercritical atomization process, CO2, a highly pressurized supercritical fluid, is used to combine the drug and coformers. By atomizing this solution with an atomizer, co-crystals are created. Co-crystals are prepared from solution using the supercritical antisolvent (SAS) method, which utilizes the antisolvent effect of supercritical fluid [59].

1.4.6 Spray drying technique

Co-crystals are made by spray drying, which involves evaporating the solvent from a solution or suspension of the drug and the coformer. This technology is the most popular because it uses a quick, continuous, and one-step process. As a result, the spray drying process will present a distinctive setting for the creation and expansion of co-crystals [60, 61].

1.5 Characterization and evaluation of co-crystals

Co-crystal characterization is an important constituent part within co-crystal research. The basic physicochemical properties of co-crystals can usually be characterized using scanning electron microscopy, Fourier transform infrared spectroscopy, differential scanning calorimetry, powder X-ray diffraction, Raman spectroscopy, solid-state nuclear magnetic resonance spectroscopy and terahertz spectroscopy.

1.5.1 Scanning calorimetry (DSC)

In this characterization method, two specimens—one serving as a sample and the other as a reference—are each subjected to the same temperature as well as a controlled-rate environment of heating or cooling. Plotting the amount of energy required to achieve a temperature difference between the two specimens that is zero leads to illuminating conclusions. Two different types of DSC are employed frequently. First up is the power compensation DSC, which keeps the two samples in various identical furnaces. By adjusting the power input, the temperature of both is brought to the same level. As a result, the energy is translated into enthalpy or heat capacity. Another type of DSC involves keeping both sample holders in the same furnace and connecting them *via* a low-resistance heat flow path. The remainder of the interpretation is unchanged. The most widely used technique for the thermal analysis of co-crystals is differential scanning calorimetry. Differential scanning calorimetry is an ideal technique for obtaining complete melting point data and additional thermal records, such as enthalpy of melting, can also be concurrently obtained. Addition to the characterization technique, DSC has presently been used as a selection tool for rapid co-crystal screening [62, 63].

1.5.2 XRD

Phase identification is used in this analytical technique to provide information on unit cell dimension. The crystalline sample and monochromatic X-ray are constructively diffracted to produce this. The cathode ray tube used to create the monochromatic ray filters and collimates the radiation to create monochromatic radiation, which is then directed at the sample. In the sample preparation scenario, the sample is finely ground to create a homogeneous sample and to analyse the average bulk composition. D-spacing analysis is performed on the sample. A set of d-spacing is produced as the sample is positioned in a random orientation. The sample is therefore examined because each mineral has a unique set of d-spacing. The sample must adhere to Bragg's law, which links the electromagnetic radiation's wavelength to the diffraction angle 2 ($n\lambda = 2d \sin \theta$), in order for any of this to occur. Co-crystals' solid-state structure can be determined at the atomic level using a characterization method called XRD. The issue is that it is not always possible to produce a single pharmaceutical co-crystal that is suitable for SXRD testing. PXRD is therefore used more often to confirm the formation of co-crystals [64].

1.5.3 Vibrational spectroscopy (IR and Raman)

For determining organic structure, electromagnetic radiation with frequencies between 4000 and 400 cm^{-1} has been one of the most powerful tools. This electromagnetic radiation is known as infrared (IR) radiation and IR spectroscopy for its use in organic chemistry. The interatomic bonds absorb the bombarded radiation. A particular chemical bond will therefore absorb various radiations at various frequencies in various environments. Thus, inferring some conclusions about the structure from their absorption data, which is provided as a spectrum, is helpful [64].

1.5.4 Scanning electron microscopy (SEM)

SEM is a kind of electron microscope that uses a raster scan model to scan an object with a high-energy electron beam to image it. The sample's surface morphology can be learned from the signals produced by the interaction of the electrons with the atoms that make up the sample. Finding the co-crystals photomicrograph and particle size is helpful [65].

1.5.5 Saturation solubility study

In accordance with the procedure described by Higuchi and Connors, saturation solubility studies were carried out in triplicate in distilled water. To reach equilibrium, excess co-crystals were added to distilled water in a screw cap tube and shaken for 24 hours at room temperature in a rotary flask shaker. An appropriate aliquot was taken out, filtered through filter paper and then analysed with a spectrophotometer. Statistics were used to validate the data from saturation solubility studies [66, 67].

1.5.6 Micromeritic properties

1.5.6.1 Bulk density (D_b)

It is the proportion of the powder's total mass to its bulk volume. The weight of the powder was measured by pouring it into a measuring cylinder, and the volume was recorded. It is calculated using a formula and expressed in gm/ml.

$$D_b = M / V_0. \qquad (1)$$

where M is the mass of powder, and V_0 is the Bulk volume of the powder.

1.5.6.2 Tapped density (D_t)

It is the proportion of the powder's total mass to its tapped volume. By tapping the powder to a fixed volume, the tapped volume was calculated. It is calculated using a formula and expressed in gm/ml,

$$D_b = M / V_t. \qquad (2)$$

1.5.6.3 Angle of repose

The angle of repose depicts a solid's ability to flow. It is a quality that has to do with how difficult it is for particles to move around one another. The surface of the powder or granule pile can only be angled away from the horizontal plane at this maximum angle.

$$\tan\theta = h / r. \qquad (3)$$

$$\theta = \tan^{-1} h / r. \qquad (4)$$

where θ = angle of repose, h = height of heap, r = radius of base of heap circle.

Method: The fix funnel method was used to calculate the angle of repose. A funnel was positioned 2–4 cm above the platform. The sample powder was gradually pushed through the funnel until the tip of the cone of sample powder that was created barely touched the stem. The height of the sample powder cone and the radius of the powder heap's circular base were then measured in order to estimate the angle of repose.

1.5.6.4 Compressibility index and Hausner's ratio

Compressibility index and the closely related Hausner's ratio have recently emerged as the most straightforward, quick and well-liked techniques for forecasting powder flow characteristics. Because all of these factors can affect the compressibility value, the compressibility index has been projected as an indirect evaluation of size and shape, surface area, bulk density, moisture content and cohesiveness of materials. By measuring the bulk density and the tapped density of crystals, the compressibility index and Hausner's ratio are estimated [68].

$$\text{Compressibility Index} = \text{Tapped density} - \text{Bulk density} / \text{Tapped density} \times 100. \text{Hausner's ratio} = \text{Tapped density} / \text{Bulk density}.$$

1.5.7 Tabletability

The crystal packing, tabletability and compaction, which are crucial factors during preformulation research, can be impacted by the co-crystallization of the drug and coformer. Co-crystals of paracetamol with trimethylglycine and oxalic acid were found to have better compaction behaviour than pure drug [38]. The formation of co-crystals with 4-aminobenzamide and isoniazid improved resveratrol's tabletability. Comparing co-crystals to conformers or pure drugs, tabletability of co-crystals was higher [24]. Co-crystallization allowed for the modification of the mechanical properties of APIs, and it demonstrated higher tabletability for vanillin isomer co-crystals than for isomers and conformer [29].

1.5.8 Dissolution studies

The dissolution study is a crucial tool for figuring out the drug's bioavailability. The dissolution test is used to determine whether an API is soluble. Dissolution studies are used to calculate the rate of drug release over time in the dissolution medium and forecast how well the formulation will work *in vivo*. The dissolution apparatus can be used to conduct dissolution studies for co-crystals. The appropriate dissolution medium is described in the drug protocol of the referred pharmacopoeia, and it can be used to conduct the dissolution studies for the co-crystals. The drug samples can be gathered in the right amount at the right time and can be examined using the right tools, like HPLC or UV [69, 70].

1.5.9 Stability

Stability study is extremely important during the development of new dosage formulation. During the development of pharmaceutical co-crystals, several stability studies should be performed such as relative humidity stress, chemical stability, thermal stability, solution stability and photostability study. In relative humidity stress, automated water sorption/desorption studies are performed to determine the effect of water on the formulation. Several researchers studied the behaviour of co-crystals under relative humidity stress conditions [71–73].

1.6 Case study of multicomponent co-crystals and drug-drug co-crystals

Fael H et al. have prepared co-crystal of norfloxacin-based solvent-mediated transformation experiment in toluene, using resorcinol as a coformer. Norfloxacin has a solubility of 0.32 ± 0.02 mg/mL, whereas the co-crystal has a solubility of 2.64 ± 0.39 mg/mL, approximately 10-fold higher [74]. Machado Cruz et al. develop a new co-crystal of the poorly water-soluble antifungal agent itraconazole. The co-crystal is stable in aqueous solution, and comparison with previously described itraconazole co-crystals revealed a relationship between the coformer's solubility and the intrinsic and powder dissolution rates. Analyses of the physical co-crystal and common excipient mixtures' dissolution behaviour were also conducted [75].

Nugrahani et al. prepared the mono- and tetrahydrate of the salt co-crystal diclofenac sodium-l-proline. Single-crystal X-ray analysis was used to characterize the hydrates, which were found to have higher solubilities and dissolution rates than the sodium salt of diclofenac acid and the anhydrous diclofenac acid-l-proline co-crystal. The salt co-crystal dissociated into a physical mixture of diclofenac acid and L-proline as a result of the release of water during drying. It is interesting that this process can be reversed. Diclofenac sodium-L-proline tetrahydrate was restored when the dried sample was maintained at 72% relative humidity and 25°C [76].

Kale et al. studied co-crystallization on the tabletability of rivaroxaban and found an improved tabletability for rivaroxaban-malonic acid. The crystal packing, specifically the presence or absence of slip planes, slip plan topology, the degree of intermolecular interactions and d-spacing, could be used to explain the tabletability of alonic acid and rivaroxaban combined with malonic acid. Slip planes with zigzag and flat-layered topologies are both present in rivaroxaban. This study's findings on the relationships between crystal structure and mechanical properties shed light on the deformation of crystals with multiple slip-plane systems [77].

Jiaxin PI et al. prepared baicalein (BE) is one of the main active flavonoids representing the variety of pharmacological effects including anticancer, anti-inflammatory and cardiovascular protective activities, but it is very low solubility, dissolution rate and poor oral absorption limit the therapeutic applications. In this study, a nano-co-crystal approach was successfully used to increase the bioavailability and dissolution rate of BE. High-pressure homogenization was used to create baicalein-nicotinamide (BE-NCT) nano-co-crystals, which were then tested both *in vitro* and *in vivo*. BE-NCT has formed the new solid phase as co-crystals, as shown by physical characterization results from scanning electron microscopy, dynamic light scattering, powder X-ray diffraction and differential scanning calorimetry [78]. Latif et al. synthesized paracetamol co-crystals to improve compaction or tabletability of paracetamol. The author created a co-crystal of paracetamol using caffeine as a conformer using techniques such as dry grinding, liquid-assisted grinding, solvent evaporation and anti-solvent addition. He then observed that the paracetamol's mechanical properties and compaction power have increased [79]. Iyan et al. developed simvastatin-nicotinamide co-crystals by solvent evaporation to improve the solubility of simvastatin by co-crystallization using nicotinamide as co-crystal agent or co-former and evaluated for solubility. When compared to raw simvastatin, saturated solubility of the co-crystal increased threefold, according to the observation [80]. Shubhangi et al. synthesized co-crystals of poorly water-soluble drug darunavir. It is a BCS Class II medication with a poor solubility. Succinic acid was used as a conformer during the cooling crystallization process that produced co crystals. By dissolving an excess amount of co-crystals in water for 24 hours on a rotary shaker and measuring the saturation solubility with a spectrophotometer, the author was able to determine the aqueous solubility of darunavir. This technique resulted in 1.92-fold increases in saturation solubility [81]. Prabhakar et al. also prepared co-crystal of piroxicam and studied for solubility. Author used various conformers such as adipic acid, benzoic acid, cinnamic acid, citric acid, glutaric acid, phydroxybenzoic acid, hippuric acid, malonic acid, resorcinol, 6 saccharine sodium, 1-hydroxy-2-napthoic acid, sodium acetate, urea, catechol, ferulic acid, aerosil-200, nicotinamide, para amino benzoic acid, anthranilic acid and succinic acid for synthesis of co-crystals and performed saturated aqueous solubility of co-crystal and found significant increase in solubility of drug after formulating as co-crystals [82]. Zheng et al. synthesized co-crystals of resveratrol with conformers 4 aminobenzamide and isoniazid and studied its enhanced solubility and tabletability. Author observed that tabletability of RES is poor and because of this even at high pressure that is 0.6 MPa and lamination of tablets, while tablets are prepared with co-crystals of resveratrol-4-aminobenzamide, and tensile strength more than 3 MPa is attained at 250 MPa compaction pressure. Author concluded that co-crystal formation improved tabletability of drug. Co-crystals of paracetamol with trimethylglycine and oxalic acid were found to have better compaction behaviour than the drug alone. The formation of co-crystals with 4-aminobenzamide and isoniazid improved resveratrol's tabletability. The tabletability of co-crystals was higher than that of coformers or pure drugs. Co-crystallization allowed for the alteration of the mechanical properties of APIs, and co-crystals of the vanillin isomers with the same coformer demonstrated greater tabletability than the isomers and conformer [65]. Muddukrishna et al. studied synthesis of paclitaxel and naringen co-crystal to improve solubility by solvent-assisted grinding method. The drug paclitaxel (PTX), which belongs to class IV, has a low solubility in water. Shake flask method was used to study the solubility of paclitaxel and naringen co-crystal for 72 hours at room temperature. HPLC analysis of the samples revealed 2.4-fold increases in the saturation solubility [83]. Pinky et al. formulated co-crystal tablet dosage form of clarithromycin to enhance the bioavailability. As clarithromycin is BCS Class II drug author prepared co-crystals by using urea as conformer by solvent evaporation method, and developed tablet formulation and evaluated for solubility, dissolution and bioavailability studies. Author concluded that the formulated tablets of clarithromycin co-crystals showed improved solubility and *in vitro* drug release profile as compared to Marketed Tablet, and thereby increase oral bioavailability and therapeutic effect [84]. Mounika et al. prepared co-crystals of fexofenadine. According to the BCS classification, fexofenadine belongs to the class II of drugs because of its high permeability and low solubility, which acts as rate-limiting factors in achieving the desired bioavailability. Therefore, by evaporating solvent, the author created co-crystals of fexofenadine using tartaric acid as a co-former, and they found that 7 of them had a higher drug release than the formulation [85]. Carmen Almansa et al. identified co-crystal of tramadol hydrochloride-celecoxib, a brand-new active pharmaceutical ingredient (API)-API co-crystal with favourable physicochemical and dissolution properties that result from the intrinsic 1:1 molecular ratio of rac-tramadol HCl and celecoxib. A medical need that is frequently met by combination therapy is the adequate treatment of pain. In comparison with individual APIs or their combination, API-API co-crystals represent a new strategy that has the potential to enhance physicochemical properties, bioavailability, stability or formulation capacity. This could result in improved pharmacokinetic profiles and clinical benefits. The single-crystal X-ray diffraction structure of ctc revealed a supramolecular 3D network in which the two active enantiomers of tramadol and celecoxib are connected by hydrogen bonds and chloride ions. Ctc also displayed a clearly defined differential scanning calorimetry profile. The saturation effect for highly insoluble celecoxib occurred at a higher concentration in ctc than in celecoxib alone, according to oversaturation studies. Celecoxib and tramadol were released from ctc more quickly and more slowly than they were from the individual APIs, respectively, according to comparative intrinsic dissolution rate studies, which suggested that ctc would have better pharmacokinetic behaviour. These data support the clinical development of ctc for the treatment of pain along with those from preclinical studies [86]. Shivarani Eesam et al. prepared drug-drug co-crystal of carvedilol with hydrochlorothiazide: A significant challenge in the discovery and development of new drugs is increasing the hydrophilicity of poorly water-soluble drugs. One method for improving the hydrophilicity of such drugs is co-crystallization. Carvedilol (CAR), a non-selective beta/alpha1 blocker with poor aqueous solubility and high permeability, is categorized as BCS class II and is used to treat mild-to-moderate congestive heart failure and hypertension. The goal of this work is to increase the solubility of CAR by creating co-crystals using the diuretic hydrochlorothiazide (HCT) as a coformer. Slurry conversion was used to create CAR-HCT (2: 0.5) co-crystals, which were then analysed using DSC, PXRD, FTIR Raman and SEM. The co-crystals were the subject of solubility, stability and dissolution (*in vitro*) studies [87]. Kang Zheng et al. presented study reports on the MNZ-PYR co-crystal, a new co-crystal of the antimicrobial drug metronidazole (MNZ) that uses pyrogallol (PYR) as a co-crystal former. Utilizing single-crystal X-ray diffraction, infrared spectroscopy, thermal analysis and density functional theory calculations, the crystal structure of the MNZ-PYR co-crystal is investigated. Due to the high-energy conformer of PYR in the co-crystal's crystal lattice, the MNZ-PYR co-crystal exhibits a higher dissolution rate than MNZ. The colour of the MNZ-PYR co-crystal changes from white (raw MNZ and PYR) to yellow as it forms, and this theoretical interpretation is based on calculations using time-dependent density functional theory. UV-vis spectroscopy is used to characterize this colour change. The findings point to the potential use of the co-crystal strategy for API colour tuning, providing opportunities for formulation development [88]. Braham Dutt et al. create aspirin (AN) and benzoic acid (BZ) co-crystal by using the solvent evaporation technique. CSD (Cambridge Structure Database) software and ΔpKa value method were used for the choice of the drug and coformer and for prediction of CC formation. Differential scanning calorimetry, Fourier transformation infrared spectroscopy and X-ray diffraction methods were used for the analysis of CCs. A total of 24 Wistar rats divided into four groups participated in *in vivo* anti-inflammatory studies [89]. Bwalya A. Witika et al. prepared co-crystal of zidovudine (AZT) and lamivudine (3TC) that are antiviral agents used orally to manage HIV/AIDS infection. The development and production of 3TC and AZT nanocrystals were carried out using a pseudo one-solvent bottom-up methodology. Rapid injections of AZT in methanol and 3TC in de-ionized water were combined with sonication at 4°C in a vessel that had been pre-cooled. A Zetasizer was used to characterize the resulting suspensions. The Zeta potential, polydispersity index and particle size were clarified. Powder X-ray diffraction, Raman spectroscopy, Fourier transform infrared spectroscopy, differential scanning calorimetry and scanning electron microscopy were all used for further characterization. The stability of the nano co-crystals and the production of nano co-crystals with particular and desirable critical quality attributes (CQA), such as particle size (PS) < 1000 nm, polydispersity index (PDI) < 0.500 and Zeta potential (ZP) < -30 mV, were evaluated for various surfactants. In the nanometer range, co-crystals were produced by all surfactants. When sodium dodecyl sulphate was used in the process, only ZP was within specification, whereas the PDI and PS are concentration-dependent for all nano co-crystals produced [90]. Dnyaneshwar P. Kale et al. presented purpose of this work is to comprehend the crystallographic underpinnings of the mechanical behaviour of rivaroxaban-malonic acid co-crystal (RIV-MAL Co) in comparison with its parent constituents, rivaroxaban (RIV) and malonic acid (MAL). By performing "out of die" bulk compaction and nanoindentation, the mechanical behaviour was assessed at both the bulk and particle levels. MAL < RIV < RIV-MAL Co was the order of tabletability for the three solids. Despite having a reasonably strong bonding strength, MAL demonstrated "lower" tabletability due to its lower plasticity (BS). This behaviour was influenced by the absence of a slip plane and "intermediate" BS. The different surface topologies of the slip planes were primarily blamed for RIV's "intermediate" tabletability. While the corrugated topology of secondary slip planes (1, 0, 2) may adversely affect the plasticity, the presence of a primary slip plane (0, 1, 1) with flat-layered topology may favour the plastic deformation of RIV. Additionally, RIV crystal's tabletability was aided by its higher elastic recovery. RIV-MAL Co's significantly "higher" tabletability compared to the other two molecular solids was caused by its greater plasticity and BS. The higher degree of intermolecular interactions, the larger separation between adjacent crystallographic layers and flat-layered topology slip across the (0, 0, 1) plane all helped RIV-MAL Co. exhibit better mechanical behaviour. It is interesting to note that the relationship between a particle level deformation parameter and a bulk-level deformation parameter, H/E (i.e. the ratio of mechanical hardness H to elastic modulus E), was found to be inverse (i.e. tensile strength at zero porosity). The co-crystal crystallographic properties of materials were highlighted in this study as having a positive impact on tabletability [91]. Ilma Nugrahani et al. prepared zwitterionic co-crystal of L-proline and diclofenac acid. This multicomponent crystal's solubility, though, was still inferior to that of diclofenac sodium salt. In order to determine whether a multicomponent crystal of diclofenac sodium hydrate could be produced using the same coformer, L-proline, which was anticipated to enhance the pharmaceutics performance, screening, solid phase characterization, structure elucidation, stability and *in vitro* pharmaceutical performance tests were among the methods used. In order to determine the molar ratio of the multicomponent crystal formation, a phase diagram screen was first performed. The single crystals were then created by slowly evaporating the material under two different conditions, yielding two different forms: one was shaped like a rod, and the other was like a flat square. The formation of the new phases was confirmed by the characterization using infrared spectroscopy, thermal analysis and diffractometry. The new salt co-crystals were finally solved structurally as stable diclofenac-sodium-proline-water (1:1:1:4) and unstable diclofenac-sodium-proline-water (1:1:1:1), known as NDPT (natrium diclofenac proline tetrahydrate) and NDPM, respectively (natrium, diclofenac, proline monohydrate). These multicomponent crystals had better solubility and dissolution rates than diclofenac sodium by itself. According to the experimental findings, this salt co-crystal can be developed further [92]. Xavier Bull et al. identified and prepared 13 co-crystals of nefiracetam, a poor water-soluble nootropic compound. The co-crystallization agents citric acid, oxalic acid and zinc chloride were used to produce three of them. The stability, solubility and rate of dissolution of the latter have all undergone thorough structural and physical characterization, and they have been compared to the original Active Pharmaceutical Ingredient (API) [93]. Prafulla P. Apshingekar et al. prepared co-crystal by ultrasound, which is known to affect crystallization; consequently, using a slurry co-crystallization method, the impact of high-power ultrasound on the ternary phase diagram has been thoroughly investigated. To comprehend how the accelerated circumstances during ultrasound-assisted co-crystallization will impact various areas of the ternary phase diagram, a thorough investigation was conducted. The ternary phase diagram was significantly affected by the use of ultrasound, especially in the regions where the co-crystals of caffeine and maleic acid were 2:1 and 1:1 (which narrowed). Additionally, the solution region was expanded in the presence of ultrasound, while the stability regions for pure caffeine and maleic acid in water were contracted. Maleic acid and caffeine solubility as well as the stability of co-crystal forms in water were found to be related to the observed effect of ultrasound on the phase diagram [94]. Dwi Setyawan et al. analysed the physicochemical characteristics and *in vitro* dissolution profile of co-crystals of quercetin and malonic acid made by solvent-drop grinding. Using the solvent-drop grinding method and 20% (w/v) ethanol addition, quercetin (Q) and malonic acid (MA) were co-crystallized in the molar ratios of 1:1 (CC1) and 1:2 (CC2) in a shaker mill that was run for 30 minutes. Differential scanning calorimetry (DSC), powder X-ray diffractometry (PXRD), scanning electron microscopy (SEM) and Fourier transform infrared (FT-IR) spectroscopy were used to identify the co-crystal phase. The paddle method was used to perform *in vitro* dissolution at 100 revolutions per minute in a medium of citrate buffer (pH 5.0 ± 0.05) containing 2.0% (w/v) sodium lauryl sulphate at 37 ± 0.5°C [95]. Agnes Nuniek Winantari et al. prepare and characterize co-crystals of acyclovir through co-crystallization of acyclovir-succinic acid (AS) for the purpose of enhancing the drug's physical properties. Using the solvent evaporation method, AS co-crystals were created. By using the polarization microscope, scanning electron microscopy (SEM), differential scanning calorimetry, powder X-ray diffraction (PXRD) and Fourier transform infrared spectroscopy, the co-crystals were characterized [96]. Jose Lopez-Cedrun et al. prepared co-crystal of tramadol–celecoxib (CTC), containing equimolar quantities of the active pharmaceutical ingredients (APIs) tramadol and celecoxib (100 mg CTC = 44 mg *rac*–tramadol hydrochloride and 56 mg celecoxib), which is a novel API-API co-crystal for the treatment of pain. In order to effectively treat acute pain following oral surgery, we sought to determine the CTC dosage. Nine Spanish hospitals participated in a phase II dose-finding, double-blind, randomized, placebo- and active-controlled study (EudraCT number: 2011-002778-21) on male and female patients under the age of ≥18 who were experiencing moderate-to-severe pain after having two or more impacted third molars that required bone removal extracted. A computer-generated list was used to randomly assign eligible patients to receive one of six single-dose treatments (CTC 50, 100, 150, 200 mg; tramadol 100 mg; and placebo). The sum of pain intensity difference (SPID) over 8 hours as measured in the per-protocol population was the main efficacy endpoint [97]. Muhammad Inam et al. designed two new co-crystals, nicotinamide and ticagrelor, have been prepared with improved solubility. An innovative co-crystallization technique has been developed to increase ticagrelor's solubility because it has a low solubility and a high rate of dissolution. This technique uses a structurally homogenous crystalline material, an active pharmaceutical ingredient (API) and co-former indefinite stoichiometric amount. A 1:1 co-crystal of ticagrelor (TICA) and nicotinamide (NCA) was created and characterized using FTIR, DSC and XRD. TICA-NCA hydrate's single-crystal structure was also examined. When compared to the solubility of a free drug, the solubility of co-crystals was investigated in pH 2 acidic medium, which was a significant improvement. Co-crystal had a higher *in vitro* dissolution rate than the commercial product [98]. Heinrich Buschmann et al. invented co-crystals of duloxetine and co-crystal formers selected from active agents preferably with analgesic activity, processes for preparation of the same and their uses as medicaments or in pharmaceutical formulations, more particularly for the treatment of pain [99]. Carlos Ramon Plata Salaman et al. invented a co-crystal of celecoxib and venlafaxine, methods for making it and its use as medications or in pharmaceutical formulations, more particularly for the treatment of pain, including chronic pain, or of depression in patients who suffer from chronic pain and/or chronic inflammation, or in patients with a chronic musculoskeletal inflammatory illness, with the inflammatory illness preferably being chosen from osteoarthritis or rheumatoid arthritis [100]. Prabhakar Panzade et al. prepared, formulated and evaluated the co-crystal of piroxicam by testing various coformers. Piroxicam co-crystals were created using the dry grinding method. The crystalline phase's melting point and solubility were established. DSC, IR and XRPD were used to characterize the potential co-crystal. Evaluations were also conducted on solubility and dissolution rate, two additional pharmaceutical properties. Piroxicam co-crystal orodispersible tablets were created, improved upon and tested using a 3^2 factorial design [101]. Mirela Nicolo et al. prepared co-crystal of betulinic acid and ascorbic acid. It has been shown that betulinic acid (BA) is a very effective anticancer agent against a variety of tumour cell lines, including those from the breast, colon, lung and brain. Betulinic acid has a strong cytotoxic effect but has a low water solubility, which is reflected in its low bioavailability. Co-crystallization emerged as a promising strategy among the many tactics used to enhance its physicochemical and pharmacokinetic profile in order to address these drawbacks. Thus, the goal of our research was to create BA and ascorbic acid co-crystals (BA+VitC) in isopropyl alcohol using a hydrothermal process. SEM, DSC, XRPD and FT-IR spectroscopy were used to characterize the newly formed co-crystals, showing that BA+VitC co-crystals were formed, and their antioxidant activity showed an additive antioxidant effect. BA+VitC co-crystals were tested on a variety of cell lines, including HeLa (cervical cancer), MCF7 and MDA-MB-231 (human breast cancer), B164A5 and B16F0 (murine melanoma), and immortalized human keratinocytes (HaCat). Results of BA on the examined tumour cell lines after co-crystallization with vitamin C showed a superior cytotoxic effect while maintaining a good selectivity index, most likely as a result of an improved BA water solubility and consequently an optimized bioavailability [102]. Abdolati Ali Mohamed Alwati et al. developed a new method for co-crystal preparation, which adhered to green chemistry principles, and provided advantages over conventional methods. It was decided that the best technology to achieve these goals was a brand-new, solvent-free, high-power ultrasound (US) technique for creating co-crystals from binary systems. Ibuprofen nicotinamide (IBU-NIC), carbamazepine-nicotinamide (CBZNIC) and carbamazepine-saccharin (CBZ-SAC) co-crystals were investigated for the use of this technology for solid-state co-crystal preparation [103].

1.7 Applications of co-crystals

1.7.1 Permeability enhancement

Drug absorption and distribution of drugs mainly depend upon the permeability of drugs across the biological membrane. The permeability of the drug is generally expected to depend upon hydrophobic interactions on the crystal surface that may interact with nonpolar cell membranes during diffusion, hydrophobic ($\pi \cdots \pi / H \cdots \pi$) and hydrophilic ($N/O \cdots H$) interactions may play an improving role in the permeability. Co-crystals improve the penetration of drugs inside the biological membrane by changing their crystalline structure [104]. Hydrochlorothiazide is a diuretic and BCS class IV drug with low solubility and low permeability, exhibiting poor oral absorption solubility and permeability [68].

Another example, 5-fluorouracil (5FU) a BCS class III drug with good solubility and poor permeability was subjected to co-crystallization with the use of coformers such as 3-hydroxybenzoic acid, 4-aminobenzoic acid and cinnamic acid. 5FU has dense packing in the crystal lattice, which may cause its poor permeability. The 5FU have disrupted and loose molecular packing during the co-crystallization process. When 5FU is co-crystallized with carboxylic acid, the hydrogen bonding sites of two components would adjust to achieve a balance, whereas new drug-coformer hetero-synthons and packing generated. This modification may change 5FU's activity and subsequently improve its permeability when across a membrane [105].

1.7.2 Stability enhancement

Stability study is very important in case of development of new dosage formulation. Stability studies of pharmaceutical co-crystals have several studies such as relative humidity stress, chemical stability, thermal stability, solution stability and photostability study. Lithium drugs have a narrow therapeutic window and are hygroscopic. Lithium co-crystals exhibit modulated pharmacokinetics compared to lithium. The co-crystals of lithium chloride (LIC) and glucose (GLU) were prepared by slow evaporation method and the physical stability of LIC-GLU was compared to lithium chloride at 50% RH and 25°C and through dynamic vapour sorption analysis. LIC-GLU co-crystals improve the physical stability of the solid form of a drug substance with respect to humidity without impacting its pharmacokinetic performance [106]. In adefovir dipivoxil-saccharin co-crystals showed thermodynamic stability at temperatures 40°C and 60°C. The change in the appearance of the samples was also visually examined. The adefovir dipivoxil started to clump together and form a cake-like structure at the first sampling time point at 60°C, whereas adefovir dipivoxil-saccharin co-crystals remained in a powder state [106]. The theophylline-oxalic acid and theophylline-caffeine co-crystals were subjected to relative humidity to check their stability in relation to crystalline theophylline anhydrate. None of the co-crystals in this study converted into a hydrated co-crystal upon storage at high relative humidity (up to 98%). Co-crystals avoid hydrate formation and improvement in the physical stability of the product [107]. Polymorphic changes can also be prevented by using the co-crystallization technique. Lowering the crystal lattice energy and increasing solvation are two mechanisms that increase the solubility of the API in a co-crystal. API solubility can be increased using either technique to varying degrees. Co-crystal solubility in non-polar solvents can be improved through a number of mechanisms, one of which is lowering the crystal lattice energy. Hydrogen bonding, van der Waals forces and electrostatic forces all affect the crystal lattice energy [108].

1.7.3 Solubility

Lowering the crystal lattice energy and increasing solvation are two mechanisms that increase the solubility of the API in a co-crystal. API solubility can be increased using either technique to varying degrees. Co-crystal solubility in non-polar solvents can be improved through a number of mechanisms, one of which is lowering the crystal lattice energy. Hydrogen bonding, van der Waals forces and electrostatic forces all affect the crystal lattice energy [109]. The solvation of the API in the co-crystal structure is the second way for enhancing solubility in co-crystals. Because hydrophobic BCS Class II drugs are frequently solubility-limited by reduced solvent-solute interactions, this is the primary method of increasing solubility in water. The incorporation of a polar, water-soluble molecule into the crystal structure can help to solvate the hydrophobic API more easily. Coformer solubility is related to co-crystal solubility. This is due to improved solvation with a conformer with a higher solubility [110]. For example, the drug-drug co-crystal of carvedilol-hydrochlorothiazide was prepared by solvent evaporation method and their solubility was significantly improved 7.3 times in 0.1 N HCl than the pure carvedilol and *in vitro* dissolution rate of co-crystals was enhanced by 2.7 times than pure carvedilol, which may lead to enhanced bioavailability [29].

1.7.4 Bioavailability

The bioavailability of an API is the fraction of the dose that reaches the system circulation in its unchanged form, as well as the rate at which the API enters the systemic circulation. The low oral bioavailability of APIs is a major challenge in the development of new formulations. The pharmaceutical co-crystal approach enhanced the aqueous solubility and oral bioavailability of the product [111]. Meloxicam-aspirin co-crystals showed better oral bioavailability as compared to pure drug and showed 12 times faster onset of action than a pure drug in rats [112]. Co-crystals of aceclofenac-nicotinamide and aceclofenac-gallic acid prepared with solvent evaporation method both co-crystals exhibited excellent dissolution rate and bioavailability increased with 1.77 and 1.37 time as compared to the pure drug [113, 114].

1.7.5 Controlled release

Co-crystallization is used to modify the product's physicochemical properties, such as solubility and dissolution rate. The dissolution rate of the API in water or a buffer solution can be increased or decreased over time, depending on the coformer that co-crystallized with the API [115]. Zonisamide-caffeine co-crystals were prepared by solvent evaporation method. It was found that the co-crystals showed lower solubility and dissolution rates and offer potential benefits in the development of sustained release of drug for the treatment of obesity [116]. Co-crystals also bear the potential to reduce the dissolution rate of the original APIs. Chen et al. used the co-crystallization approach to sustain the dissolution behaviour of ribavirin, a water-soluble antiviral drug. The most useful hydrogen bonding group of ribavirin is the amide functionality, which is known to form robust hydrogen bonding interactions with carboxylic acids and amide compounds. The ribavirin-gallic acid forms co-crystals with reduced release rate [117].

1.7.6 Multidrug co-crystals

Combining multiple active pharmaceutical ingredients (APIs) into one unit dose is a new approach for patient compliance. It becomes a popular trend in drug formulation industries, the need to target multiple receptors for the effective treatment of complex disorders such as HIV/AIDS, cancer, and diabetes. Multiple APIs have been combined in a single delivery system using salts, mesoporous complexes, co-amorphous systems and co-crystals [113]. Multidrug co-crystals (MDCs) have an advantage over co-amorphous systems in terms of enhanced stability and reduced payload compared to mesoporous and cyclodextrin complexes [118]. As dissociable solid crystalline supramolecular complexes, multidrug co-crystals contain two or more therapeutically beneficial components in a stoichiometric ratio within the same crystal lattice, where the components may predominantly interact *via* non-ionic interactions and rarely *via* hybrid interactions (a combination of ionic and non-ionic interactions involving partial proton transfer and hydrogen bonding) with or without the presence of solvate molecules. MDC has potential advantages over pure drug components such as increased solubility, dissolution, bioavailability, improved stability of unstable APIs *via* intermolecular interactions, increased mechanical strength and flowability [118–122]. Techniques generally used for formulation multidrug co-crystals are solvent evaporation, neat and liquid-assisted grinding, slurry reaction, melting and cooling crystallization. MDC formulations are evolving day by day exploring different combinations of APIs. But still more efforts are required for medically relevant APIs, which could be beneficial to the patients and pharmaceutical industry. Much more steps in terms of MDCs still have to be taken for improved and evolved formulation [123].

1.7.7 Mechanical properties enhancement (Tablatability)

Because of its numerous technical and economic advantages, tablets are the most commonly used pharmaceutical dosage form. Among these advantages are low manufacturing costs, high production throughput, ease of consumption, storage and handling. Several deficiencies caused by poor flowability and mechanical properties, on the other hand, have always been a challenge in the path to successful tablet production [124]. Some of these techniques include adding silicon dioxide to improve tablet mechanical strength and magnesium stearate to improve flowability. Co-crystallization has also been studied as a technique for improving the chemical and physical properties of powders, such as mechanical strength and flow properties [125]. Co-crystallization with theophylline, oxalic acid, naphthalene and phenazine conformers, for example, improved the compression properties of paracetamol form I [126].

1.7.8 Taste masking

Oral disintegrating tablets require fast disintegrating tablets with rapid dissolution. This strategy allows the use of tablets without the need for chewing or water intake, broadening the range of drug users to include geriatric, paediatric and travelling patients who do not have access to water. To improve the patient experience, readily disintegrating tablets require the use of taste masking agents. So far, the main approach has been to use sugar excipients. Co-crystallization could be a good strategy to improve dissolution rate using sugar-based coformers such as sucralose as coformer for preparing co-crystals with hydrochlorothiazide. The formed co-crystals provide the benefits of increased dissolution rate and taste masking of the product [127]. Another example, theophylline with the bitter taste was masked by formulating co-crystals with artificial sweeteners such as sodium glutamate, sodium saccharin and d-sorbitol. In 1:1 stoichiometric ratio *via* liquid-assisted grinding, the prepared co-crystal showed enhanced dissolution and sweet taste, which was detected by automated sweetness tasting machine [128].

1.7.9 Generation/extension of intellectual property

Intellectual property (IP) is vital for pharmaceutical companies. The intellectual property (IP) protection of new ideas, inventions, processes or products grants exclusivity over the manufacturing process and products. Patents, copyright and trademarks, for example, are legal mechanisms that allow individuals or organizations/ companies to gain recognition or financial benefit from their work or investment in a creation. A total of 138 patents are granted to recognize an invention that meets the criteria of global novelty, non-obviousness and industrial application. Pharmaceutical companies must deal with drug or drug product patent life cycle management to keep their pharmaceuticals on the market for as long as possible. Screening of novel solid dosage forms of marketed drugs, such as polymorphs, salts and co-crystals, provides the opportunity to grant new IP and extend the patent life cycle of those drugs. Pharmaceutical co-crystals have regulatory and intellectual property advantages that provide them with unique possibilities, benefits and challenges. From a regulatory standpoint, drugs containing a novel co-crystal are considered similar to a new polymorph of the API. This guidance takes novel co-crystals to be considered as a new drug substance, which promotes their independent patentability as novel solid forms [129].

1.7.10 Melting point

Melting point is the physical property of solids, which is used to determine the purity of the product [130]. The high melting point of the new materials demonstrates their thermodynamical stability; that is, the thermal stability of an API can be increased by selecting a coformer with a higher melting point. When working with thermolabile drugs, co-crystals with low melting points can also be useful. The melting point of pharmaceutical co-crystals can be managed by judicious selection of the coformers. Melting point contributes to a major consideration during the formulation of co-crystals. Co-crystals with high melting points are usually needed but they have poor aqueous solubility, whereas low melting point co-crystals have problems with processing, drying and stability, so further study within this area is required [130].

1.7.11 pH-independent solubility

In pharmaceutical co-crystal design and screening in most cases the API is uncharged. There are very few reports on the co-crystallization of charged APIs. Co-crystals constitute an important class of pharmaceutical solids for their ability to modulate solubility and pH dependence of water-insoluble drugs [131]. Co-crystals with acidic coformers, indomethacin–saccharin (IND – SAC) carbamazepine–saccharin (CBZ – SAC), not only enhance aqueous solubility but also impart a pH sensitivity than the drugs. IND – SAC exhibited solubilities 13 to 65 times higher than IND at pH values of 1 to 3, whereas CBZ – SAC exhibited a 2 to 10 times higher solubility than CBZ dihydrate in acidic pH values of 1 to 3 [132]. Gabapentin is shown to form co-crystal with 3-hydroxy benzoic acid and salts with salicylic acid, 1-hydroxy-2-napthoic acid and RS-mandelic acid. There is partial proton transfer from 4-hydroxy benzoic acid to gabapentin. Multicomponent crystals gabapentin-3-hydroxybenzoic acid (1:1), gabapentin-4-hydroxybenzoic acid (1:1), gabapentin-salicylic acid (1:1), gabapentin-1-hydroxy-2-napthoic acid (1:1) and gabapentin-RS-mandelic acid (1:1) are thermodynamically more stable and equal or less soluble than gabapentin hydrate and carboxylic acid coformers in pure water. Gabapentin-3-hydroxy benzoic acid co-crystal is stable at pH 4.0 and 5.7. This indicates that gabapentin3HBA co-crystal is less soluble at pH 4.0 and 5.7, while co-crystal is more soluble at pH 2.6 [133].

1.7.12 Hygroscopicity reduction

The ability of a solid substance that absorbs moisture from its surroundings is known as hygroscopic material. Hygroscopicity is a term that refers to materials that easily absorb water in a non-structured way. Thus, the adsorbed water is reversible and not structured inside a crystal lattice. The categorization of hygroscopic and non-hygroscopic materials in pharmaceuticals are regarded as hygroscopic if they absorb more than 5% of their mass in RH between 40 and 90% at 25°C. Non-hygroscopic materials are those that absorb less than 1% moisture under the same conditions. If the critical RH of a hygroscopic material is lower than that of the surrounding atmosphere, it may deliquesce (where adsorbed water starts to solvate molecules of the solid) [134]. Co-crystals of levofloxacin (LVFX) and N-acetyl-meta-aminophenol (AMAP) using a grinding and heating approach crystallized from a eutectic melting of the 2 drugs after water desorption from an LVFX hydrate. Levofloxacin monohydrate contains one ½ H2O, while co-crystal formation coformer metacetamol contains OH group at meta position, which binds with LVFX through hydrogen bonds leaving no binding site for H2O to make compound hygroscopic. This co-crystal exhibited dramatic improvements in physicochemical properties of LVFX, including hygroscopicity, physical stability and photostability, while retaining its good dissolution characteristics and chemical stability under various temperature and humidity conditions [133]. Co-crystal of metoclopramide HCl (MCPHCl), with oxalic acid (OXA), is acting as the coformer. The crystal structure of metoclopramide HCl-oxalic acid (MCPHCl–OXA) co-crystal was determined by single-crystal X-ray crystallography. The salt co-crystal has higher stability than its parent drug against high humidity and dissociation in an aqueous environment. These properties are attributed to the utilization of all hydrogen bond donors and acceptors of MCP, suggesting the OXA acts as a substitute for a water molecule in the structure, which makes it less hygroscopic. In addition, the salt co-crystal is promising for extended-release drug formulation by exhibiting a lower dissolution rate compared to the parent drug. These findings demonstrate the utility of salt [134]. The amide groups of individual nicotinamide molecules are all involved in intermolecular hydrogen bonding in co-crystals of ibuprofen-nicotinamide and flurbiprofen-nicotinamide, leaving the pyridine nitrogen free to interact with the environmental water vapour molecules, contributing to its hygroscopic nature. However, in co-crystal form with IBU or FLU, all of nicotinamide's pyridine nitrogen forms hydrogen bonds with the profens' carboxylic hydrogens and is thus unavailable for bonding with water, resulting in a decrease in moisture sorption at relatively low RHs [135–140].

2. Conclusion

Co-crystals enable a wide range of APIs to be used in pharmaceutical therapy. Some of the most appealing properties of co-crystallized APIs are increased solubility and chemical and physical stability. Because of their patentability, they are also appealing from an economic and legal standpoint. Several difficulties arise when attempting to create co-crystals. The prediction of the crystal structure of larger molecules is time consuming and difficult. The predicted structure will not always match the experimental result. Even though methods such as liquid-assisted grinding are very efficient in the lab, they are economically unfavourable in large-scale synthesis. Overall, because of improved drug delivery performance, stability and an important intellectual property status, co-crystals are expected to play an important role in future drug development.

Author details

Raju Thenge[1*], Vaibhav Adhao[1], Gautam Mehetre[1], Nishant Chopade[1], Pavan Chinchole[1], Ritesh Popat[1], Rahul Darakhe[1], Prashant Deshmukh[1], Nikesh Tekade[2], Bhaskar Mohite[3], Nandu Kayande[4], Nilesh Mahajan[5] and Rakesh Patel[6]

1 Dr. Rajendra Gode College of Pharmacy, Malkapur, Maharashtra, India

2 SGSPS Institute of Pharmacy, Akola, Maharashtra, India

3 Anuradha College of Pharmacy, Chikhali, Maharashtra, India

4 Thakur Shivkumar College of Pharmacy, Burhanpur, MP, India

5 Dadasaheb Balpande College of Pharmacy, Nagpur, Maharashtra, India

6 Dr. A.P.J. Abdul Kalam University, Indore, MP, India

*Address all correspondence to: rajuthenge11@gmail.com

References

[1] Mohd Y, Mohd A, Kumar A, Aggrawal A. Biopharmaceutical classification system: An account. International Journal of Pharmaceutical Tech Research. 2010;**2**(3):1681-1690

[2] Reddy BB, Karunakar S. Biopharmaceutics classification system: A regulatory approach. Dissolution Technology. 2011;**5**(5):31-37

[3] Chowdary KPR, Kumar P. Recent research on formulation development of BCS class II drugs: A review. International Research Journal of Pharmacy and Applied Sciences. 2013;**3**(1):173-181

[4] Wagh MP, Patel JS. Biopharmaceutical classification system: Scientific basis for biowaiver extensions. International Journal of Pharmaceutics. 2010;**2**(1):12-19

[5] Amidon GL, Lennernaes H, Shah VP, Crison JR. A theoretical basis for a biopharmaceutic drug classification: The correlation of in vitro drug product dissolution and in vivo bioavailability. Pharmaceutical Research. 1995;**12**:413-420

[6] Katariya MK, Bhandari A. Biopharmaceutics drug deposition classification syatem: An extension of biopharmaceutics classification system. International Research Journal of Pharmacy. 2012;**3**(3):5-10

[7] Aakeroy CB, Forbes S, Desper J. Using co-crystals to systematically modulate aqueous solubility and melting behavior of an anticancer drug. Journal of the American Chemical Society. 2009;**131**:17048-17049

[8] Washington DC, Iii P, Elie WW, Matzger SC. Polymorphism in carbamazepine Co-crystals. Crystal Growth & Design. 2008;**8**:14-16

[9] Ramanathan T. Mass Spectrometry in Drug Metabolism and Pharmacokinetics. Hoboken, NJ: John Wiley & Sons, Inc; 2009. pp. 1-4

[10] Blagdan N, Matas D, Gavan M, York P. Crystal engineering of active pharmaceutical ingredients to improve solubility and dissolution rates. Advanced Drug Delivery Reviews. 2007;**59**:617-630

[11] Cho E, Cho W, Cha KH, Park J. Enhanced dissolution of megestrol acetate microcrystals prepared by Antisolvent precipitation process using hydrophilic additives. International Journal of Pharmaceutics. 2010;**396**:91-98

[12] Umeda Y, Fukami T, Furuishi T, Suzuki T, Tanjoh K, Tomono K. Characterization of multicomponent crystal formed between indomethacin and lidocaine. Drug Delivery and Industrial Pharmacy. 2009;**35**:843-851

[13] Rasenack N, Hartenhauer H, Muller BW. Microcrystals for dissolution rate enhancement of poorly water-soluble drugs. International Journal of Pharmaceutics. 2003;**254**:137-145

[14] Hong JY, Kim JK, Song YK, Park JS, Kim CK. A new self-emulsifying formulation of itraconazole with improved dissolution and oral absorption. Journal of Controlled Release. 2006;**110**:332-338

[15] Amin K, Dannenfelser RM, Zielinski J, Wang B. Lyophilization of polyethylene glycol mixtures. Journal of Pharmaceutical Sciences. 2004;**93**:2244-2249

[16] Torchilin V. Micellarnano carriers: Pharmaceutical perspectives. Pharmacy Research. 2007;**24**:1-16

[17] Yue X, Qiao Y, Qiao N, Guo S, Xing J. Amphiphilic methoxy poly (ethylene glycol)-b-poly (−caprolactone)-b-poly (2-dimethylaminoethyl methacrylate) cationic copolymer nanoparticles as a vector for gene and drug delivery. Biomacromolecules. 2010;**11**:2306-2312

[18] Huang LF, Tong WQ. Impact of solid state properties on developability assessment of drug candidates. Advanced Drug Delivery Reviews. 2004;**56**:321-334

[19] Schultheiss N, Newman A. Pharmaceutical Co-crystals and their physicochemical properties. Crystal Growth & Design. 2009;**9**:2950-2967

[20] Shan N, Zaworotko MJ. The role of Co-crystals in pharmaceutical science. Drug Discovery Today. 2008;**13**:440-446

[21] Vishweshwar P, McMahon JA, Bis JA, Zaworotko MJ. Pharmaceutical Co-crystals. Journal of Pharmaceutical Sciences. 2006;**95**:499-516

[22] Yadav AV, Shete AS, Dabke AP, Kulkarni PV, Sakhare SS. Co-crystals: A novel approach to modify physicochemical properties of active ingredients. Indian Journal of Pharmaceutical Sciences. 2009;**71**:359-370

[23] Mirza S, Miroshnyk I, Heinamaki J, Yliruusi J. Co-crystals: An emerging approach for enhancing properties of pharmaceutical solids. Dosis. 2008;**24**:90-96

[24] Basavoju S, Bostrom D, Velaga S. Indomethacin–saccharin co-crystals: Design, synthesis and preliminary pharmaceutical characterization. Pharmaceutical Research. 2008;**25**:530-541

[25] Khan M, Enkelmann V, Brunklaus G. Crystal engineering of pharmaceutical Co-crystals: Application of methyl paraben as molecular hook. Journal of the American Chemical Society. 2010;**132**:5254-5263

[26] Bis JA, Vishweshwar P, Weyna D, Zaworotko MJ. Hierarchy of supramolecular synthons: Persistent hydroxyl pyridine hydrogen bonds in Co-crystals that contain a cyano acceptor. Molecular Pharmaceutics. 2007;**4**:401-416

[27] He GW, Jacob C, Guo LF, Chow PS, Tan RBH. Screening for Cocrystallization tendency: The role of intermolecular interactions. Journal of Physical Chemistry. 2008;**112**:9890-9895

[28] Weyna DR, Shattock T, Vishweshwar P, Zaworotko MJ. Synthesisand structural characterization of Co-crystals and pharmaceutical Co-crystals: Mechanochemistry vs. slow evaporation from solution. Crystal Growth & Design. 2009;**9**:1106-1123

[29] Trask AV, Motherwell WDS, Jones W. Physical stability enhancement of theophylline via Cocrystallization. International Journal of Pharmaceutics. 2006;**320**:114-123

[30] Oswald IDH, Allan DR, McGregor PA, Motherwell DWS, Parsons S, Pulham CR. The formation of paracetamol (acetaminophen) adducts with hydrogen-bond acceptors. Acta Crystallography Section. 2002;**58**:1057-1066

[31] Miroshnyk I, Mirza S, Sandler N. Pharmaceutical Co-crystals-an opportunity for drug product enhancement. Expert Opinion on Drug Delivery. 2009;**6**:333-341

[32] Walsh RDB, Bradner MW. Crystal engineering of the composition of

pharmaceutical phases. Chemical Communications. 2003;**68**:186-187

[33] Cincic D, Friscic T, Jones W. Iso-structural materials achieved by using structurally equivalent donors and acceptors in halogen-bonded Co-crystals. Chemical European Journal. 2008;**14**:747-753

[34] Horst JH, Deij MA, Cains PW. Discovering new Co-crystals. Crystal Growth & Design. 2009;**9**:1531-1537

[35] Padrela L, Rodrigues MA, Velaga SP, Fernandes AC. Screening for pharmaceutical Co-crystals using the supercritical fluid enhanced atomization process. Journal of Supercritical Fluids. 2010;**53**:156-164

[36] Aakeroy CB, Salmon DJ. Building co-crystals with molecular sense and supramolecular sensibility. Crystal Eng Communication. 2005;7:439-448

[37] Almarsson O, Zaworotko MJ. Crystal engineering of the composition of pharmaceutical phases. Do pharmaceutical Co-crystals represent a new path to improved medicines? Chemical Communications. 2004;**17**:1889-1896

[38] McNamara DP, Childs SL, Giordano J, Iarriccio A, Cassidy J. Use of a glutaric acid Co-crystals to improve oral bioavailability of a low solubility API. Pharmaceutical Research. 2006;**23**:1888-1897

[39] Ning Q, Mingzhong L, Angela D, Gary T. Pharmaceutical Co-crystals: An overview. International Journal of Pharmaceutics. 2011;**419**:1-11

[40] Dhumal RS. Ultrasound assisted engineering of lactose. Crystals. Pharmaceutical Research. 2008;**25**(12):2835-2844

[41] Bermejo M, Gonzalez-Alvarez I. How and where are drugs absorbed? In: Gad SC, editor. Preclinical Development Handbook: ADME and Biopharmaceutical Properties. Hoboken: John Wiley & Sons, Inc; 2007. pp. 249-280

[42] Shiraki K, Takata N, Takano R, Hayashi Y, Terada K. Dissolution improvement and the mechanism of the improvement from Cocrystallization of poorly water-soluble compounds. Pharmaceutical Research. 2008;**25**:2581-2592

[43] Desiraju GR. Supramolecular synthons in crystal engineering-a new organic synthesis. Chemical International Edition. England. 1995;**34**:2311-2327

[44] Remenar RF, Morissette SL, Peterson ML, Moulton B, MacPhee JM. Crystal engineering of novel Co-crystals of a triazole drug with 1, 4-dicarboxylic acids. Journal of the American Chemical Society. 2003;**125**:8456-8457

[45] Mohammad MA, Alhalaweh A, Velaga SP. Hansen solubility parameter as a tool to predict Co-crystals formation. International Journal of Pharmaceutics. 2011;**40**:63-71

[46] Shargel L, Yu AB. Applied Biopharmaceutics & Pharmacokinetics. 4th ed. New York: McGraw-Hill; 1999. p. 289

[47] Gao Y, Gao J, Liu Z, Kan H, Zu H, Sun W. Coformer selection based on degredation pathway of drugs: A case study of adefovirdipivoxil-saccharin and adefovirdipivoxil-nicotanamide Co-crystals. Indian Journal of Pharmaceutical Sciences. 2012;**438**:327-335

[48] Dale SH, Elsegood MRJ, Hemmings M, Wilkinson AL. The

Cocrystallization of pyridine with benzene polycarboxylic acids: The interplay of strong and weak hydrogen bonding motifs. Crystal Engineering Communication. 2004;**6**:207-214

[49] Variankaval N, Wenslow R, Murry J, Hartman R, Helmy R. Preparation and solid-state characterization of nonstoichiometric Co-crystals of a phosphodiesterase-IV inhibitor and l-tartaric acid. Crystal Growth & Design. 2006;**6**:690-700

[50] Zhang GZ. Efficient co-crystal screening using solution-mediated phase transformation. Journal of Pharmaceutical Sciences. 2007;**96**(5):990-995

[51] Alhalaweh A, Velaga P. Formation of Co-crystals from stoichiometric solutions of incongruently saturating systems by spray drying. Crystal Growth & Design. 2010;**10**(8):3302-3305

[52] Braga D, Grepioni F. Reactions between or within molecular crystals. Chemical International. Edition. 2004;**43**(31):4002-4011

[53] Mohammed M, Joshu SB, Snowden MJ, Dennis D. A review of hot-melt extrusion. Process Technology to Pharmaceutical Products, International Journal Pharmaceutics. 2008;**28**:1-9

[54] Chaudhari PD, Uttekar PS. Melt sonocrystalllization: A novel particle engineering technique for solubility enhancement. International Journal of PharmTech. Research. 2009;**1**(1):111-120

[55] Yadav S, Gupta PC, Sharma N, J, Kumar J. Co-crystals: An alternative approach to modify physicochemical properties of drugs. International Journal of Pharmaceutics. 2015;**5**(2):427-436

[56] Grossjohann C, Serrano DR, Paluch KJ. Polymorphism in sulfadimidine/4-aminosalicylic acid Co-crystals: Solid-state characterization and physicochemical properties. Journal of Pharmaceutical Sciences. 2015;**104**:1385-1398

[57] Lin HL, Hsu PC, Lin SY. Theophylline-citric acid Co-crystals easily induced by DSC-FTIR microspectroscopy or different storage conditions. Asian Journal of Pharmaceutical Sciences. 2013;**8**:19-27

[58] Tauk TK, Lin SY, Lin HL, Y. T. Huang YT. Simultaneous DSC-FTIR microspectroscopy used to screen and detect the Co-crystals formation in real time. Bioorganic Medical and Chemical Letter. 2011;**21**:3148-3151

[59] Lu E, Rodriguez-Hornedo N. A rapid thermal method for Co-crystals screening. Crystal Engineering Communication. 2008;**10**:665-668

[60] Yamashita H, Hirakura Y, Yuda M, Terada K. Coformer screening using thermal analysis based on binary phase diagram. Pharmaceutical Research. 2014;**31**:1946-1957

[61] Vaghela P, Tank HM, Jalpa P. Co-crystals: A novel approach to improve the physicochemical and mechanical properties. Indo American Journal of Pharmaceutical Research. 2014;**4**(10):5055-5065

[62] Steed JW. The role of co-crystals in pharmaceutical design. Trends in Pharmaceutical Sciences. 2013;**34**(3):185-193

[63] Rajurkar VG, Sunil NA, Ghawate V. Tablet formulation and enhancement of aqueous solubility of Efavirenz by solvent evaporation Co-crystal technique. Medicinal Chemistry. 2015;**2**(8):112-121

[64] Maeno Y, Fukami T, Kawahata M, Yamaguchi K, Tagami T. Novel

pharmaceutical Co-crystals consisting of paracetamol and trimethylglycine, a new promising Co-crystals former. International Journal of Pharmaceutics. 2014;**473**:179-186

[65] Zhou Z, Li W, Sun WJ, Lu T, Tong HHY. Resveratrol Co-crystals with enhanced solubility and tabletability. International Journal of Pharmaceutics. 2016;**509**:391-399

[66] Krishna GR, Shi L, Bag PP, Sun CC, Reddy CM. Correlation among crystal structure, mechanical behaviour and tabletability in co-crystals of vanillin isomers. Crystal Growth & Design. 2015;**15**:1827-1832

[67] Li J, Liu P, Liu JP, Zhang WL. Novel Tanshinone II A ternary solid dispersion pellets prepared by a single-step technique: In vitro and in vivo evaluation. European Journal of Pharmaceutics and Biopharmaceutics. 2012;**80**(2):426-432

[68] Gurunath S, Nanjwade BK, Patil PA. Enhanced solubility and intestinal absorption of candesartan cilexetil solid dispersions using everted rat intestinal sacs. Saudi Pharmaceutical Journal. 2014;**22**(3):246-257

[69] Yan YD, Sung JH, Kim KK, Kim JW, Lee BJ, Choi HG. Novel valsartan-loaded solid dispersion with enhanced bioavailability and no crystalline changes. International Journal of Pharmaceutics. 2012;**422**:202-210

[70] Challa VR, Ravindra Babu P, Challa SR, Johnson B, Maheswari C. Pharmacokinetic interaction study between quercetin and valsartan in rats and in vitro models. Drug Delivery and Industrial Pharmacy. 2013;**39**:865-872

[71] Muller P, Flesch G, Gasparo M, Gasparini M. Pharmacokinetics and pharmacodynamic effects of the angiotensin II antagonist valsartan at steady state in healthy, normotensive subjects. European Journal of Clinical Pharmacology. 1997;**52**(6):441-449

[72] Flesch G, Muller P, Lloyd P. Absolute bioavailability and pharmacokinetics of valsartan, an angiotensin II receptor antagonist, in man. European Journal of Clinical Pharmacology. 1997;**52**(2):115-120

[73] Gunaratna C, Cregor M, Kissinger C. Pharmacokinetic and pharmacodynamic studies in rats using a new method of automated blood sampling. Current Separations. 2000;**18**(4):153-157

[74] Fael H, Barbas R, Prohens R, Ràfols C, Fuguet E. Synthesis and characterization of a new Norfloxacin/resorcinol co-crystal with enhanced solubility and dissolution profile. Pharmaceutics. 2022;**4**:49

[75] Machado Cruz R, Boleslavská T, Beránek J, Tieger E, Twamley B, Santos-Martinez MJ, et al. Identification and pharmaceutical characterization of a new itraconazoleterephthalic acid co-crystal. Pharmaceutics. 2020;**12**:741

[76] Nugrahani I, Kumalasari RA, Auli WN, Horikawa A, Uekusa H. Salt co-crystal of diclofenacSodium-L-Proline: Structural, Pseudopolymorphism, and pharmaceutics performance study. Pharmaceutics. 2020;**12**:690

[77] Kale DP, Puri V, Kumar A, Kumar N, Bansal AK. The role of cocrystallizationmediated altered crystallographic properties on the tabletability of rivaroxaban and malonic acid. Pharmaceutics. 2020;**12**:546

[78] Jiaxinpi SW, Li W, DerejeKebebe YZ, Zhang B, Qi D, Guo P, et al. A

nano-cocrystal strategy to improve the dissolution rate and oral bioavailability of baicalein. Asian Journal of Pharmaceutical Sciences. 2018;**2008**:154-164

[79] Latif S, Abbas N, Hussain A, Arshad MS, Bukhari NI, Afzal H, et al. Development of paracetamol-caffeine co-crystals to improve compressional, formulation and in vivo performance. Drug Development and Industrial Pharmacy. 2018;**44**(7):1099-1108

[80] Sopyan I, Fudholi A, Muchtaridi M, SariIP.Simvastatin-nicotinamideco-crystal: Design, preparation and preliminary characterization. Tropical Journal of Pharmaceutical Research. 2017;**16**(2):297-303

[81] Bagde SA, Upadhye KP, Dixit GR, Bakhle SS. Formulation and Evaluation of Co-Crystals of Poorly Water Soluble Drug. IJPSR. 2017;**7**(12):4988-4997

[82] Rajbhar P, Sahu AK, Gautam SS, Prasad RK, Singh V, Nair SK. Formulation and evaluation of clarithromycin Co-crystals tablets dosage forms to enhance theBioavailability. The Pharma Innovation Journal. 2016;**5**(6):05-13

[83] Muddukrishna BS, Dengale SJ, Shenoy GG, Bhat. Preparation, solid state characterisation of paclitaxel and NaringenCo-crystals with improved solubility. International Journal of Applied Pharmaceutics. 2016;**8**(4):32-37

[84] Rajbhar P, Sahu AK, Gautam SS, Prasad RK, Singh V, Nair SK. Formulation and evaluation of clarithromycin co-crystals tablets dosage forms to enhance the bioavailability. The Pharma Innovation Journal. 2016;**5**(6):05-13

[85] Mounika P, Vijaya Raj S, Divya1 G. A. Preparation and characterization of novel Co-crystal forms of fexofenadine. international Journal of Innovative Pharmaceutical Research. 2015;**6**(1):458-463

[86] Almansa C, Merce R, Tesson N, Farran J. Co-crystal of tramadol hydrochloride-celecoxib (ctc): A novel API-API Co-crystal for the treatment of pain. Crystal Growth & Design. 2021;**17**:1021

[87] Eesam S, Bhandaru JS, Naliganti C, Bobbala RK, Akkinepally RR. Solubility enhancement of carvedilol using drug–drug cocrystallization with hydrochlorothiazide. Eesam, Future Journal of Pharmaceutical Sciences. 2020;**77**:1-13

[88] Zheng K, Gao S, Chen M, Li A, Weiwei W, Qian S, et al. Color tuning of an active pharmaceutical ingredient through cocrystallization: A case study of a metronidazole–pyrogallol cocrystal. CrystEngComm. 2020;**22**(8):1404-1413

[89] Dutt B, Choudhary M, Budhwar V. Preparation, characterization and evaluation of aspirin: Benzoic acid co-crystals with enhanced pharmaceutical properties. Future Journal of Pharmaceutical Sciences. 2020;**10**:1186

[90] Witika BA, Smith VJ, Walker RB. Quality by design optimization of cold Sonochemical synthesis of zidovudine lamivudine Nanosuspensions. Pharmaceutics. 2020;**12**(4):367

[91] Kale DP, Puri V, Kumar A, Kumar N, Bansal AK. The role of Cocrystallization-mediated altered crystallographic properties on the Tabletability of rivaroxaban and malonic acid. Pharmaceutics. 2020;**12**(6):546

[92] Nugrahani I, Kumalasari RA, Auli WN, Horikawa A, Uekusa H. Salt Cocrystal of diclofenac sodium-L-Proline: Structural,

Pseudopolymorphism, and pharmaceutics performance study. Pharmaceutics. 2020;**12, 7**:690

[93] Bull X, Robeyns K, Garrido CC, Tumanov N, Collard L, Wouters J, et al. Improving Nefiracetam dissolution and solubility behavior using a Cocrystallization approach. Pharmaceutics. 2020;**12**(7):653

[94] Winantari AN, Setyawan D, Siswodihardjo S, Soewandhi SN. Cocrystallization acyclovir-succinic acid using solvent evaporation. Methods. 2017;**10**:6

[95] Apshingekar PP, Aher S, Kelly AL, Brown EC, Paradkar A. Synthesis of caffeine/maleic acid Co-crystal by ultrasound-assisted slurry co-crystallization. Journal of Pharmaceutical Sciences. 2016;**1-5**

[96] Setyawan D, Jovita RO, Iqbal M, Paramanandana A, Yusuf H, Lestari MLAD. Co-crystalization of quercetin and malonic acid using solvent-drop grinding method. Tropical Journal of Pharmaceutical Research June. 2018;**17**(6):997-1002

[97] JoseLopez-Cedrun SV, Burgueno M, Juaez I, AboulHosn S, Martin-Granizo R, Grau J, et al. Co-crystal of Tramadol–Celecoxib in Patients with Moderate to Severe Acute Post-surgical Oral Pain: A Dose-Finding, Randomised, Double-Blind, Placebo- and Active-Controlled, Multicentre, Phase II Trial. Drugs. 2018;**2**:137-148

[98] Inam M, Jiajia W, Shen J, Phan CU, Tang G, Hu X. preparation and characterization of novel pharmaceutical Co-crystals: Ticagrelor with nicotinamide. MDPI Crystals. 2018;**8**(10):336

[99] Buschmann HH, Carandell LS, Buchholz JB. Co-crystals of duloxetine and naproxen. Patent. 2019;**2**(291):345

[100] Salaman CRP, Videla S, Tesson N, Castano MT. Co-crystals of venlafaxine and celecoxib. Esteve Pharmaceuticals SA. 2017;**2**(340):818

[101] Panzade P, Shendarkar G, Shaikh S, Rathi PB. Pharmaceutical co-crystal of Piroxicam: Design, formulation and evaluation. Advanced Pharmaceutical Bulletin. 2017;**7**(3):399-408

[102] Nicolov M, Ghiulai RM, Voicu M. Cocrystal formation of Betulinic acid and ascorbic acid: Synthesis, Physico-chemical assessment, antioxidant, and Antiproliferative activity. Medicinal and Pharmaceutical Chemistry Editor's. 2019;**7**(92):10

[103] Alwati AAM. Ultrasound assisted processing of solid state pharmaceuticals. Faculty of Life Sciences University of Bradford. 2017;**129**:172-181

[104] Jung M-S, Kim J-S, Kim M-S, Alhalaweh A, Cho W, Hwang S-J, et al. Bioavailability of indomethacin–saccharin cocrystal. Journal of Pharmaceutical Pharmacology. 2010;**62**:1560-1568

[105] Sathali AA, Selvaraj V. Enhancement of solubility and dissolution rate of racecadotril by solid dispersion methods. Joural of Current Chemical Pharmaceutical Science. 2012;**2**(3):209-225

[106] Sanphui P, Devi VK, Clara D, Malviya N, Ganguly S, Desiraju GR. Co-crystals of hydrochlorothiazide: Solubility and diffusion/permeability enhancements through drug-coformer interactions. Molecular Pharmaceutics. 2015;**12**(5):1615-1622

[107] Dai XL, Li S, Chen JM, Lu TB. Improving the membrane permeability of 5-fluorouracil via Cocrystallization. Crystal Growth & Design. 2016;**16**(8):4430-4438

[108] Mannava MKC, Gunnam A, Lodagekar A, Shastri NR, Nangia AK, Solomon KA. Enhanced solubility, permeability, and tabletability of nicorandil by salt and cocrystal formation. CrystEngComm. 2021;**23**(1):227-237

[109] Duggirala NK, Smith AJ, Wojtas Ł, Shytle RD, Zaworotko MJ. Physical stability enhancement and pharmacokinetics of a lithium ionic cocrystal with glucose. Crystal Growth & Design. 2014;**14**(11):6135-6142

[110] Gao Y, Zu H, Zhang J. Enhanced dissolution and stability of adefovir dipivoxil by cocrystal formation. The Journal of Pharmacy and Pharmacology. 2011;**63**(4):483-490

[111] Pagire SK, Jadav N, Vangala VR, Whiteside B, Paradkar A. Thermodynamic investigation of CarbamazepineSaccharin Co-crystal polymorphs. Journal of Pharmaceutical Science. 2017;**106**:2009-2014

[112] Bethune SJ, Huang N, Jayasankar A, Rodríguez-Hornedo N. Understanding and predicting the effect of cocrystal components and pH on cocrystal solubility. Crystal Growth & Design. 2009;**9**:3976-3988

[113] Aitipamula S, Banerjee R, Bansal AK, Biradha K, Cheney ML, Choudhury AR, et al. Polymorphs, salts, and co-crystals: What's in a name? Crystal Growth & Design. 2012;**12**(5):2147-2152

[114] Cheney ML, Weyna DR, Shan N, Hanna M, Wojtas L, Zaworotko MJ. Coformer selection in pharmaceutical cocrystal development: A case study of a meloxicam aspirin cocrystal that exhibits enhanced solubility and pharmacokinetics. Journal of Pharmaceutical Sciences. 2011;**100**:2172-2181

[115] Verma S, Arun Nanda SP, Basu. Improvement of solubility and bioavailability of aceclofenac using cocrystallization. Drug Invention Today. 2019;**11**(1):59-63

[116] Karimi-Jafari M, Padrela L, Walker G, Croker D. Creating Co-crystals: A review of pharmaceutical Cocrystal preparation routes and applications. Crystal Growth & Design. 2018;**18**(10):6370-6387

[117] Aitipamula S, Cadden J, Chow P. Co-crystals of zonisamide: Physicochemical characterization and sustained release solid forms. CrystEngComm. 2018;**20**(21):2923-2931

[118] Sanphui P, Goud NR, Khandavilli UR, Nangia A. Fast dissolving curcumin co-crystals. Crystal Growth & Design. 2011;**11**(9):4135-4145

[119] Aitipamula S, Chow PS, Tan RB. Trimorphs of a pharmaceutical cocrystal involving two active pharmaceutical ingredients: Potential relevance to combination drugs. CrystEngComm. 2009;**11**(9):1823-1827

[120] Chadha R, Saini A, Arora P, Jain DS, Dasgupta A, Guru Row TN. Multicomponent solids of lamotrigine with some selected coformers and their characterization by thermoanalytical, spectroscopic and Xray diffraction methods. CrystEngComm. 2011;**13**(20): 6271-6284

[121] Luszczki JJ, Czuczwar M, Kis J, Krysa J, Pasztelan I, Swiader M, et al. Interactions of lamotrigine with Topiramate and first-generation antiepileptic drugs in the maximal electroshock test in mice: An Isobolographic analysis. Epilepsia. 2003;**44**(8):1003-1013

[122] Patil SP, Modi SR, Bansal AK. Generation of 1: 1 carbamazepine:

Nicotinamide co-crystals by spray drying. European Journal of Pharmaceutical Sciences. 2014;**62**:251-257

[123] Perumalla SR, Sun CC. Enabling tablet product development of 5-Fluorocytosine through integrated crystal and particle engineering. Journal of Pharmaceutical Sciences. 2014;**103**(4):1126-1132

[124] Karki S, Friscic T, Fabian L, Laity PR, Day GM, Jones W. Improving mechanical properties of crystalline solids by cocrystal formation: New compressible forms of paracetamol. Advanced Materials. 2009;**21**(38-39):3905-3909

[125] Maeno Y, Fukami T, Kawahata M, Yamaguchi K, Tagami T, Ozeki T, et al. Novel pharmaceutical cocrystal consisting of paracetamol and trimethylglycine, a new promising cocrystal former. International Journal of Pharmaceutics. 2014;**473**(1):179-186

[126] Aitipamula S, Wong AB, Kanaujia P. Evaluating suspension formulations of theophylline co-crystals with artificial sweeteners. Journal of Pharmaceutical Sciences. 2017;**2017**:30670-30676

[127] Newman A, Wenslow R. Solid form changes during drug development: Good, bad, and ugly case studies. AAPS Open. 2016;**2**(1):2

[128] Trask AV. An overview of pharmaceutical Co-crystals as intellectual property. Molecular Pharmaceutics. 2007;**4**(3):301-309

[129] Gadade DD, Pekamwar SS. Pharmaceutical co-crystals: Regulatory and strategic aspects, design and development. Advanced Pharmaceutical Bulletin. 2016;**6**(4):479-494

[130] Abourahma H, Cocuzza DS, Melendez J, Urban JM. Pyrazinamide co-crystals and the search for polymorphs. CrystEngComm. 2011;**13**:1-22

[131] Batisai E, Ayamine A, Kilinkissa OEY, Bathori N. Melting point-solubility-structure correlations in multicomponent crystal containing fumaric or adipic acid. CrystEngComm. 2014;**16**:9992-9998

[132] Mohammad MA, Alhalaweh A, Velaga SP. Hansen solubility parameter as a tool to predict cocrystal formation. International Journal of Pharmaceutics. 2011;**407**:63-71

[133] Alhalaweh A, Roy L, Rodríguez-Hornedo N, Velaga S. pH-dependent solubility of indomethacin–saccharin and carbamazepine–saccharin co-crystals in aqueous media. Molecular Pharmaceutics. 2012;**9**(9):2605-2612

[134] Reddy L, Bethune S, Kampf J, Rodríguez-Hornedo N. Co-crystals and salts of gabapentin: pH dependent cocrystal stability and solubility. Crystal Growth & Design. 2008;**9**(1):378-385

[135] Ford JL, Willson R. Thermal analysis and calorimetry of pharmaceuticals. Handbook of Thermal Analysis and Calorimetry: From Macromolecules to Man. 1999;**4**:923-1016

[136] Chen Y, Li L, Yao J, Ma YY, Chen JM, Lu TB. Improving the solubility and bioavailability of Apixaban via ApixabanOxalic acid cocrystal. Crystal Growth & Design. 2016;**16**:2923-2930

[137] Chen J-M, Li S, Lu T-B. Pharmaceutical Co-crystals of ribavirin with reduced release rates. Crystal Growth & Design. 2014;**14**(12):6399-6408

[138] Dhumal RS, Kelly AL, York P, Coates PD, Paradkar A. Cocrystalization

and simultaneous agglomeration using hot melt extrusion. Pharmaceutical Research. 2010;**27**(12):2725-2733

[139] Ogata T, Tanaka D, Ozeki T. Enhancing the solubility and masking the bitter taste of propiverine using crystalline complex formation. Drug Development and Industrial Pharmacy. 2014;**40**(8):1084-1091

[140] Kumar S, Nanda A. Pharmaceutical co-crystals: An overview. Indian Journal of Pharmaceutical Sciences. 2017;**79**(6):858-871

Chapter 13

Co-Crystallization Techniques for Improving Nutraceutical Absorption and Bioavailability

Asmita Gajbhiye, Debashree Das and Shailendra Patil

Abstract

Nutraceuticals is an umbrella term for therapeutic leads derived from plants, animals and/or microbial species. Being synthesized in nature's own laboratory a nutraceuticals have structural and functional features for interacting with an array of physiological targets. However, because of this very structural complexity and diversified nature, nutraceuticals often suffer from diminished gastrointestinal (GI) absorption and limited systemic bioavailability. Thus, in-spite of having an obvious edge over synthetic molecules, pharmaceutical applicability of nutraceuticals play second fiddle in the present pharmaceutical prospective. In this regard, co-crystallization of nutraceuticals have evolved as an attractive prospect. Co-crystallization causes stoichiometric non-covalent binding between nutraceutical API (active pharmaceutical ingredient) and a pharmaceutically acceptable co-former creating a single-phase crystalline material. Nutraceutical co-crystals thus created possess excellent absorption and bioavailability attributes. The principal aim of the current chapter is to highlight co-crystallization as the means of nutraceutical ascendancy over toxic synthetic drugs currently dominating the pharmaceutical market. In the current chapter the authors provide a detail exposition on the methods and application of co-crystallization in context of nutraceutical absorption and bioavailability. Herein, we discuss in detail about the constituents, characteristics, mechanism of action and protocol for preparation of nutraceutical co-crystals with relevant references from current and past studies.

Keywords: co-crystals, bioavailability, absorption, stability, solubility, nutraceutical, nano co-crystals

1. Introduction

Nature is the ultimate chemist; it houses a vast repertoire of medicinal molecules. Most of the works done by early physicians are based on the principle of *Medicatrix naturae* or the healing power of nature. With the advent of modern research, the scientific fraternity have perfected the means to isolate nutraceutical APIs (active pharmaceutical ingredients) from plants, animals, and even microbial species. The period between 1981 and 2014, can be claimed as the most promising era of nutraceutical drug discovery. During this time major portion of small molecule ligands to gain USFDA (US Food and Drug Administration) approval were of natural origin. Even against the COVID-19 pandemic the most potent arsenal interred was a nutraceutical obtained from the blue blood of a horseshoe crab. Time and again it has been proven that, despite having made significant strides in synthetic medicine, nutraceuticals still dominate the healthcare market [1]. Patients for most part prefer non-toxic natural alternatives to synthetic drugs. The origin of nearly half of all human pharmaceuticals can be traced back to natural sources [2].

Widely used OTC (over the counter) aspirin is a popular analgesic obtained from bark of willow tree, vincristine and vinblastine are potent anticancer agents isolated from rosy periwinkle [3], aggrastat a highly recommended anticoagulant is extracted from an afrotropic native the saw-scaled viper [4], these are some of the popular examples of drugs culminated from the nature's repertoire. Nevertheless, despite holding cure to the most intractable of human maladies [5], a very low percentage of marketed medicine is formulated using nutraceutical pharmacophores [6].

Poor absorption from the GI (gastrointestinal) tract and the consequent limitation in systemic bioavailability are predominant roadblocks in pharmaceutical use of nutraceuticals. A fact that is also supported by restrictive solubility profile of nutraceutical molecules. Irrespective of its source of origin, the major contributors of unsuccessful pharmaceutical formulations, are diminished gastro-intestinal (GI) absorption and less than the required systemic bioavailability [7]. The definition of bioavailability defines the fraction of dose following administration that reaches the systemic circulation. It is also a representation of the bio-efficacy or in other words the therapeutic utility of any medicinal compounds [8]. Factors responsible for low bioavailability include molecular instability, poor aqueous solubility and pitiable rate of dissolution and absorption in systemic physiology. Therefore, for exploiting the efficacy of nutraceuticals in active pharmaceutical use, we must concentrate on improving their GI absorption and bioavailability [9]. Several strategies targeting to improve, GI absorption and bioavailability of the therapeutic lead have although been developed, drug modification via co-crystallization is presently the rage of the hour. Like co-crystals of synthetic molecules, nutraceutical co-crystals are crystalline solid composed of a nutraceutical API and a pharmaceutically acceptable excipient also known as the co-former non-covalently bonded in a stoichiometric ratio [10].

The cardinal imperative of the current chapter is to provide an overview of the concept of co-crystallization in modulating the absorption and bioavailability of nutraceutical ligands. Since the ascendency of crystal engineering, co-crystallization has proven to be of immense use in modifying the physicochemical attributes of APIs. The principal advantage of employing co-crystallization strategies is that co-crystals improve the solubility and absorption characteristics of the target API without alternating in any way the intrinsic pharmacological activity of the molecule. In subsequent sections of the current chapter a lot of interesting insights can be gained regarding the properties, strategies, advancement and prospects of co-crystallization in accentuating the use of nutraceuticals in pharmaceutical drug designing.

2. Need for co-crystallization of nutraceuticals

Evolutionary biomechanics have helped to create a vast reservoir of naturally occurring therapeutic compounds. Alkaloids, flavonoids, terpenoids, and steroids are principal categories of nutraceuticals having a wide range of pharmacological properties [11]. Natural pharmacophores have rigid confirmations, complex molecular architecture, and well-defined stereochemistry. These in turn aid the nutraceuticals to bind with a variety of physiological targets and thereby increase their bio-efficacy [12]. Nevertheless, because of poor solubility and dissolution characteristics leading to limited gastro-intestinal absorption and restrictive bioavailability, the bio-efficacy of a nutraceutical scafold is significantly compromised (**Figure 1**) [13]. Furthermore, nutraceuticals are often annotated with functional groups that allow them to bind with a variety of biological targets. But these very groups are also often responsible for the undesirable solubility and stability characteristics of the nutraceutical pharmacophores. Consequently, even though natural products are endowed with an amazingly wide therapeutic window, they have taken a back seat in active clinical use [14].

Naturally occurring therapeutic molecules are essentially cost-effective. Also, in comparison to synthetic drugs, nutraceuticals are way less likely to cause toxic manifestations in systemic physiology. That being so, currently the major focus of the pharmaceutical industry is to explore various means of improving the absorption and bioavailability of nutraceuticals for the purpose of producing effective pharmaceutical formulations [7]. The energetics in crystalline solids dictates that the atoms in a standalone crystal on attaining minimum potential energy will attain maximum stability [15]. Therefore, by converting into their crystalline form, nutraceutical APIs can be made more stable soluble, absorbable and consequently more bioavailable [16].

Crystallization procedures are widely employed by the pharmaceutical industry for the extraction, separation, and purification of drug leads from natural resources [17]. By crystallizing nutraceuticals, they can be converted into a more thermodynamically stable and highly soluble molecule with much greater percentage purity than their amorphous counterparts [18]. Solubility, bioavailability, as well as the

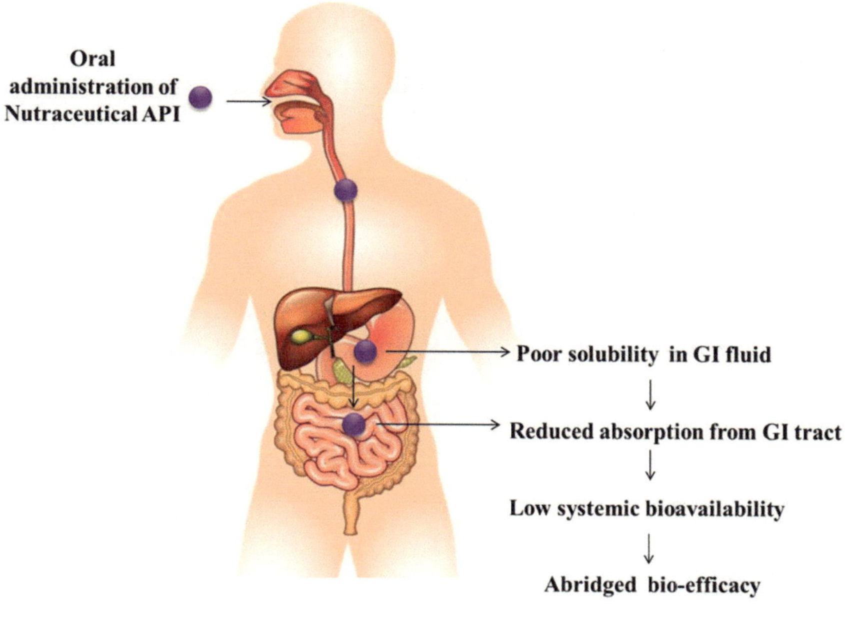

Figure 1.
Schematic representation of relation between solubility, GI (gastrointestinal) absorption, bioavailability and bio-efficacy of nutraceuticals.

shelf-life of an API are all influenced by the purity, size, and shape distribution of the crystal lattice. Pharmaceutical crystallization has evolved a lot since its inception [19]. Currently, polymorphs, salts, hydrates, solvates, and co-crystals are some of the commonly envisaged pharmaceutically crystals. Polymorphs are diverse crystalline shapes of the same atom or molecules. On the other hand, in conjugation with the drug molecule, either an organic solvent, or water and/or a crystalline co-former is required for producing solvates, hydrates, and co-crystals respectively. However, each crystal form has its own limitations. For example, isolated chemical hydrates and solvates eventually lose stability due to the loss of the solvent or water molecule [20]. Besides, using an appropriate co-former, co-crystals of both synthetic as well as nutraceutical APIs can be efficiently created. For this reason, procuring palatable formulations of challenging molecules can be achieved by employing the strategy of co-crystallization. Pharmaceutical co-crystals can also produce salts and display polymorphism and solvatomorphism, which broadens the range of solid-state forms for a particular API. Pharmaceutically acceptable components and nutraceutical API are combined in co-crystals in a stoichiometric ratio through non-covalent interactions like hydrogen bonds, van der Waals forces, and stacking interactions [21].

Since it was realized that by using co-crystal engineering one may be able to improve the physicochemical properties of nutraceuticals, a significant number of studies highlighting the use of crystal engineering and supramolecular synthons as excellent means for designing pharmaceutical-based co-crystals have been archived. This has further encouraged the development of the co-crystal approach to improve the performance of nutraceuticals [22]. As co-crystal research has grown, a wide range of application areas for co-crystal creation to manipulate physical properties have become available. Furthermore, co-crystallization is suitable for changing the permeability of candidate molecules across cell membranes as well as for increasing the dissolving characteristics of nutraceutical API [23]. The scope of the current chapter is dedicated to improving nutraceutical absorption and bioavailability by means of co-crystallization. Herein the authors, have attempted to state all the plausible factors pertaining to the application of co-crystallization in mitigating poor gastrointestinal absorption and bioavailability of nutraceuticals.

3. Components of nutraceutical co-crystals

Essentially, a nutraceutical co-crystal is made up of naturally occurring API and the conformer required to induce co-crystallization. In **Figure 2** we have illustrated the composition of a typical nutraceutical co-crystal. Nutraceuticals are strong candidates for co-crystallization [24]. The term nutraceutical was coined by conjoining

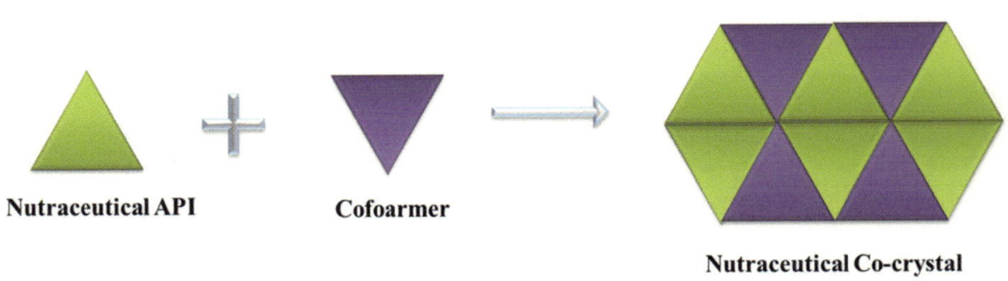

Figure 2.
Components of nutraceutical co-crystals.

two terms "nutrition" and "pharmaceutics." It was originally described by DeFelice in 1989 as food (or component of a food) that gives medicinal or health benefits, including the prevention and/or treatment of an illness [25]. Since the definition appeared to be extremely generalized, a definition citing differences between dietary supplements, nutraceuticals, and functional foods were stated [26]. In the light of this, nutraceuticals were defined to included compounds obtained from minerals, vitamins, amino acids, therapeutic herbs or other botanicals, dietary substances, concentrates, metabolites, isolates, extricates, or any combinations of the aforementioned. Subsequently, nutraceuticals became an umbrella term for naturally occurring molecules that are employed for both their nutritional value as well as therapeutic efficacy [27]. Currently, a vast number of nutraceuticals are used for their therapeutic and prophylactic properties in both allopathic as well as alternative systems of medicine [28]. The major impediment in active use of APIs of natural origin is the lack the characteristics essential for viable drug formulation. Nutraceuticals are often observed to have diminished aqueous solubility, decreased dissolution rate, poor permeation, and low absorption through biological membranes [29].

Co-crystals can overcome the absorption and bioavailability issue associated with nutraceutical API. However, formation of co-crystals depends in large on the co-former employed for the co-crystallization. The co-former of appropriate choice is preferably selected by in accordance with the GRAS list. GRAS or generally regarded as safe, is a list issued by the USFDA. It consists of more than 3000 co-formers such as succinic acid, benzoic acid, nicotinamide, isonicotinamide, picolinic acid, betaine, saccharin, maleic acid, and proline [30]. The choice of appropriate co-formers is of extreme importance. Several reasons, including but not limited to lack of complementarity in hydrogen bonding, preferred packing patterns, conformational flexibility, molecular shape and size, and stability can impede binding of the co-former with the API. However, if the co-former exhibits strong intermolecular interactions with the nutraceutical even systems seemingly immiscible in nature can form co-crystals. Nonetheless, miscibility of the components is considered as an advantage in formulation of co-crystals. Consequently, it is of immense importance that a lot of experimental effort is put into the selection of an appropriate co-former [31].

To select the correct co-former, as well as to characterize the nutraceutical co-crystals, information-based systems are employed. Examples of these systems include hydrogen-bonding penchant, synthonic building, supramolecular compatibility test, Cambridge Structure Database (CSD), pKa-based models, Fabian's strategy, Cross section vitality calculation, the conductor-like screening show for genuine solvents (COSMO-RS), Hansen dissolvability parameter, virtual co-crystal screening (based upon atomic electrostatic potential surfaces-MEPS), warm investigation, measuring immersion temperature, Kofler contact strategy and coordinating [32].

For example, the PKa based tool utilizes the difference between pKa of nutraceutical and its co-former to predicts co-crystallization. If the difference between the co-crystal components i.e. $\delta pKa < 1$ flawless formation of co-crystal takes place. If $\delta pKa > 1$ the system will lead tend to form salts [33]. Cambridge structural database is used to predict the intermolecular hydrogen bonding between co-crystal starting materials. Also, single crystal X-ray crystallography can be used to characterize the crystal structure of a compound [34]. Hansen solubility parameter is used to assess the miscibility between cocrystal components based on the difference in solubility parameters. Usually, the difference in solubility parameters of components $<7\ MPa^{1/2}$ predicts co-crystal formation [35]. Supramolecular synthon approach is yet another tool screening co-formers for co-crystallizaion. It is classified into supramolecular homosynthon and supramolecular heterosynthon approaches. Supramolecular homosynthon approach is observed between similar functional group while the heterosynthon approach is observed between different functional groups [36]. The binary and ternary phase diagrams are used for evaluating the ease of solubility between drug and co-former, and between the drug, co-former, and solvent respectively. It has been observed that typically the 'W' shaped phase diagram preludes co-crystal formation and a 'V' shaped diagram predicts the formation of eutectic mixture [37]. Conductor-like screening model for real solvents or CSMO-RS is a computational screening technique which works on the difference in enthalpy between co-crystal components. For co-crystal formation to be favored, enthalpy of the drug-co-former complex must be more than the enthalpy of the parent components [38].

4. Mechanism of co-crystallization

Co-crystallization of nutraceuticals defines the incorporation of a nutraceutical API and a co-former inside the same crystal lamella. Of essential importance is the nature of the solvent used for co-crystallization. Also, to be noted is the stoichiometric proportion in which the co-former will interact with the nutraceutical API to form non-covalent bond. For inducing co-crystallization, the co-former must have a certain degree of melt miscibility with the nutraceutical. Both the constituents of the co-crystal must exhibit similar repeat unit chemistry and similar crystal unit cell lattice [39]. Besides factors including temperature, blending and pH are also compelling parameters instrumental to the biomechanics of co-crystallization [40]. The rules of hydrogen holding, synthons, and chart sets are included in planning co-crystal frameworks. Co-crystallization is an empirical and multistage process [41]. **Figure 3** shows the schematic of the co-crystal formation. As observed in certain, cases for example in co-crystals containing naphthalene, the diffusion of solids and vapor is also an essential factor in defining co-crystallization parameters. As opposed to it, in heavier aromatic hydrocarbons, surface diffusion is of much importance in staging the co-crystal arrangement [42].

By employing an intermediate liquid at ambient temperature, formation of solid co-crystals in the liquid phase can be achieved. Eutectic formation in co-crystal synthesis is also an increasingly significant mechanism in co-crystal formation. The co-crystal formation at the interface of two colorless crystals of diphenylamine and

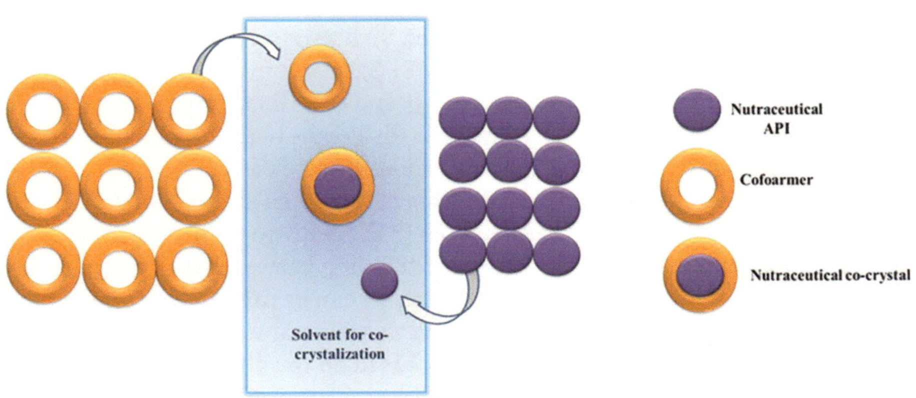

Figure 3.
Mechanism of co-crystallization.

benzophenone was revealed by microscopic observation, where the contact surface was converted into liquid [43]. Furthermore, eutectic-mediated co-crystallization in conjugation with grinding increases the fresh reactant surfaces for the eutectic formation while improving the co-crystal nucleation in the eutectic phase [44].

For instances with no conceivable mass exchange, for example in fluid or gaseous stage, co-crystallization occurs through the arrangement of amorphous intermediates. This is mostly observed when molecular solids with strong intermolecular hydrogen bonding undergoes co-crystallization. Even the choice of appropriate co-formers relies on the functional groups inclined to form complementary hydrogen bonding with the nutraceutical API. Owing to their directional interactions, hydrogen bonds most emphatically impact molecular recognition [45]. To further emphasize the significance of hydrogen bonding in co-crystallization, certain guidelines have been created to anticipate the consequences of hydrogen bond interactions in co-crystallization. These guidelines include: (1) the hydrogen bonding in any crystal structure will include all acidic hydrogen atoms, (2) all good hydrogen bond acceptors will participate in hydrogen bonding if there is an adequate supply of hydrogen bond donors, (3) hydrogen bonds will preferentially form between the best proton donor and acceptor, and (4) intramolecular hydrogen bonds in a six-membered ring will form in preference to intermolecular hydrogen bonds [46].

Apart from hydrogen bonding, the stereochemistry and competing interactions between molecules are also required to be taken into consideration. Electrostatic energies and free volume of the co-crystal are important constraints in the biomechanics of co-crystallization. For a stable co-crystal to form it is important to maintain a low level of electrostatic energies and free volume inside the crystal [47]. Furthermore, temperatures of co-crystallization are yet another factor of consequence. Below the glass transition temperature of the reactants results in amorphous phase formation; however, higher than glass temperature results in metastable polymorphic forms [48]. For liquid-assisted grinding, it is yet not possible to correctly define the mechanism of co-crystal formation. However, in some instances, it is observed that the liquid phase acts as a lubricating medium to induce molecular diffusion [49]. The co-crystals resulting from both heat and liquid-assisted grinding are thermodynamically stable. Therefore, it can be stated that the low solvent fraction used in the process of liquid-assisted grinding is not a sole reliant in controlling the outcome of the process. The same is also true for slurry co-crystallization. Moreover, the nature of the liquid phase used in grinding can be significantly influential during mechanochemical co-crystallization. The mentioned mechanisms are the ones mostly involved with mechanochemical synthesis of co-crystals [50].

5. Impact of co-crystallization on gastro-intestinal absorption and bioavailability of nutraceuticals

Nutraceuticals have also held special significance in drug discovery and design. Despite having developmentally evolved structural and physicochemical properties those very properties also impedes their bench-to-beside translation. Molecular complexity, poor aqueous solubility, functional group reactivity, and general instability are the cardinal constraints in achieving viable nutraceutical formulation [51]. For these reasons nutraceuticals do not make it to the frontline in active therapy.

The low absorption of nutraceuticals from gastro-intestinal tract is because of inherent impairment in aqueous solubility and permeability. Consequently, nutraceuticals in therapeutic use are needed to be administered frequently and in large doses [52]. Gastro-intestinal absorption defines the amount of drug that gets absorbed from the gastro-intestinal tract post oral administration of a drug molecule. Bioavailability on the other hand is the concentration of administered dose that reaches the systemic circulation. Gastrointestinal absorption and bioavailability are interdependent phenomenon. After oral administration, the lead compound gets disintegrated and dissolved in the gastric fluid. For effective absorption, API needs to be present in an aqueous solution at the site of absorption. Thus, for increasing GI absorption, it is of utmost importance that the aqueous solubility of the nutraceutical API must be improved [53].

By far the most prolific utility of co-crystals to date has been to improve the solubility of the starting material, particularly when that starting material is an active pharmaceutical ingredient. Low aqueous solubility is a barrier to satisfactory drug delivery and, as such, often prevents a medicine from being fit for its purpose. Inherently, a co-crystal will have a different solubility than that of the starting materials due to the altered underlying crystal structure. The solubility alteration can be in either direction. Enhanced solubility is desirable, as it will improve the bioavailability of the drug, but excessive enhancement can be problematic as it can lead to undesirable precipitation of the starting material due to the generation of a supersaturated solution. This has been characterized for co-crystal materials as a "spring and parachute" effect [44].

A 'spring' can be a formulation of the API of thermodynamical higher energy providing faster dissolution and thus a higher rate and extent of absorption. However, a limiting factor of this improved dissolution profile can be rapid recrystallization of a more stable and less soluble form. Thus, an excipient or co-former or a process which retards the rate of recrystallization is needed. This is called the 'parachute'. For every poorly water-soluble drug an individual concept combining the benefits of 'spring and parachute' is needed to accomplish a supersaturated solution of the drug [54].

Thus, co-crystals bear the potential to enhance the delivery and clinical performance of drug products by modulating drug solubility, pharmacokinetics, and bioavailability. Particularly, using cocrystals to improve oral drug absorption of BCS class II and IV drugs has been a strong focus of several case studies published in the literature. Stanton et al. have compared the improvement on the solubility and pharmacokinetics of AMG 517, a potent and selective transient receptor vanilliod 1 (TRPV1) antagonist, when co-crystallizing this drug with carboxylic acid (cinnamic acid and benzoic acid and amide co-formers are used). All four AMG517 cocrystals showed faster intrinsic and powder dissolution rates in fasted simulated intestinal fluid than the free base of AMG 517. The results on the pharmacokinetics showed a 2.4- to 7.1-fold increase in the area under the concentration-time curve in rat PK investigations, which highlights the improvement in bioavailability of AMG 517 when in a cocrystalline form. Other studies have demonstrated the efficiency of cocrystallization in improving the solubility and bioavailability of poorly soluble APIs such as indomethacin, baicalein and quercetin [55].

6. Applications of co-crystallization in improving nutraceutical solubility and bioavailability

Nutraceutical APIs are of vital importance in all areas of modern drug development. Pharmacophores of natural origin not only improve drug development but can also be conjugated to enhance the physicochemical properties of already approved drugs. However, a relatively large percentage of nutraceuticals of therapeutic value exhibit poor water solubility and bioavailability [56]. Literary evidence cites numerous examples of nutraceuticals such as flavonoids and other essential nutrients as candidates for co-crystallization studies. For example, on formulating as a co-crystal, absorption and bioavailability of Protocatechuic acid a nutraceutical antioxidant was found to significantly enhance. This was achieved by employing pharmaceutical grade co-formers. Examples of pharmaceutical co-formers include caprolactam, isonicotinamide, isonicotinic acid, theophylline, nicotinamide, and theobromine. The process employed for co-crystallization of Protocatechuic acid was accomplished by gradually evaporating stoichiometric amounts of the nutraceutical and a co-former in a suitable solvent. Following which the co-crystals were extracted out from the mother liquors prior to evaporation of the entire solvent [57].

Another extensively envisaged class of nutraceuticals is the Flavonoid family. Of which quercetin is an important member. It is known to possess potent therapeutic properties. Quercetin is documented for its properties of free radical scavenging, enzyme inhibition (ornithine carboxylase, protein kinase, calmodulin), vasodilatation and platelet disaggregation. Despite having significant therapeutic priviledge, quercetin fails to achieve its required in vivo potency. Mostly because, in pure form quercetin is limited by, primarily due to its low solubility and consequent poor absorption in the gut and diminished bioavailability [58]. Also it was observed that on forming co-crystals with succinic acid, solubility and dissolution profile of quercetin was found to improve significantly [59]. The nutraceutical compound Hesperetin, is a well acclaimed antioxidant, antiallergic, antimutagenic, and anti-cancer agent [60]. Co-crystallization of hesperitin to improve its bio-efficacy is an extensively documented endeavor. Hesperetin was co-crystallized using pharmaceutically acceptable co-formers such as isonicotinamide and nicotinic acid. Co-crystallization of hesperetin with isonicotinamide forms a supramolecular synthon wherein isonicotinamide binds with the hesperitin nutraceutical by forming an OH---N hydrogen bond. Crystallization of hesperetin with nicotinic acid results in two 1:1 cocrystals in which the nicotinic acid exists as a zwitterionic state [61].

The nutraceutical molecule Pterostilbene is a popular component of traditional system of medicine. It is found expressed in several tree barks and a variety of berries, such as grapes. The physical stability and in-turn pharmaceutical viability of Pterostilbene can be significantly improved by co-crystallizing it with either caffeine or carbamazepine [62]. The co-crystals thus formed were of a 1:1 stoichiometric molar ratio. For characterization crystallographic (XRPD, single crystal) and thermoanalytical (TGA, DSC) techniques were used. Physical stability of the reported nutraceutical co-crystals with respect to relative humidity was also established [62].

Efficacy of the nutraceutical compound P-coumaric acid was improved by co-crystallizing it with nicotinamide. The co-former is a member of the vitamin B complex family. The consequent 2:1 (p-coumaric acid-nicotinamide) co-crystals were characterized by X-ray powder diffraction, thermal analyses, and spectroscopic techniques [63]. Derived from *Curcuma longa*, curcumin, is a pharmaceutically viable nutraceutical with excellent therapeutic attributes. However, as in context of most nutraceuticals, curcumin also suffers from poor water solubility, which limits its bioavailability. Co-crystallization of curcumin have been reported as excellent means of improving the molecules aqueous solubility. For the purpose salicylic acid and hydroxyquinol were employed as co-formers. It was observed that the curcumin-salicylic acid system forms an eutectic mixture, whereas the curcumin-hydroxyquinol system forms cocrystals. The reason for this predicament was attributed to the weak intramolecular hydrogen bonding interactions in salicylic acid and strong hydrogen bonding interactions between hydroxyl −OH groups present in hydroxyquinol molecule and curcumin molecule. However, both curcumin-salicylic acid eutectic as well as curcumin-hydroxyquinol cocrystals demonstrated improved powder dissolution, absorption and bioavailability rates than parent curcumin [64].

Citric acid is an alpha acid that is naturally found concentrated in citrus fruits. Citric acid is commonly used as a food additive to provide acidity and sour taste to foods and beverages. It is also employed as prophylaxic for kidney stones by making urine more alkaline. Because of its excellent aqueous solubility, it is used as a co-former in pharmaceutical co-crystallization [65]. Many examples of citric acid has been cited in literature. For example, citric acid improves the solubility and dissolution profile of the poorly water-soluble drug, simvastatin [66]. Synthesis of atorvastatin calcium co-crystals for solubility enhancement was also achieved by employing citric acid and nicotinamide as co-formers [67]. Gossypol is a natural product occurring as biphenolic compound derived from the cotton plant (genus *Gossypium*). It is extensively envisaged for its pharmacological applications such as anticancer, antimicrobial, and antiviral properties. The nutraceutical is however limited because of high toxicity. This adverse effect of gossypol can be avoided by increasing the bioavailability of the compound so that the desired therapeutic effect can be achieved in a smaller dose. For the purpose, (−)-gossypol co-crystals with a C1–8 carboxylic acid or C1–8 sulfonic acid which are inhibitors of anti-apoptotic Bcl-2 family proteins have been created [68]. In recent years nutraceutical co-crystallization has achieved new heights. In a study, it was reported that conjugating cardiotonic drug milrinone with nutraceuticals such as syringic acid and gallic acid improves the *in-vitro* and *in-vivo* performances of cardiotonic drug milrinone [69].

7. Conclusions

Co-crystallization is a promising approach for improving the physicochemical properties of APIs. For years the research fraternity has worked tirelessly to develop numerous methodologies for the preparation of pharmaceutically acceptable co-crystals. The co-crystallization protocol includes lab-scale synthetic methodology as well as large-scale production methods. In the current chapter, we have aimed to provide standard descriptions and various examples of established and emerging co-crystal preparations in context of nutraceutical co-crystals. Also in the chapter, we have provided detailed insight into the proposed mechanisms of co-crystallization in different techniques. As co-crystals continue to gain interest and prove their value, the range of demonstrated co-crystal application areas continues to expand. The current chapter also highlights the increasing application of pharmaceutical co-crystals. It is anticipated that co-crystals will become more and more routine in pharmaceutical development as their benefits continue to be demonstrated and routine routes of manufacturing are proven. Since the early 2000s, it was realized that cocrystal engineering may be a potential approach to improve the physicochemical properties of pharmaceuticals, which was contributed to several representative pharmaceutical cocrystal publications. In conclusion, the current chapter emphasizes the role of crystal engineering in pharmaceutical-based cocrystal design. Also by virtue of the current chapter the authors encourage researchers to explore the possibility of creating novel nutraceutical co-crystal for bringing naturally occurring molecules to the forefront of drug designing and development paradigms.

Conflict of interest

The authors declare no conflict of interest.

Author details

Asmita Gajbhiye[1], Debashree Das[1] and Shailendra Patil[2]*

1 Department of Pharmaceutical Sciences, Dr. Harisingh Gour Central University, Sagar, Madhya Pradesh, India

2 SVN Institute of Pharmaceutical Sciences, Swami Vivekanand University, Sagar, Madhya Pradesh, India

*Address all correspondence to: drasmitapatil27@gmail.com

References

[1] Nejatian M, Darabzadeh N, Bodbodak S, Saberian H, Rafiee Z, Kharazmi MS, et al. Practical application of nanoencapsulated nutraceuticals in real food products; a systematic review. Advances in Colloid and Interface Science. 2022:102690

[2] Atanasov AG, Zotchev SB, Dirsch VM, Supuran CT. Natural products in drug discovery: Advances and opportunities. Nature Reviews Drug Discovery. 2022;**20**(3):200-216

[3] Diyabalanage T. 2 plant secondary metabolites as prospective pharmaceuticals and cosmeceuticals. Chemistry of Natural Products: Phytochemistry and Pharmacognosy of Medicinal Plants. 2022;**19**:19

[4] Moore GW. Snake venoms in diagnostic hemostasis and thrombosis. In: Seminars in Thrombosis and Hemostasis. Vol. 48(02). New York, NY, USA: Thieme Medical Publishers, Inc; 2022. pp. 145-160

[5] Dzobo K. The role of natural products as sources of therapeutic agents for innovative drug discovery. Comprehensive Pharmacology. 2022:408. DOI: 10.1016/B978-0-12-820472-6.00041-4

[6] Calixto JB. The role of natural products in modern drug discovery. Anais da Academia Brasileira de Ciências. 2019;**3**:91

[7] Paroha S, Dewangan RP, Dubey RD, Sahoo PK. Conventional and nanomaterial-based techniques to increase the bioavailability of therapeutic natural products: A review. Environmental Chemistry Letters. 2020;**18**(6):1767-1778

[8] Rein MJ, Renouf M, Cruz-Hernandez C, Actis-Goretta L, Thakkar SK, da Silva PM. Bioavailability of bioactive food compounds: A challenging journey to bioefficacy. British Journal of Clinical Pharmacology. 2013;**75**(3):588-602

[9] Da Silva FL, Marques MB, Kato KC, Carneiro G. Nanonization techniques to overcome poor water-solubility with drugs. Expert Opinion on Drug Discovery. 2020;**15**(7):853-864

[10] Guo Z. The modification of natural products for medical use. Acta Pharmaceutica Sinica B. 2017;**7**(2):119-136

[11] Shakya AK. Medicinal plants: Future source of new drugs. International Journal of Herbal Medicine. 2016;**4**(4):59-64

[12] Koehn FE, Carter GT. The evolving role of natural products in drug discovery. Nature Reviews Drug Discovery. 2005;**4**(3):206-220

[13] Sut S, Baldan V, Faggian M, Peron G, DallAcqua S. Nutraceuticals, a new challenge for medicinal chemistry. Current Medicinal Chemistry. 2016;**23**(28):3198-3223

[14] Paterson I, Anderson EA. The renaissance of natural products as drug candidates. Science. 2005;**310**(5747):451-453

[15] Selivanova IA, Terekhov RP. Crystal engineering as a scientific basis for modification of physicochemical properties of bioflavonoids. Russian Chemical Bulletin. 2019;**68**(12):2155-2162

[16] Censi R, Di Martino P. Polymorph impact on the bioavailability and stability of poorly soluble drugs. Molecules. 2015;**20**(10):18759-18776

[17] Wangchuk P, Loukas A. Techniques and technologies for the biodiscovery of novel small molecule drug lead compounds from natural products. In: Natural Products and Drug Discovery. Elsevier Ltd.; 2018. pp. 435-465

[18] Belca LM, Ručigaj A, Teslič D, Krajnc M. The use of ultrasound in the crystallization process of an active pharmaceutical ingredient. Ultrasonics Sonochemistry. 2019;**58**:104642

[19] Gao Y, Zhang T, Ma Y, Xue F, Gao Z, Hou B, et al. Application of PAT-based feedback control approaches in pharmaceutical crystallization. Crystals. 2021;**11**(3):221

[20] Abramov YA, Sun G, Zeng Q. Emerging landscape of computational modeling in pharmaceutical development. Journal of Chemical Information and Modeling. 2022;**62**(5):1160-1171

[21] Panzade PS, Shendarkar GR. Pharmaceutical cocrystal: A game changing approach for the administration of old drugs in new crystalline form. Drug Development and Industrial Pharmacy. 2020;**46**(10):1559-1568

[22] Thakuria R, Sarma B. Drug-drug and drug-nutraceutical cocrystal/salt as alternative medicine for combination therapy: A crystal engineering approach. Crystals. 2018;**8**(2):101

[23] Bolla G, Sarma B, Nangia AK. Crystal engineering of pharmaceutical cocrystals in the discovery and development of improved drugs. Chemical Reviews. 2022;**122**(13):11514-11603

[24] Zaworotko MJ, Clarke H, Kapildev A, Kavuru P, Shytle RD, Pujari T, et al. Nutraceutical co-crystal compositions. 2019. Patent Number: 10376521

[25] Santini A, Novellino E. Nutraceuticals-shedding light on the grey area between pharmaceuticals and food. Expert Review of Clinical Pharmacology. 2018;**11**(6):545-547

[26] Gopi S, Balakrishnan P, editors. Handbook of Nutraceuticals and Natural Products. John Wiley & Sons, Inc.; 2022

[27] Nwosu OK, Ubaoji KI. Nutraceuticals: History, classification and market demand. In: Functional Foods and Nutraceuticals. Cham: Springer; 2020. pp. 13-22

[28] Malik A, Rana S, Alam MS, Kumar M, Singh R, Kumar P, et al. The potential role of nutraceutical in health and disease. International Journal of Pharmacy and Biological Sciences-IJPBS. 2019;**9**(1):763-771

[29] Manocha S, Dhiman S, Grewal AS, Guarve K. Nanotechnology: An approach to overcome bioavailability challenges of nutraceuticals. Journal of Drug Delivery Science and Technology. 2022;**18**:103418

[30] Thipparaboina R, Kumar D, Chavan RB, Shastri NR. Multidrug co-crystals: Towards the development of effective therapeutic hybrids. Drug Discovery Today. 2016;**21**(3):481-490

[31] Yarlagadda DL, Anand VS, Nair AR, Sree KN, Dengale SJ, Bhat K. Considerations for the selection of co-formers in the preparation of co-amorphous formulations. International Journal of Pharmaceutics. 2021;**602**:120649

[32] Qiao N, Li M, Schlindwein W, Malek N, Davies A, Trappitt G. Pharmaceutical cocrystals: An overview. International Journal of Pharmaceutics. 2011;**419**(1-2):1-1

[33] Vemuri VD, Lankalapalli S. Insight into concept and progress on pharmaceutical co-crystals: An overview. Indian Journal of Pharmaceutical Education and Research. 2019;**53**:522-538

[34] Wood PA, Feeder N, Furlow M, Galek PT, Groom CR, Pidcock E. Knowledge-based approaches to co-crystal design. CrystEngComm. 2014;**16**(26):5839-5848

[35] Nagy S, Pál S, Széchenyi A. Reliability of the Hansen solubility parameters as co-crystal formation prediction tool. International Journal of Pharmaceutics. 2019;**558**:319-327

[36] Srirambhatla VK, Kraft A, Watt S, Powell AV. Crystal design approaches for the synthesis of paracetamol co-crystals. Crystal Growth & Design. 2012;**12**(10):4870-4879

[37] Blagden N, Berry DJ, Parkin A, Javed H, Ibrahim A, Gavan PT, et al. Current directions in co-crystal growth. New Journal of Chemistry. 2008;**32**(10):1659-1672

[38] Gao Z, Rohani S, Gong J, Wang J. Recent developments in the crystallization process: Toward the pharmaceutical industry. Engineering. 2017;**3**(3):343-353

[39] Gallagher PK, Cheng SZ. Applications to Polymers and Plastics. Amsterdam: Elsevier Science BV; 2002

[40] Ngilirabanga JB, Samsodien H. Pharmaceutical co-crystal: An alternative strategy for enhanced physicochemical properties and drug synergy. Nano Select. 2021;**2**(3):512-526

[41] Nadkarni A. Development of high-throughput approaches for the phage display generation and production of recombinant antibody fragments for macromolecular co-crystallization [doctoral dissertation]. University of Georgia;

[42] Marin L, Bejan A, Shova S. Phenothiazine based co-crystals with enhanced luminescence. Dyes and Pigments. 2020;**175**:108164

[43] Mazzeo PP, Prencipe M, Feiler T, Emmerling F, Bacchi A. On the mechanism of cocrystal mechanochemical reaction via low melting eutectic: A time-resolved in situ monitoring investigation. Crystal Growth & Design. 2022;**22**(7):4260-4267

[44] Thayyil AR, Juturu T, Nayak S, Kamath S. Pharmaceutical co-crystallization: Regulatory aspects, design, characterization, and applications. Advanced Pharmaceutical Bulletin. 2020;**10**(2):203

[45] Kuminek G, Cao F, de Oliveira B, da Rocha A, Gonçalves Cardoso S, Rodríguez-Hornedo N. Cocrystals to facilitate delivery of poorly soluble compounds beyond-rule-of-5. Advanced Drug Delivery Reviews. 2016;**101**:143-166

[46] Etter MC. Encoding and decoding hydrogen-bond patterns of organic compounds. Accounts of Chemical Research. 1990;**23**(4):120-126

[47] Şen N, Dursun H, Hope KS, Nazir H, Acar N, Atakol O. Towards low-impact-sensitivity through crystal engineering: New energetic co-crystals formed between picric acid, trinitrotoluene and 9-Vinylanthracene. Journal of Molecular Structure. 2020;**1219**:128614

[48] Karimi-Jafari M, Padrela L, Walker GM, Croker DM. Creating cocrystals: A review of pharmaceutical cocrystal preparation routes and applications. Crystal Growth & Design. 2018;**18**(10):6370-6387

[49] Friscic T, Jones W. Recent advances in understanding the mechanism of cocrystal formation via grinding. Crystal Growth and Design. 2009;**9**(3):1621-1637

[50] Chezanoglou E, Goula AM. Co-crystallization in sucrose: A promising

method for encapsulation of food bioactive components. Trends in Food Science & Technology. 2021;**114**:262-274

[51] Press NJ, Joly E, Ertl P. Natural product drug delivery: A special challenge? In: Progress in Medicinal Chemistry. Vol. 58. Elsevier B.V.; 2019. pp. 157-187

[52] Jain H, Chella N. Methods to improve the solubility of therapeutical natural products: A review. Environmental Chemistry Letters. 2021;**19**(1):111-121

[53] Li Z, Zhao T, Li J, Yu Q, Feng Y, Xie Y, et al. Nanomedicine based on natural products: Improving clinical application potential. Journal of Nanomaterials. 2022;**2022**

[54] Mannava MC, Bommaka MK, Dandela R, Solomon KA, Nangia AK. Fluorobenzoic acid co-formers to improve the solubility and permeability of the BCS class IV drug naftopidil. Chemical Communications. 2022;**58**(37):5582-5585

[55] Mureşan-Pop M, Chiriac LB, Martin F, Simon S. Novel nutraceutical Myricetin composite of enhanced dissolution obtained by co-crystallization with acetamide. Composites Part B: Engineering. 2016;**89**:60-66

[56] Muthukrishnan L. Nanonutraceuticals—Challenges and novel nano-based carriers for effective delivery and enhanced bioavailability. Food and Bioprocess Technology. 2022:1-30

[57] Chadha R et al. Cocrystallization in nutraceuticals. In: Glebovsky V, editor. Recrystallization in Materials Processing. London: IntechOpen; 2015. DOI: 10.5772/59365

[58] Formica JV, Regelson W. Review of the biology of quercetin and related bioflavonoids. Food and Chemical Toxicology. 1995;**33**(12):1061-1080

[59] Athiyah U, Kusuma PA, Tutik T, Lestari ML, Isadiartuti D, Paramita DP, et al. Crystal engineering of quercetin by liquid assisted grinding method. Jurnal Teknologi. 2019;**81**(1)

[60] de Oliveira JM, Santos C, Fernandes E. Therapeutic potential of hesperidin and its aglycone hesperetin: Cell cycle regulation and apoptosis induction in cancer models. Phytomedicine. 2020;**73**:152887

[61] Chadha K, Karan M, Bhalla Y, Chadha R, Khullar S, Mandal S, et al. Cocrystals of hesperetin: Structural, pharmacokinetic, and pharmacodynamic evaluation. Crystal Growth & Design. 2017;**17**(5):2386-2405

[62] Bethune SJ, Schultheiss N, Henck JO. Improving the poor aqueous solubility of nutraceutical compound pterostilbene through cocrystal formation. Crystal Growth & Design. 2011;**11**(7):2817-2823

[63] Bevill MJ, Vlahova PI, Smit JP. Polymorphic cocrystals of nutraceutical compound p-coumaric acid with nicotinamide: Characterization, relative solid-state stability, and conversion to alternate stoichiometries. Crystal Growth & Design. 2014;**14**(3):1438-1448

[64] Sathisaran I, Dalvi SV. Crystal engineering of curcumin with salicylic acid and hydroxyquinol as co-formers. Crystal Growth & Design. 2017;**17**(7):3974-3988

[65] Sanphui P, Goud NR, Khandavilli UBR, Nangia A. Fast dissolving curcumin cocrystals. Crystal Growth & Design. 2011;**11**(9):4135-4145

[66] Khan FM, Ahmad M, Batool F. Enhancement of solubility and release profile of simvastatin by co-crystallization with citric acid. Tropical Journal of Pharmaceutical Research. 2019;**18**(12):2465-2472

[67] Naqvi A, Ahmad M, Minhas MU, Khan KU, Batool F, Rizwan A. Preparation and evaluation of pharmaceutical co-crystals for solubility enhancement of atorvastatin calcium. Polymer Bulletin. 2020;**77**(12):6191-6211

[68] Hall AV, Chambers LI, Musa OM, Steed JW. Cocrystals, co-amorphous phases and coordination complexes of γ- and ε-lactams. In: Handbook of Pyrrolidone and Caprolactam Based Materials: Synthesis, Characterization and Industrial Applications. Vol. 6. 2021. pp. 1171-1237

[69] Liu L, Yu YM, Bu FZ, Li YT, Yan CW, Wu ZY. The first co-crystallization of milrinone with nutraceuticals: The adjusting effects of hydrophilicity/hydrophobicity in cavities on the *in-vitro/in-vivo* properties of the cocrystals. Crystal Growth & Design. 2022;**22**(3):1623-1637

Chapter 14

Co-Crystallization of Plant-Derived Antimalarial Drugs: An Alternate Technique for Improved Physicochemical Qualities and Antimalarial Drug Synergy

Zakio Makuvara

Abstract

Malaria is a complex disease associated with a variety of epidemiology and clinical symptoms worldwide. Despite the availability of a variety of antimalarial medications, national policies of many countries advocate for a single-medication first-line therapy for the majority of clinical malaria symptoms. However, the studies revealed that using multiple first-line medicines against malaria works more effectively. In this scenario, single-target monotherapy approaches have difficulties since malaria symptoms are seldom caused by single molecular entities. The current work is based on the critical literature review and primary sources as well as secondary databases. The chapter outline is as follows: (1) main antimalarial plant-derived active pharmaceutical ingredients (APD-APIs), (2) limitations of single APD-APIs and shift to multiple first-line therapies in malaria treatment, (3) techniques in the development and properties of APD-APIs co-crystals. The search for novel plant-derived antimalarial medicines and the development of antimalarial co-crystals are essential in the fight against antimalarial drug resistance.

Keywords: antimalarial drugs, mono-therapy, multiple first-line treatments, co-crystallization, plant-derived antimalarial drugs

1. Introduction

Malaria deaths and cases have decreased dramatically in the last 15 years, yet it remains one of the leading tropical diseases in terms of reported deaths [1]. Accordingly, the World Health Organization (WHO) recorded up to 216 million cases of malaria and about 445,000 deaths in 2016 only [1]. Development of antimalarial medicine resistance, as well as dramatically diminished sensitivity to artemisinin combination therapy (ACT), is the primary cause of this trend [2–6]. Apart from

IntechOpen

that, the chemotherapeutic choices for treating and preventing malaria are limited [4]. In light of these circumstances, novel antimalarial drug discovery, particularly medicines associated with multiple mode of action and versatility in terms of efficacy against resistant *Plasmodia* spp., is critical. Surprisingly, due to poor physicochemical characteristics and pharmacokinetic profiles, many novel prospective antimalarial medicines are overlooked [7, 8]. In accordance with this, novel studies are being performed on the prospect of producing antimalarial salts and co-crystals [4]. The fundamental goal of these investigations is to enhance the physiochemical characteristics of antimalarial medicines without interfering with their bioactivity [9–11].

The search for APD-APIs is motivated by previous studies, which have revealed the existence of two important plant-based antimalarial drugs (1) quinine and (2) artemisinin from *Cinchona* spp. stem bark and *Artemisia annua*, respectively [12–14]. It is envisaged that bioprospecting of existing enormous plant biodiversity can come up with novel antimalarial drugs. More importantly, the quest for novel plant-based antimalarial drugs is based on ethnopharmacological studies, which are critical in drug development and discovery [15]. The basic idea in an ethnopharmacological study in this case is to come up with inexpensive and easily used antimalarial therapies, which subsequently limit the cost of drug discovery and development research [16–18]. However, only approximate of 6 and 15% of all land plants have been analyzed for pharmacological activity and have an elucidated phytochemistry, respectively [17]. The main reasons for considering APD-APIs in malaria treatment include low cost, effectiveness, easy availability, safety, and cultural preferences [19].

Interestingly, plants are important sources of APIs, which can be utilized in treatment and prevention many human health problems including malaria [17]. Generally, up to 25% of known plant species are exploited in medicine production worldwide and approximately 65% of the global population count on plants for their basic health care [20, 21]. These plants have been identified as rich sources of template compounds for synthesis of other important drugs and in the prevention as well as fight against many infectious diseases including malaria. In the case of malaria, two lead antimalarial drugs, quinine and artemisinin, have been utilized as derivatives of chloroquine and artemether, respectively. Additionally, antimalarial drugs such as primaquine, amodiaquine, and mefloquine are synthesized based on quinine and in antimalarial drugs including arteether, and sodium artesunate, where artemisinin is the lead compound [7, 22]. Plants are associated with potential antimalarial APIs classified into major groups including flavonoids, alkaloids, glycosides, terpenoids, and phenolic acids [23].

Co-crystals are solid compounds that show promise in drug development, particularly in terms of improving physicochemical properties such as drug solubility. Generally, co-crystals are formed due to the interactions between (1) active pharmaceutical ingredients (APIs) and (2) co-crystals forming agents (normally solid under ambient conditions) [24, 25]. Normally, H-bond holds the two components of co-crystals, and this is facilitated by functional groups of APIs, e.g., carboxylic acid functional group. Moreover, APIs are associated with other function groups such as amine and amide groups [26]. Co-crystallization is performed under relatively mild reaction conditions. The techniques for preparing co-crystals are classified into (1) solid-state and (2) solution-based [27–30].

Despite the various studies that have been conducted on a wide range of pharmacological molecules, plant-derived antimalarial drug molecules appear to have been neglected [10]. Many current antimalarial drugs are becoming ineffective owing to the drug resistance. For instance, *Plasmodium spp.* and *Plasmodium falciparum* have shown resistance to the antimalarial quinine derivatives such as chloroquine and an increase in resistance to the artemisinin-based therapies, respectively [2, 3]. The aim of this chapter is to explore multicomponent crystal structures utilization in antimalarial treatment and review the literature that addresses the feasibility of this therapeutic option. Up to date, there is no structured literature that relates to the co-crystallization of APD-APIs. Therefore, this chapter identifies the research gaps and outlines (1) APD-APIs, (2) limitations of single APD-APIs in the treatment of malaria, (3) techniques in the development and properties of APD-APIs co-crystals.

2. Summary of main APD-APIs

According to Ungogo [31], statistics for pharmaceuticals authorized by the U.S Food and Drug Administration (1981–2010) suggested that around 35% of approved new medicines were derived from natural sources, with plants-derived drugs contributing 25%. Phenolics, quinones, alkaloids, saponins, terpenes, and their derivatives are examples of APD-APIs. Notably, these APD-APIs can be utilized as both crude phytomedicines and pure pharmaceuticals. They can, nevertheless, serve as basis for the production of synthetic pharmacologically complex active compounds, models for designing lead molecules, and taxonomic markers for the discovery of novel drugs [31].

2.1 Alkaloids

Alkaloids are a group of diverse plant secondary metabolites characterized by a basic nitrogen associated with a carbon ring [32]. The classification of these APD-APIs is on the basis of the principal C-N skeleton, and in certain instances, classification is according to biological origin. Using the first classification system, alkaloids are classified into 13 classes: pyrroles, pyrrolines, pyrrolidines, pyrrolizidines, indoles, pyridines, pyrimidines, piperidines, quinolones, isoquinolines, quinolizidines, tropanes, and imidazoles [31]. Antimalarial alkaloids have been reported in several studies, for instance, Iwu and keayman [33] isolated alkaloids (which are antimalarial) from *Picralima nitida* fruits. The authors reported IC50 values in the range 1.6–2.4 μg/ml when crude dichloromethane extracts were tested for antiplasmodial action. Additionally, indole alkaloids including akuammicine and alstonine were isolated with aid of chromatographic technique, and these alkaloids were inhibitory against *P. falciparum* strains (1) D6 and (2) W2 as indicated by IC50 values ranging from 0.01 to 0.9 μg/ml [5]. More recently, *Holarrhena africana* bark and leaves' alkaloid fractions showed antiplasmodial activity (**Figure 1**) [34].

2.2 Terpenoids

Terpenoids are compounds of plant essential oils and terpene hydrocarbons derivatives, and according to [35], these APD-APIs are classified into eight categories: monoterpenoids, diterpenoids, triterpenoids, tetraterpenoids, hemiterpenoids, sesquiterpenoids, sesterterpenoids, and polyterpenoids. Notably, in several studies, terpenoids were identified in antimalarial plant essential oils [35–38], and most of the plants from which essential oils are extracted have been exploited as traditional antimalarial and antipyretic medicines [39]. One of the most common antimalarial terpenoids is artemisinin, which is classified as sesquiterpenoid. This sesquiterpenoid (artemisinin) as well as bioactive compounds derived from this antimalarial is highly antimalarial especially against *P. falciparum* that is chloroquine-resistant.

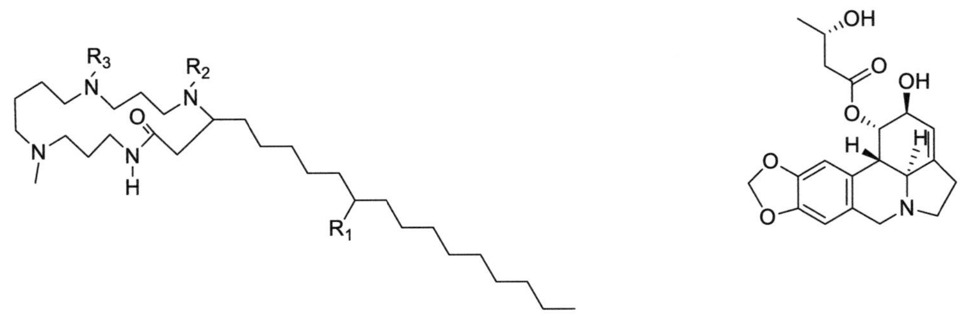

Figure 1.
Some examples of the antimalarial alkaloids.

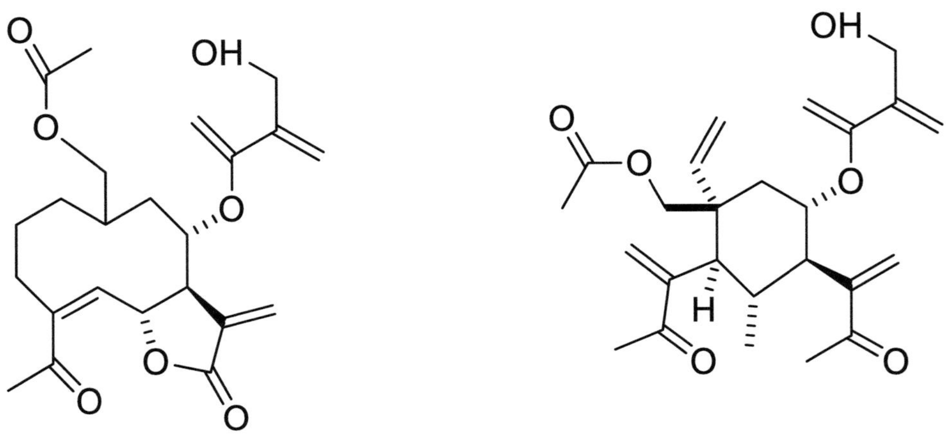

Figure 2.
Some examples of the antimalarial terpenoids.

A study by [40] identified several diterpenoids, for example, (13S)-ent-7β-hydroxy3-cleroden-15-oic acid and (13S)-ent-18-(E)-coumaroyloxy-8(17)-labden-15-oic acid from a plant, *Nuxia sphaerocephala* in Madagascar. The identified diterpenoids were antiplasmodial as indicated by IC50 values ranging from 4.3 to 21.0 μgml^{-1} against FcB1 *P. falciparum*. Several studies have identified different classes of plant derived terpenoids and their antimalarial activities (**Figure 2**) [40–45].

2.3 Quinones

Quinones are normally classed on the basis of their molecular structure, and accordingly, they are classified into three major groups: anthraquinones, benzoquinones, naphthoquinones. The three classes of quinones are aromatic ring based where anthraquinones, benzoquinones, and naphthoquinones have linear/angular anthracene ring, benzene ring, and naphthalenic ring, respectively [46]. Benzoquinones were isolated and had a substantial *in vitro* antimalarial action especially against strains of *P. falciparum* in a number of studies [47–49]. Recent studies on antimicrobial activity of quinones-rich *Aspidosperma nitidum* indicated strong *in vitro* antimalarial efficacy against W2 strain of *P. falciparum* and *P. berghei* in vivo respectively [50].

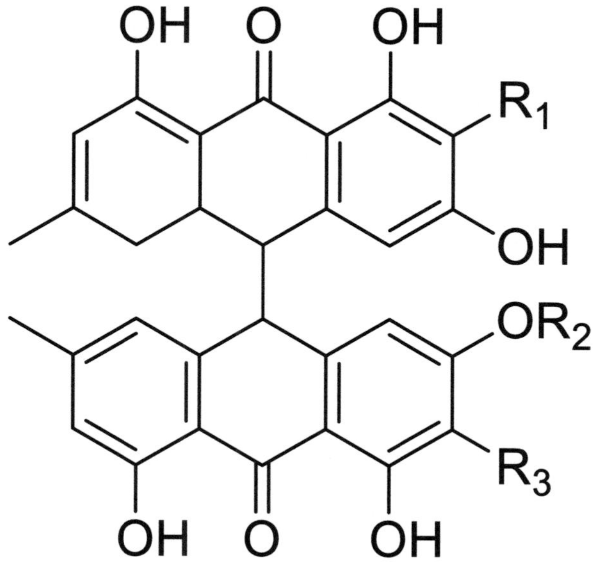

Figure 3.
Some examples of the antimalarial quinones.

Naphthoquinones such as atovaquone were identified and have shown antimalarial activity due to their quinonic nature [51, 52]. Plant-based quinones including 2-acetylnaphtho-[2,3b]-furan-4,9-dione and plumbagin high activity against *P. berghei* (IC50 = 0.002 μgml^{-1}) and *P. falciparum* (IC50 = 0.05 μgml^{-1}) respectively (**Figure 3**) [50, 53, 54].

2.4 Phenolics

Phenolic compounds are considered highly abundant group of plant metabolites. These metabolites are classified into three major groups: flavonoids (polyphenolic compounds, which exist as aglycones, methylated derivatives, and glucosides in plants), phenolic acids (e.g., hydroxybenzoic and hydroxycinnamic acids), and polyphenols [55, 56]. Additionally, these APD-APIs are characterized by a hydroxyl group bonded to an aromatic hydrocarbon group, with the most basic being a phenol (C_6H_5OH). Phenolics include lignins and tannins (polyphenolic compounds with high molecular weight) such as hydrolyzable and condensed tannins. Classification of phenolics is normally based on three methods: (1) number of hydroxylic groups, (2) chemical composition, and (3) number of aromatic rings as well as number of carbon atoms in the side chain [56]. Generally, phenolic compounds are rarely in a free form in plants, and therefore, they exist as glycosylates and polyphenols [55–57]. Phenolic compounds such as ellagic acid have shown significant degree of activity against malaria parasites, for example, [58] reported antimalarial activity of ellagic acid against *Plasmodium vinckei*. The presence of the phenolics in plants used traditionally against malaria has been noted in several of experimental reports [59–61]. The *Artocarpus styracifolius* (Moraceae) ethyl acetate extract (10 μg/ml) containing flavonoids (polyphenol) inactivated FcB1 *P. falciparum* significantly [62, 63]. According to [62], prenylated flavonoids including artoheterophyllin displayed high activity against *P. falciparum* strain FcB1 (IC50 = 4.797 μM) (**Figure 4**).

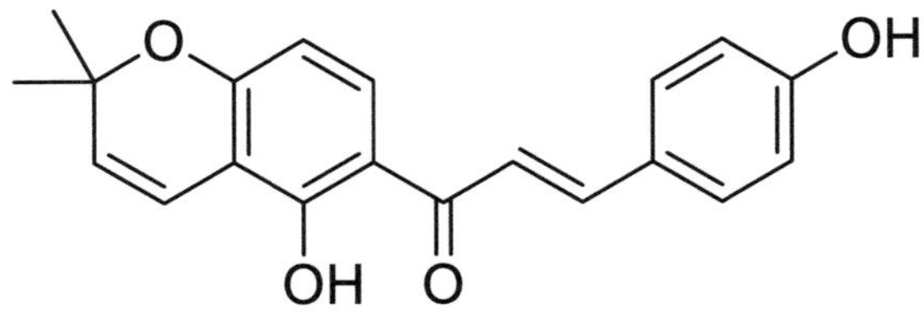

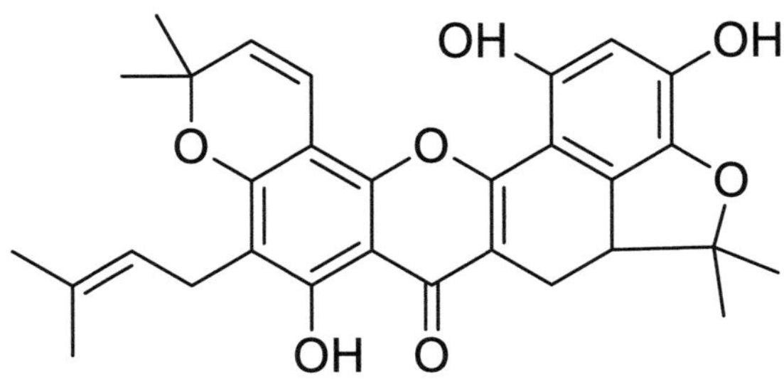

Figure 4.
Structural summary of some of the antimalarial phenolics.

3. Limitations of single APD-APIs and shift to multiple first-line therapies in the treatment of malaria

3.1 Limitations of single APD-APIs in malaria treatment

The treatment of malaria is basically based on natural products, for example, APD-APIs, semisynthetic and synthetic compounds. Effective and safe antimalarial drugs are broadly classified into three main categories: (1) quinoline derivatives, (2) antifolates, and (3) artemisinin derivatives [64]. The first identified and widely used APD-APIs was quinine, an alkaloid. Notably, quinine was extracted from the *Cinchona calisaya* bark [65] and was used as first-line monotherapy. However, this antimalarial drug was exploited in the synthesis of a number of derivatives including 8-aminoquinoline (primaquine) and 4-aminoquinoline (chloroquine) [65, 66]. These derivatives of quinine were shown to eliminate malaria parasites through preventing biotransformation of heme, into nontoxic pigment granules, and therefore allowing heme to accumulate and promote cell lysis as well as Plasmodia auto-digestion [66]. Though quinine was an effective APD-API, development of resistance among *P. falciparum* strains and high toxicity has significantly contributed to its limited use. Additionally, this alkaloid (quinine) has a fairly short pharmacological half-life [66, 67]. However, use of quinine combined with other antimalarial drugs (in order to improve therapeutic efficacy) against malaria has been reported [12, 64].

The derivative of quinine, 8-aminoquinoline (primaquine), was utilized as a monotherapy against malaria during the first part of the twentieth century. However, it was disregarded due to abnormally elevated toxicity associated with highly reduced activity [64]. The other antimalarial drugs, which were widely exploited as first-monotherapy after abandonment of primaquine, include quinacrine, a derivative of acridine. Another derivative of quinine, a 4-aminoquinoline, chloroquine was later used as a first-line monotherapy against malaria for several years due to its efficacy, low as well as manageable side effects, and low cost [68]. Being the first-line monotherapy for a long period of time, chloroquine has led to *P. falciparum* strains, which are chloroquine-resistant [36]. Other quinine derivatives used as first-line monotherapies and are linked to several adverse effects and emergence of resistance include pyronaridine and mefloquine [69]. Although chloroquine significantly reduced malaria-related mortality and morbidity, its prolonged use has resulted in spread of resistance. For instance, cases of chloroquine resistance were reported in countries including Brazil, Thailand, and Vietnam by 1964 [70, 71]. Furthermore, according WHO reports of 1979 and 1981, chloroquine resistance was reported to have covered most parts of North-East India, South America, and Southeast Asia by 1980 [71].

Though not plant-derived, pyrimethamine was widely utilized as an antimalarial monotherapy in early 1950 and late 1960 as a prophylactic and treatment drug. Due to resistance of malarial parasite against pyrimethamine, pyrimethamine was combined with sulfadoxine to produce a more efficient antimalarial drug, sulfadoxine-pyrimethamine (SP) [71]. This antimalarial drug was recommended as a first-line drug in many countries associated with chloroquine inactivity [72, 73]. Although for some time, resistance to pyrimethamine was inhibited by sulfadoxine, inactivity of sulfadoxine to malaria parasites was finally reported in African and Asian countries [71–73]. This prompted the use of artemisinin, an antimalarial drug, which was discovered from an important plant, *Artemisia annua* in the year 1972 [74]. Artemisinin is an APD-API classified under terpenoids and is specifically a sesquiterpene lactone [75]. This APD-API has been identified to be effective against blood as well as *P. falciparum* gametocyte stages [76].

The use of artemisinin as monotherapy has been noted in many regions including western part of Cambodia, and clinical studies in these regions have shown emerging *P. falciparum* strains, which are resistant to artemisinin [77]. Apart from reports of resistance of *P. falciparum* strains to artemisinin, artemisinin is inherently linked to solubility and bioavailability challenges [78, 79]. This, therefore, has resulted in the synthesis of quite a number of artemisinin derivatives with varying degrees of solubilities in oil and water [78–80]. The most common synthetic artemisinin derivatives include artemether, dihydroartemisinin, artesunate, and arteether. Based on their solubilities in water and oil, they are administered into the patient using different routes, for instance, artemether and dihydroartemisinin, which are oil- and water-soluble, are intramuscularly and administered orally administered, respectively [78]. In the face of this improvement, artemisinin derivatives are quickly absorbed, distributed, and metabolized.

Artemisinin and its derivatives including artesunate are characterized by being quick-acting and rapid blood parasite reduction. However, this effectiveness is hampered by a rise of artemisinin-resistant *P. falciparum* as described in nations including western Cambodia, Myanmar, Viet Nam, and Thailand [5, 78, 81]. Additionally, reports of decreased sensitivity to artemisinin of *P. falciparum* isolates have been made in Nigeria and Madagascar [82]. A number of malaria patients from countries such as Sierra Leone, India, and western Thailand took time to respond to artemisinin derivatives including artesunate and artemether [78, 83, 84]. Furthermore, the use of these antimalarial drugs as first-line monotherapy is associated with maintenance of an effective drug concentration for a short period after drug administration. In addition to this, short oral treatment courses have contributed to increased rates of recrudescence [66, 71, 85]. An increase in the number days of days of treatment to 7 has significantly reduced recurrent parasitemia, when artemisinin or its derivatives are utilized as monotherapy [74, 77, 85]. Generally, insensitivity to conventional antimalarial monotherapy including artemisinin as well as artemisinin-derived drugs has contributed significantly to antimalarial monotherapies being overlooked and disregarded [86]. Thus, a number of techniques are being explored globally to enhance potency of antimalarial drugs especially plant-derived ones and significantly interrupt parasite resistance to these drugs.

3.2 Shift to multiple first-line therapies in malaria treatment

Shift from monotherapy to multiple first-line therapies in malaria treatment, e.g., use of artemisinin-based combination therapy (ACTs) has been exploited as an intervention to alleviate resistance to several antimalarial monotherapies [87], and according to [88], the adoption of ACTs was as a result of occurrence of resistance to oral artemisinin monotherapies. ACTs are produced by combining artemisinin derivatives with complimentary partner drugs, and the net effects of combining these drugs are: (1) rapid action and short period of treatment due to artemisinin derivatives and (2) prevention of recrudescence due to the partner drug [71, 89, 90]. It is against this background that WHO recommended the use of ACTs in the early 2000s in countries that had prevalence of *Plasmodium falciparum* strains that were highly resistant to the conventional available antimalarials [85, 91]. To date, ACTs continue to be among the most effective globally and remain a highly acclaimed first-line treatment for all cases of basic malaria [92]. The recommended ACTs include artemether/lumefantrine and dihydroartemisinin/piperaquine [93]. The efficacy of the artemisinins has been reported to be based on their activity, which have been improved by utilized synthetic artemisinin dimers, trimers, as well as tetramers without interfering with the peroxide bridge [94]. Generally, improving ACTs activity improves efficacy and postpone the development of resistance to malarial parasites. Although ACTs have been characterized with high curative activity, reports of *P. falciparum* strains with elevated resistance to ACTs have been presented in the Greater Mekong Region [95]. Faced with resistance against ACTs, some regions have adopted triple artemisinin-based combination therapy (TACT against multidrug resistant *P. falciparum* while awaiting registration of novel antimalarial drugs [96]. The efficacy of TACT is based on molecular antimalarial resistance mechanisms, which indicate counter-selection of antimalarial resistance by frequently utilized drugs, (1) piperaquine and (2) mefloquine [93].

4. Techniques in the development and properties of APD-APIs co-crystals

4.1 Techniques for development of co-crystals

Despite the fact that there are several APD-APIs, they lack key pharmacological activities due to poor physicochemical qualities such as low bioavailability, stability, and solubility [97]. Nanoparticles, co-crystallization, liposomal formulations, chemical changes, and changing ADP-APIs into solids such as polymorphs, salts, and hydrates are just a few of the strategies that may be employed to improve physical characteristics of ADP-APIs [98]. Co-crystallization has been praised for its effectiveness in increasing the pharmacological characteristics of APD-APIs. The use of co-crystallization to adjust the physical features of APD-APIs is excellent since co-crystals are not considered as new medications by the US Food and Drug Administration, but rather pro-drugs [99]. Although co-crystallization of APD-APIs improves their biopharmaceutical and physicochemical traits, there is need to screen APD-APIs based co-crystals. The screening of co-crystals efficiency is basically based on emerging techniques including quantitative structure-activity, Hansen solubility parameters calculation, and pKa rule [100, 101].

Co-crystallization involves dissolving APIs and respective coformers in an appropriate solvent at a predetermined stoichiometric ratio and the solvent is then removed to saturate of solutes for co-crystal production [25, 26]. This therefore implies that co-crystallization is based on slow solvent evaporation as well as reaction co-crystallization and slurry and antisolvent diffusion [12, 28]. Basically, co-crystallization is dependent on strong H-bonds between APIs and their respective coformers, thereby facilitating co-crystal formation [27, 29]. Notably, co-crystallization under the solution-based technique can be effectively achieved if the least soluble component is prevented from sole precipitation, and co-crystals' purity can be improved by selecting APIs and coformers with congruent solubilities [28–30]. In addition to this, other factors such as solvent systems, stoichiometric ratio, and crystallization temperature influence co-crystallization process [29]. Costa et al. [102] reported that co-crystal structures from APIs and coformers with similar shapes and polarities co-crystallize easily with each other.

In addition to solution-based technique, solid-state grinding can be applied, and this involves homogenizing APIs and coformers in mortar to prepare co-crystals using mechanical techniques [29, 102]. Solid-state grinding techniques (SSGTs) are based on and depend on molecular mobility and existence complementarity between APIs and coformers [26–30]. Preparation of co-crystals may involve addition of small quantities of solvents before grinding of APIs and coformers, where the solvent facilitates co-crystal formation. This technique is called liquid-assisted method and is highly efficient in the formation of co-crystals [26–30]. APIs (bioactive compounds) generated from antimalarial plants are essential and have received attention in drug discovery and development. However, due to their poor physicochemical and biological qualities, such as solubility, stability, and dissolution performance, the large proportion of antimalarial plant-derived APIs (APD-APIs), such as alkaloids, flavonoids, phenolic acids, and terpenoids, are disregarded [19, 21, 23]. These PDADs-APIs supply a lot of hydrogen bond donors and acceptors for co-crystal formation, which makes it possible for APD-APIs and coformers to interact [29, 102]. Co-crystallization of these APD-APIs with coformers provides distinct advantages in terms of modulating physicochemical features of these compounds while avoiding covalent interactions that might compromise their therapeutic potential [27–29]. These PDADs-APIs supply a lot of hydrogen bond donors and acceptors for co-crystal formation, which makes it possible for APD-APIs and coformers to interact [102].

Co-crystallization can be applied to the production of multicomponent solids with more than two APIs. This combination of APIs has recently improved physical properties of individual APIs and reduced the number of doses given to a patient [103, 104]. It has, however, noted that formulation of APIs-APIs combinations is associated with inherent challenges including chemical interactions, instability, and variations in solubility of different APIs [105]. Though APIs-APIs combinations could potentially address the issues around antimalarial resistance, there is dearth of published information on APIs-APIs co-crystals. As indicated for other APIs-APIs co-crystals, APD-APIs- APD-APIs combinations are presumed to have synergistic as well as additive effects and enhanced bioavailability, among other advantages of biopharmaceuticals (**Figure 5**).

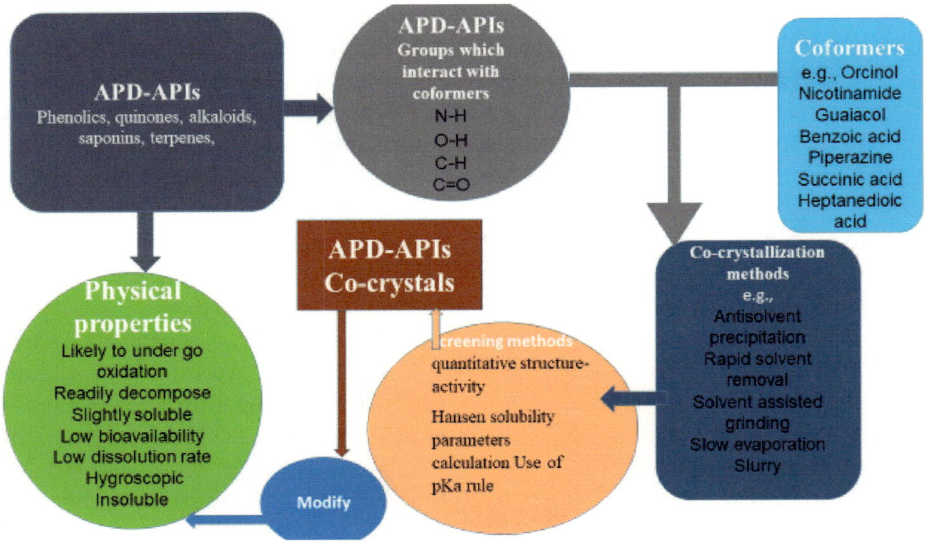

Figure 5.
Theoretical outline of the formation of APD-APIs co-crystals.

4.2 Properties of APD-APIs co-crystals

APD-APIs have poor physicochemical qualities, and their combination with coformers to produce co-crystals considerably improves a variety of attributes including thermal stability, solubility, and hygroscopicity [106]. The alteration of these APD-APIs affects therapeutic action while retaining pharmacological properties [97]. An overview of the key attributes of both APD-APIs and APD-APIs co-crystals is outlined in this section.

4.2.1 Thermal stability

Thermal stability is a critical feature for any APD-API or APD-API co-crystal. However, most APD-APIs have low thermal stability, and modifying these APD-APIs into APD-API co-crystals has demonstrated to enhance overall stability [107]. Notably, APD-APIs that easily sublime at room temperature inevitably result in drug loss during manufacture and storage. According to Lu et al. [108], the conversion of APD-APIs into APD-API co-crystals such as 2,6-dihydroxybenzoic acid has greatly increased thermal stability, as evidenced by results of study using differential scanning calorimetry and the thermogravimetric analysis method. When compared with APD-API, dihydroartemisinin, which sublimes at a relatively low temperature, co-crystals such as 2,6-dihydroxybenzoic acid have a higher sublimation temperature above 100°C, indicating a better degree of thermal stability [108].

4.2.2 Solubility

APD-APIs are often either slightly soluble or insoluble, which limits their application as biopharmaceuticals. The modification of these APD-APIs into co-crystals may be crucial, as several studies have shown that co-crystals can maintain stability while also enhancing solubility [109]. In most circumstances, it has been noted that selecting highly soluble coformers can increase co-crystal solubility. For example, in the production of certain APD-APIs co-crystals, extremely soluble coformers such as succinic acid and benzoic acid have been used [110].

4.2.3 Hygroscopicity

Because of the presence of free functional groups such as hydroxyl groups, most APD-APIs, including phenols, are very unstable at high relative humidity (have high hygroscopicity) [111]. Wong et al. [112], on the other hand, claim that the interaction between APD-API and their respective coformers during crystallization processes increases stability at high relative humidity. Curcumin-resorcinol co-crystals, for example, have been demonstrated to be very stable at high (95%) relative humidity as compared with curcumin, which quickly absorbs moisture at 75% relative humidity [113]. The interaction between the APD-API functional groups and those of the coformers, resulting in intermolecular interactions, is correlated to the stability of APD-API co-crystals at high (95%) relative humidity (low hygroscopicity) [114]. The presence of these intermolecular connections in APD-API co-crystals inhibits the interaction between moisture and APD-API functional groups [111]. This basically means that when the interactions between coformers and APD-APIs increase, the barrier to moisture absorption of APD-API co-crystals falls dramatically.

NB the other important properties of APD-APIs, which are modified in order to improve their efficacy through co-crystallization production, include bioavailability, dissolution, and tabletability [112].

5. Challenges and opportunities associated with development of co-crystallized antimalarial drugs from APD-APIs

Notably, APD-APIs are divided into two categories: (1) potential compounds for natural medicine production and (2) templates for artificially synthesized pharmaceuticals [115]. The quest for novel plant-derived antimalarial drugs, as well as the development of phytomedicines in general, is, however, inherently associated with two major obstacles, (1) existence of extremely active plant compounds with complicated molecular structures, where no feasible industrial production is envisaged, and (2) presence of APD-APIs with relatively reduced activity yet with relatively simple molecular structures, for which artificial production could be conducted [115, 116]. With notable examples of naturally occurring ADP-APIs, the development of novel antimalarial drugs is without. Although various powerful plant-derived antiplasmodial compounds have been documented, the majority of them have only been assessed in vitro, with few being evaluated for toxicity and even fewer being evaluated in vivo [117, 118]. Furthermore, most of them seem to be present in low quantities in plants and are frequently found as part of complicated composites, making separation and processing extremely costly. Among other factors, scientific evaluation of traditional ADP-APIs is limited by paucity of ethnobotany information [115, 117].

6. Conclusion and outlook

Though co-crystallization is a critical technique of improving therapeutic potential of pharmaceutically poor APD-APIs, there are several changes associated with APD-APIs co-crystal production including identification of suitable coformers and appropriate methods of production. However, like any other co-crystals, APD-APIs co-crystals are presumed to improve physical and pharmaceutical properties of ADP-APIs. APD-APIs such as phenolic acids and terpenoids have been shown to provide important functional groups, which allows for the formation of non-covalent intermolecular associations with a number of coformers during co-crystallization processes. In this chapter, information on pharmaceutical applications of APD-APIs co-crystals is summarized. With more research and clinical studies, co-crystallization of APD-APIs into single and multi-component molecules could provide the basis for malaria treatment.

Conflict of interest

The authors declare no conflict of interest.

Author details

Zakio Makuvara[1,2]

1 School of Natural Sciences, Great Zimbabwe University, Masvingo, Zimbabwe

2 Department of Physics, Geography and Environmental Sciences, Great Zimbabwe University, Masvingo, Zimbabwe

*Address all correspondence to: zmakuvara@gzu.ac.zw; zkmakuvara@gmail.com

References

[1] WHO, World Malaria Report 2020: 20 Years of Global Progress and Challenges. WHO. 2020.

[2] Arya A et al. Artemisinin-based combination therapy (ACT) and drug resistance molecular markers: A systematic review of clinical studies from two malaria endemic regions–India and sub-Saharan Africa. International Journal for Parasitology: Drugs and Drug Resistance. 2021;**15**:43-56

[3] Erhunse N, Sahal D. Protecting future antimalarials from the trap of resistance: Lessons from artemisinin-based combination therapy (ACT) failures. Journal of Pharmaceutical Analysis. 2021;**11**(5):541-554

[4] Nordmann T, Borrmann S, Ramharter M. Drug-induced hypersensitivity to artemisinin-based therapies for malaria. Trends in Parasitology. 2021;**38**(2):136-146

[5] Ouji M et al. Plasmodium falciparum resistance to artemisinin-based combination therapies: A sword of Damocles in the path toward malaria elimination. Parasite. 2018;**25**:24. DOI: 10.1051/parasite/2018021

[6] Ross LS, Fidock DA. Elucidating mechanisms of drug-resistant plasmodium falciparum. Cell Host & Microbe. 2019;**26**(1):35-47

[7] Edwin GT, Korsik M, Todd MH. The past, present and future of anti-malarial medicines. Malaria Journal. 2019;**18**(1):1-21

[8] Katsuno K et al. Hit and lead criteria in drug discovery for infectious diseases of the developing world. Nature Reviews Drug Discovery. 2015;**14**(11):751-758

[9] Bilia AR et al. Vesicles and micelles: Two versatile vectors for the delivery of natural products. Journal of Drug Delivery Science and Technology. 2016;**32**:241-255

[10] Kazi M et al. Enhancing oral bioavailability of apigenin using a bioactive self-nanoemulsifying drug delivery system (bio-SNEDDS): In vitro, in vivo and stability evaluations. Pharmaceutics. 2020;**12**(8):749

[11] Noonan TJ et al. A preformulation co-crystal screening case study: Polymorphic co-crystals of an imidazopyridazine antimalarial drug lead with the coformer succinic acid. Journal of Molecular Structure. 2020;**1204**:127561

[12] Achan J et al. Quinine, an old anti-malarial drug in a modern world: Role in the treatment of malaria. Malaria Journal. 2011;**10**(1):1-12

[13] Ceravolo IP et al. Studies on activities and chemical characterization of medicinal plants in search for new antimalarials: A ten year review on ethnopharmacology. Frontiers in Pharmacology. 2021;**12**:734263. DOI: 10.3389/fphar.2021.734263

[14] Krettli AU et al. The search for new antimalarial drugs from plants used to treat fever and malaria or plants ramdomly selected: A review. Memórias do Instituto Oswaldo Cruz. 2001;**96**(8):1033-1042

[15] Brusotti G et al. Isolation and characterization of bioactive compounds from plant resources: The role of analysis in the ethnopharmacological approach. Journal of Pharmaceutical and Biomedical Analysis. 2014;**87**:218-228

[16] Ashraf MA. Phytochemicals as potential anticancer drugs: Time to ponder nature's bounty. BioMed Research International. 2020;**2020**:8602879. DOI: 10.1155/2020/8602879

[17] Atanasov AG et al. Discovery and resupply of pharmacologically active plant-derived natural products: A review. Biotechnology Advances. 2015;**33**(8):1582-1614

[18] Leonti M. The future is written: Impact of scripts on the cognition, selection, knowledge and transmission of medicinal plant use and its implications for ethnobotany and ethnopharmacology. Journal of Ethnopharmacology. 2011;**134**(3):542-555

[19] Noronha M et al. A literature review on traditional herbal medicines for malaria. South African Journal of Botany. 2020;**128**:292-303

[20] Anyinam C. Ecology and ethnomedicine: Exploring links between current environmental crisis and indigenous medical practices. Social Science & Medicine. 1995;**40**(3):321-329

[21] Mazid M, Khan TA, Mohammad F. Medicinal plants of rural India: A review of use by Indian folks. Indo Global Journal of Pharmaceutical Sciences. 2012;**2**(3):286-304

[22] Kumari A et al. Current scenario of artemisinin and its analogues for antimalarial activity. European Journal of Medicinal Chemistry. 2019;**163**:804-829

[23] Nwodo JN et al. Exploring cancer therapeutics with natural products from African medicinal plants, part II: Alkaloids, terpenoids and flavonoids. Anti-Cancer Agents in Medicinal Chemistry (Formerly Current Medicinal Chemistry-Anti-Cancer Agents). 2016;**16**(1):108-127

[24] Ancheria RK et al. An overview of pharmaceutical co-crystal. Asian Journal of Pharmaceutical Research and Development. 2019;7(2):39-46

[25] Conceicao J et al. Cyclodextrins as drug carriers in pharmaceutical technology: The state of the art. Current Pharmaceutical Design. 2018;**24**(13):1405-1433

[26] Kavanagh ON, Walker G, Lusi M. Graph-set analysis helps to understand charge transfer in a novel ionic cocrystal when the Δp K a rule fails. Crystal Growth & Design. 2019;**19**(9): 5308-5313

[27] Blagden N, Coles S Berry D. Pharmaceutical co-crystals–are we there yet? CrystEngComm. 2014;**16**(26):5753-5761

[28] Dalpiaz A, Pavan B, Ferretti V. Can pharmaceutical co-crystals provide an opportunity to modify the biological properties of drugs? Drug Discovery Today. 2017;**22**(8):1134-1138

[29] Duggirala NK et al. Pharmaceutical cocrystals: Along the path to improved medicines. Chemical Communications. 2016;**52**(4):640-655

[30] Huang S et al. Simultaneously improving the physicochemical properties, dissolution performance, and bioavailability of apigenin and daidzein by co-crystallization with theophylline. Journal of Pharmaceutical Sciences. 2019;**108**(9):2982-2993

[31] Ungogo MA et al. A review of the antimalarial, antitrypanosomal, and antileishmanial activities of natural compounds isolated from Nigerian flora. Frontiers in Chemistry. 2020;**8**(617448):1221

[32] Kurek J editor. Alkaloids: Their Importance in Nature and Human Life. Intechopen; 2019. p.1-8

[33] Iwu MM, Kiayman DL. Evaluation of the in vitro antimalarial activity of Picralima nitida extracts. Journal of Ethnopharmacology. 1992;**36**(2):133-135

[34] Nnadi CO et al. Potent antitrypanosomal activities of 3-aminosteroids against African trypanosomes: Investigation of cellular effects and of cross-resistance with existing drugs. Molecules. 2019;**24**(2):268

[35] Chaturvedi D. Sesquiterpene Lactones: Structural Diversity and Their Biological Activities, In-Opportunity, Challanges and Scope of Natural Products in Medicinal Chemistry. ISBN: 978-81-308-0448-4. Trivandrum: Research Signpost; 2011. pp. 313-334

[36] Kaur K et al. Quinolines and structurally related heterocycles as antimalarials. European Journal of Medicinal Chemistry. 2010;**45**(8): 3245-3264

[37] Khamsan S et al. A new isoflavonc from Jacaranda obtusifolia HBK ssp. rhombifolia (GFW Meijer) gentry. Acta Pharmaceutica Sciencia. 2011;53(2):181-188

[38] Nogueira CR, Lopes LM. Antiplasmodial natural products. Molecules. 2011;**16**(3):2146-2190

[39] Titanji VP, Zofou D, Ngemenya MN. The antimalarial potential of medicinal plants used for the treatment of malaria in Cameroonian folk medicine. African Journal of Traditional, Complementary, and Alternative Medicines. 2008;**5**(3):302

[40] Mahmout Y et al. 15ème colloque sur la Pharmacopée et la Médecine Traditionnelles Africaines. Conseil Africain et Malgache pour l'Enseignement Supérieur (CAMES). 2008:**1**

[41] Ajaiyeoba E et al. Antiplasmodial compounds from Cassia siamea stem bark extract. Phytotherapy Research: An International Journal Devoted to Pharmacological and Toxicological Evaluation of Natural Product Derivatives. 2008;**22**(2):254-255

[42] Mbah J et al. Antiplasmodial triterpenes from the stem bark of Baillonella toxisperma. ISESCO Journal of Science and Technology. 2011;**7**(12):84-87

[43] Talontsi FM et al. Antibacterial and antiplasmodial constituents of Beilschmiedia cryptocaryoides. Journal of Natural Products. 2013;**76**(1):97-102

[44] Zofou D et al. Hypericum lanceolatum (Hypericaceae) as a potential source of new anti-malarial agents: A bioassay-guided fractionation of the stem bark. Malaria Journal. 2011;**10**(1):1-7

[45] Zofou D et al. Antimalarial drug interactions of compounds isolated from Kigelia africana (Bignoniaceae) and their synergism with artemether, against the multidrug-resistant W2mef plasmodium falciparum strain. Parasitology Research. 2012;**110**(2):539-544

[46] Santos AG et al. A simple, comprehensive, and miniaturized solvent extraction method for determination of particulate-phase polycyclic aromatic compounds in air. Journal of Chromatography A. 2016;**1435**:6-17

[47] Ichino T et al. Nonadiabatic effects in the photoelectron spectrum of the pyrazolide-d 3 anion: Three-state interactions in the pyrazolyl-d 3 radical.

The Journal of Chemical Physics. 2006;**125**(8):084312

[48] Radwan MM et al. Non-cannabinoid constituents from a high potency Cannabis sativa variety. Phytochemistry. 2008;**69**(14):2627-2633

[49] Tasdemir D et al. Antitrypanosomal and antileishmanial activities of flavonoids and their analogues: in vitro, in vivo, structure-activity relationship, and quantitative structure-activity relationship studies. Antimicrobial Agents and Chemotherapy. 2006;**50**(4):1352-1364

[50] do Nascimento Brandão DL et al. Estudo in silico de diterpenos isolados de Portulaca pilosa L e sua correlação com estudos etnobotânicos. Research, Society and Development. 2020;**9**(11):e99491110635-e99491110635

[51] Vale VV et al. Naphthoquinones isolated from Eleutherine plicata herb: In vitro antimalarial activity and molecular modeling to investigate their binding modes. Medicinal Chemistry Research. 2020;**29**(3):487-494

[52] Waller RF, McFadden GI. The apicoplast: A review of the derived plastid of apicomplexan parasites. Current Issues in Molecular Biology. 2005;**7**(1):57-80

[53] Gómez-Estrada H et al. In vitro antimalarial activity of fractions and constituents isolated from Tabebuia billbergii. Revista Cubana de Plantas Medicinales. 2012;**17**(2):172-180

[54] Moreira CM et al. A systematic review of sub-microscopic plasmodium vivax infection. Malaria Journal. 2015;**14**(1):1-10

[55] Mamede L et al. Natural phenolic compounds and derivatives as potential antimalarial agents. Planta Medica. 2020;**86**(09):585-618

[56] Saxena M et al. Phytochemistry of medicinal plants. Journal of Pharmacognosy and Phytochemistry. 2013;**1**(6):168-182

[57] Bekono BD et al. The potential of anti-malarial compounds derived from African medicinal plants: A review of pharmacological evaluations from 2013 to 2019. Malaria Journal. 2020;**19**(1):1-35

[58] Soh PN et al. In vitro and in vivo properties of ellagic acid in malaria treatment. Antimicrobial Agents and Chemotherapy. 2009;**53**(3):1100-1106

[59] Aldulaimi O et al. A characterization of the antimalarial activity of the bark of Cylicodiscus gabunensis harms. Journal of Ethnopharmacology. 2017;**198**: 221-225

[60] Banzouzi J-T et al. In vitro antiplasmodial activity of extracts of Alchornea cordifolia and identification of an active constituent: Ellagic acid. Journal of Ethnopharmacology. 2002;**81**(3):399-401

[61] Reddy MK et al. Antioxidant, antimalarial and antimicrobial activities of tannin-rich fractions, ellagitannins and phenolic acids from Punica granatum L. Planta Medica. 2007;**53**(05):461-467

[62] Davis RA et al. Antimalarial activity of pyrroloiminoquinones from the Australian marine sponge Zyzzya sp. Journal of Medicinal Chemistry. 2012;**55**(12):5851-5858

[63] Tajuddeen N, Van Heerden FR. Antiplasmodial natural products: An update. Malaria Journal. 2019;**18**(1):1-62

[64] Pinheiro L et al. Current antimalarial therapies and advances in the development of semi-synthetic artemisinin derivatives. Anais da Academia Brasileira de Ciências. 2018;**90**:1251-1271

[65] Lee M. Plants against malaria. Part 1: Cinchona or the Peruvian bark. The Journal of the Royal College of Physicians of Edinburgh. 2002;**32**(3):189-196

[66] Karunamoorthi K et al. Role of traditional antimalarial plants in the battle against the global malaria burden. Vector-Borne and Zoonotic Diseases. 2013;**13**(8):521-544

[67] Muregi FW, Ishih A. Next-generation antimalarial drugs: Hybrid molecules as a new strategy in drug design. Drug Development Research. 2010;**71**(1):20-32

[68] Teixeira C et al. "Recycling" classical drugs for malaria. Chemical Reviews. 2014;**114**(22):11164-11220

[69] Nosten F, Phillips-Howard PA, Kuile FOT. Other 4-methanolquinolines, amyl alcohols and phentathrenes: Mefloquine, lumefantrine and halofantrine. In: Staines HM, Sanjeev KS, editors. Treatment and Prevention of Malaria. Springer Nature; 2011. pp. 95-111

[70] Moore DV, Lanier JE. Observations on two plasmodium falciparum infections with an abnormal response to chloroquine. American Journal of Tropical Medicine and Hygiene. 1961;**10**(1):5-9

[71] Rasmussen C, Alonso P, Ringwald P. Current and emerging strategies to combat antimalarial resistance. Expert Review of Anti-Infective Therapy. 2022;**20**(3):353-372

[72] Roper C et al. Intercontinental spread of pyrimethamine-resistant malaria. Science. 2004;**305**(5687):1124-1124

[73] Vinayak S et al. Origin and evolution of sulfadoxine resistant plasmodium falciparum. PLoS Pathogens. 2010;**6**(3):e1000830

[74] Tu Y et al. Studies on the constituents of Artemisia annua L. Acta Pharmaceutica Sinica. 2015;**57**(1):366-370

[75] Mohammadi S et al. Medicinal plants used in the treatment of malaria: A key emphasis to Artemisia, Cinchona, Cryptolepis, and Tabebuia genera. Phytotherapy Research. 2020;**34**(7):1556-1569

[76] Duffy S, Avery VM. Identification of inhibitors of plasmodium falciparum gametocyte development. Malaria Journal. 2013;**12**(1):1-15

[77] White NJ. Qinghaosu (artemisinin): The price of success. Science. 2008

[78] Adebayo J et al. Enhancing the antimalarial activity of artesunate. Parasitology Research. 2020;**119**(9): 2749-2764

[79] Memvanga PB, Préat V. Formulation design and in vivo antimalarial evaluation of lipid-based drug delivery systems for oral delivery of β-arteether. European Journal of Pharmaceutics and Biopharmaceutics. 2012;**82**(1): 112-119

[80] de Carvalho LP, Kreidenweiss A, Held J. The preclinical discovery and development of rectal artesunate for the treatment of malaria in young children: A review of the evidence. Expert Opinion on Drug Discovery. 2021;**16**(1):13-22

[81] Thu AM et al. Combating multidrug-resistant Plasmodium falciparum malaria. The FEBS Journal. 2017;**284**(16):2569-2578

[82] Randrianarivelojosia M et al. Madagascan isolates of plasmodium falciparum showing low sensitivity to artemether in vitro. Annals of

Tropical Medicine & Parasitology. 2001;**95**(3):237-243

[83] Gogtay N et al. Probable resistance to parenteral artemether in plasmodium falciparum: Case reports from Mumbai (Bombay), India. Annals of Tropical Medicine & Parasitology. 2000;**94**(5):519-520

[84] Sahr F et al. Apparent drug failure following artesunate treatment of plasmodium falciparum malaria in Freetown, Sierra Leone: Four case reports. Annals of Tropical Medicine & Parasitology. 2001;**95**(5):445-449

[85] Group, I.A.S. Artesunate combinations for treatment of malaria: meta-analysis. The Lancet. 2004;**363**(9402):9-17

[86] Newton PN et al. Poor quality vital anti-malarials in Africa-an urgent neglected public health priority. Malaria Journal. 2011;**10**(1):1-22

[87] Kavishe RA, Koenderink JB, Alifrangis M. Oxidative stress in malaria and artemisinin combination therapy: Pros and cons. The FEBS Journal. 2017;**284**(16):2579-2591

[88] Bosman A, Mendis KN. A major transition in malaria treatment: the adoption and deployment of artemisinin-based combination therapies. In: Defining and Defeating the Intolerable Burden of Malaria III: Progress and Perspectives: Supplement to Volume 77 (6) of American Journal of Tropical Medicine and Hygiene. 2007. Available from: https://www.ncbi.nlm.nih.gov/books/NBK1715/

[89] Jiang J-B et al. Antimalarial activity of mefloquine and qinghaosu. The Lancet. 1982;**320**(8293):285-288

[90] Nigam M et al. Bioactive compounds and health benefits of Artemisia species. Natural Product Communications. 2019;**14**(7):1934578X19850354

[91] WHO. Monitoring antimalarial drug resistance: Report of a WHO consultation, Geneva, Switzerland, 3-5 December 2001. World Health Organization; 2002

[92] Khan AQ et al. Surveillance of genetic markers associated with plasmodium falciparum resistance to artemisinin-based combination therapy in Pakistan, 2018-2019. Malaria Journal. 2020;**19**(1):1-9

[93] Bassat Q et al. Challenges in the clinical development pathway for triple and multiple drug combinations in the treatment of uncomplicated falciparum malaria. Malaria Journal. 2022;**21**(1):1-8

[94] Fröhlich T et al. Synthesis of artemisinin-derived dimers, trimers and dendrimers: Investigation of their antimalarial and antiviral activities including putative mechanisms of action. Chemistry–A European Journal. 2018;**24**(32):8103-8113

[95] Leang R et al. Evidence of plasmodium falciparum malaria multidrug resistance to artemisinin and piperaquine in western Cambodia: Dihydroartemisinin-piperaquine open-label multicenter clinical assessment. Antimicrobial Agents and Chemotherapy. 2015;**59**(8):4719-4726

[96] van der Pluijm RW et al. Triple artemisinin-based combination therapies for malaria—A new paradigm? Trends in Parasitology. 2021;**37**(1):15-24

[97] Gupta D et al. Salts of therapeutic agents: Chemical, physicochemical, and biological considerations. Molecules. 2018;**23**(7):1719

[98] Kalepu S, Nekkanti V. Insoluble drug delivery strategies: Review

of recent advances and business prospects. Acta Pharmaceutica Sinica B. 2015;**5**(5):442-453

[99] Thayyil AR et al. Pharmaceutical co-crystallization: Regulatory aspects, design, characterization, and applications. Advanced Pharmaceutical Bulletin. 2020;**10**(2):203

[100] Gadade DD, Pekamwar SS. Pharmaceutical cocrystals: Regulatory and strategic aspects, design and development. Advanced pharmaceutical bulletin. 2016;**6**(4):479

[101] Mswahili ME et al. Cocrystal prediction using machine learning models and descriptors. Applied Sciences. 2021;**11**(3):1323

[102] Costa RN et al. Optimization and comparison of statistical tools for the prediction of multicomponent forms of a molecule: The antiretroviral nevirapine as a case study. CrystEngComm. 2020;**22**(43):7460-7474

[103] Ngilirabanga JB, Samsodien H. Pharmaceutical co-crystal: An alternative strategy for enhanced physicochemical properties and drug synergy. Nano Select. 2021;**2**(3):512-526

[104] Patole T, Deshpande A. Co-crystallization-atechniqueforsolubility enhancement. International Journal of Pharmaceutical Sciences and Research. 2014;**5**(9):3566

[105] Thipparaboina R et al. Multidrug co-crystals: Towards the development of effective therapeutic hybrids. Drug Discovery Today. 2016;**21**(3):481-490

[106] Karagianni A, Malamatari M, Kachrimanis K. Pharmaceutical cocrystals: New solid phase modification approaches for the formulation of APIs. Pharmaceutics. 2018;**10**(1):18

[107] Bandaru RK et al. Recent advances in pharmaceutical cocrystals: From bench to market. Frontiers in Pharmacology. 2021;**12**:780582. DOI: 10.3389/fphar.2021.780582

[108] Lu J et al. Characterization and pseudopolymorphism of L-phenylalanine anhydrous and monohydrate forms. African Journal of Pharmacy and Pharmacology. 2012;**6**(4):269-277

[109] Kesisoglou F, Wu Y. Understanding the effect of API properties on bioavailability through absorption modeling. The AAPS Journal. 2008;**10**(4):516-525

[110] Kuminek G et al. Cocrystals to facilitate delivery of poorly soluble compounds beyond-rule-of-5. Advanced Drug Delivery Reviews. 2016;**101**:143-166

[111] Han S et al. Hygroscopicity of organic compounds as a function of organic functionality, water solubility, molecular weight, and oxidation level. Atmospheric Chemistry and Physics. 2022;**22**(6):3985-4004

[112] Wong SN et al. Cocrystallization of curcumin with benzenediols and benzenetriols via rapid solvent removal. Crystal Growth & Design. 2018;**18**(9):5534-5546

[113] Vemuri VD, Lankalapalli S. Insight into concept and progress on pharmaceutical co-crystals: An overview. Indian Journal of Pharmaceutical Education and Research. 2019;**53**:522-538

[114] Sanphui P et al. Fast dissolving curcumin cocrystals. Crystal Growth & Design. 2011;**11**(9):4135-4145

[115] Bero J, Frédérich M, Quetin-Leclercq J. Antimalarial compounds

isolated from plants used in traditional medicine. Journal of Pharmacy and Pharmacology. 2009;**61**(11):1401-1433

[116] Lahlou M. The success of natural products in drug discovery. Pharmacology & Pharmacy. 2013;**4**(3A):5

[117] Laryea MK, Borquaye LS. Antimalarial efficacy and toxicological assessment of extracts of some Ghanaian medicinal plants. Journal of Parasitology Research. 2019;**2019**:1630405. DOI: 10.1155/2019/1630405

[118] Oliveira AB et al. Plant-derived antimalarial agents: New leads and efficient phythomedicines. Part I. alkaloids. Anais da Academia Brasileira de Ciencias. 2009;**81**(4):715-740